Biopsy Pathology of the Prostate

Biopsy Pathology Series

General Editors

Professor A. Munro Neville
PhD, DSc, MD, FRCPath,
Ludwig Institute for Cancer Research,
London, UK

Professor F. Walker
MD, PhD, FRCPath,
Department of Pathology,
University of Aberdeen, UK

Dr Clive R. Taylor MD PhD
Department of Pathology and Laboratory Medicine,
USC School of Medicine,
Los Angeles, CA, USA

Editor Emeritus

Leonard S. Gottlieb MD, MPH,
Department of Pathology and Laboratory Medicine,
Boston University Medical Center, Boston, MA, USA

Titles in the series

1. Biopsy Pathology of the Small Intestine
   F.D. Lee and P.G. Toner

3. Brain Biopsy
   J.H. Adams, D.I. Graham and D. Doyle

4. Biopsy Pathology of the Lymphoreticular System
   D.H. Wright and P.G. Isaacson

6. Biopsy Pathology of Bone and Bone Marrow
   B. Frisch, S.M. Lewis, R. Burkhardt and R. Bartl

7. Biopsy Pathology of the Breast
   J. Sloane

9. Biopsy Pathology of the Bronchi
   E.M. McDowell and T.F. Beals

10. Biopsy Pathology in Colorectal Disease
    I.C. Talbot and A.B. Price

11. Biopsy Pathology and Cytology of the Cervix
    D.V. Coleman and D.M.D. Evans

12. Biopsy Pathology of the Liver (2nd edn)
    R.S. Patrick and J.O'D. McGee

13. Biopsy Pathology of the Pulmonary Vasculature
    C.A. Wagenvoort and W.J. Mooi

14. Biopsy Pathology of the Endometrium
    C.H. Buckley and H. Fox

15. Biopsy Pathology of Muscle (2nd edn)
    M. Swash and M.S. Schwartz

16. Biopsy Pathology of the Skin
    N. Kirkham

17. Biopsy Pathology of Melanocytic Disorders
    W.J. Mooi and T. Krausz

18. Biopsy Pathology of the Thyroid and Parathyroid
    O. Ljungberg

19. Biopsy Pathology of the Oesophagus, Stomach and Duodenum (2nd edn)
    D.W. Day and M.F. Dixon

20. Biopsy Pathology of the Prostate
    D.G. Bostwick and P.A. Dundore

21. Biopsy Pathology of the Eye and Ocular Adnexa
    N.A. Rao

Biopsy Pathology of the Prostate

David G. Bostwick MD
Consultant and Professor of Pathology, Department of
Laboratory Medicine and Pathology, Mayo Clinic and Mayo
Medical School, Rochester, Minnesota, USA

and

Paul A. Dundore MD
Senior Associate Consultant in Pathology, Department of
Laboratory Medicine and Pathology, Mayo Clinic,
Jacksonville, Florida, USA

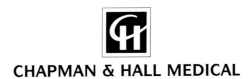

CHAPMAN & HALL MEDICAL
London · Weinheim · New York · Tokyo · Melbourne · Madras

Published by Chapman & Hall, 2–6 Boundary Row, London SE1 8HN, UK

Chapman & Hall, 2–6 Boundary Row, London SE1 8HN, UK

Chapman & Hall GmbH, Pappelallee 3, 69469 Weinheim, Germany

Chapman & Hall USA, 115 Fifth Avenue, New York, NY 10003, USA

Chapman & Hall Japan, ITP-Japan, Kyowa Building, 3F, 2-2-1 Hirakawacho, Chiyoda-Ku, Tokyo 102, Japan

Chapman & Hall Australia, 102 Dodds Street, South Melbourne, Victoria 3205, Australia

Chapman & Hall India, R. Seshadri, 32 Second Main Road, CIT East, Madras 600 035, India

First edition 1997

© 1997 David G. Bostwick and Paul A. Dundore.

Typeset by Type Study, Scarborough, North Yorkshire
Printed in Hong Kong

ISBN 0 412 75510 6

A catalogue record for this book is available from the British Library

Library of Congress Catalog Card Number: 96-086621

To Dr George M. Farrow, Consultant in Pathology and Professor of Pathology, Mayo Clinic and Mayo Medical School

CONTENTS

PREFACE

The lowly prostate, an oft-forgotten walnut-sized organ buried deep in the pelvis, breaks its silence late in life by enlarging and blocking urine flow or launching life-threatening cancer cells from hidden primary nests within the gland to distant sites such as bone and lymph nodes. Prostatic nodular hyperplasia and adenocarcinoma are enormous public health issues, accounting for more than 1 million surgical specimens annually in the US. The incidence of prostate cancer has tripled during the past decade, chiefly as a result of early detection efforts with serum PSA and digital rectal examination.

This massive diagnostic burden for pathologists is compounded by a number of recent events which have increased the difficulty in prostate needle biopsy interpretation. First, the size of contemporary needle biopsy cores is considerably narrower than traditional Vim–Silverman and Tru-Cut biopsies, providing about 36% of the width of each core for pathological examination. Second, many patients now undergo biopsy with elevated serum PSA but no other clinical evidence of cancer, resulting in an enormous number of biopsies that contain only a small suspicious focus. Third, numerous diagnostic pitfalls and mimics of prostate cancer have recently been described or refined, including atypical adenomatous hyperplasia, sclerosing adenosis, post-atrophic hyperplasia and prostatic intraepithelial neoplasia. The great number of prostate biopsy specimens being generated magnifies the risk of encountering rare or unusual lesions and the potential for misinterpretation of small foci. Finally, sextant biopsies (three from each side) have largely replaced the single bilateral cores of a decade ago, providing multiple specimens from each patient.

This prostate biopsy interpretation book was prepared with the practicing pathologist as the foremost consideration. It is hoped that this text and collection of tables and photomicrographs will materially aid in continuing efforts to recognize, understand and accurately interpret the light-microscopic findings in the increasing number of difficult prostate biopsy specimens. This book is not intended to replace comprehensive textbooks of urological pathology or other original sources of information, but rather to complement them as a practical aid.

We are indebted to many individuals who have been involved in the preparation of this book. Mrs Annette Bjorheim provided expert and invaluable secretarial assistance throughout this project. Drs Antonio Lopez-Beltran and Anna Pacelli carefully reviewed the text. The encouragement and cooperation of our colleagues in the Division of Anatomic Pathology at Mayo Clinic

Rochester are sincerely appreciated, with special thanks to the Division Chief, Dr Jeffrey Myers. Mr Nicholas Dunton of Chapman & Hall has been a tireless champion of this effort. To our wives and children, we owe a particular debt of gratitude for their understanding and patience.

We earnestly solicit constructive criticism from colleagues so that the utility of this text can be expanded and improved to its maximum potential.

David G. Bostwick and Paul A. Dundore
Rochester, Minnesota and Jacksonville, Florida, June 1996

1

NORMAL ANATOMY AND HISTOLOGY

1.1 ANATOMY AND HISTOLOGY OF THE PROSTATE

1.1.1 Prostatic urethra and verumontanum

The urethra serves as a reference landmark for the study of prostatic anatomy (Figures 1.1 and 1.2) (McNeal and Bostwick, 1990).

There is a single 35° bend in the center of the prostatic urethra, creating proximal and distal segments of equal length. The verumontanum bulges from the posterior wall at the urethral bend and tapers distally to form the crista urethralis. Most prostatic ducts and the ejaculatory ducts empty into the urethra in this part of the mid and distal prostatic urethra, whereas the small periurethral glands have ducts throughout the length of the urethra. Just proximal to the verumontanum is a müllerian remnant, the utricle, a small 0.5 cm long epithelium-lined cul-de-sac.

A circumferential sleeve of muscle surrounds the entire urethra. This muscular layer includes a proximal preprostatic smooth muscle sphincter which prevents retrograde ejaculation and a distal sphincter of striated and smooth muscle at the apex which is important in control of micturition.

1.1.2 Zones of the prostate

The prostate is composed of three zones: the peripheral zone, central zone and transition zone (Table 1.1).

The peripheral zone contains about 70% of the volume of the prostate, and is the most common site of prostatic intraepithelial neoplasia (PIN) and carcinoma. Peripheral zone acini are simple, round to oval, and set in a loose stroma of smooth muscle and collagen (Figure 1.3). Digital rectal examination often includes a description of the left and right 'lobes' based on palpation of the median furrow in the midline which divides the peripheral zone into left and right halves.

The central zone is a cone-shaped area that includes the entire base of the prostate and encompasses the ejaculatory ducts; it comprises about 25% of the volume of the prostate. Central zone acini are large and complex, with intraluminal ridges, papillary infoldings, and occasional epithelial arches and cribriform glands mimicking PIN (Figure 1.4) . The ratio of epithelium to stroma is higher in the central zone than the rest of the prostate, and the stroma is composed of compact interlacing smooth muscle bundles.

The transition zone contains the smallest volume of the normal prostate, about 5%, but

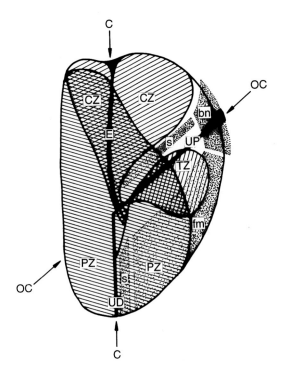

Figure 1.1 Sagittal diagram of the distal prostatic urethral segment (UD), proximal urethral segment (UP) and ejaculatory ducts (E), showing their relationships to a sagittal section of the anteromedial non-glandular tissues — bladder neck (bn), anterior fibromuscular stroma (fm), preprostatic sphincter (s), distal striated sphincter (s). These structures are shown in relation to a three-dimensional representation of the glandular prostate — central zone (CZ), peripheral zone (PZ), transition zone (TZ). The coronal plane (C) and the oblique coronal plane (OC) are indicated by arrows. (Source: redrawn from McNeal and Bostwick, 1990).

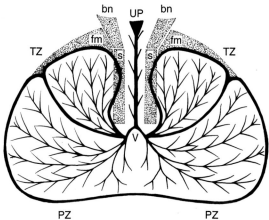

Figure 1.2 Oblique coronal section diagram of the prostate showing location of the peripheral zone (PZ) and transition zone (TZ) in relation to the proximal urethral segment (UP), verumontanum (V), preprostatic sphincter (s), bladder neck (bn) and periurethral region with periurethral glands. The branching pattern of the prostatic ducts is indicated; medial transition zone ducts penetrate into the sphincter. (Source: redrawn from McNeal and Bostwick, 1990).

can enlarge together with the anterior fibromuscular stroma to massive size as a result of benign prostatic hyperplasia and dwarf the remainder of the prostate. Transition zone glands tend to be simple, small and round, similar to those in the peripheral zone, but are embedded in a compact stroma that forms a distinctive boundary with the loose stroma of

Figure 1.3 Normal peripheral zone **(a)**, consisting of simple acini and a loose stroma of smooth muscle and collagen. The epithelium **(b)** is columnar, with small round basal nuclei and an inconspicuous flattened basal cell layer.

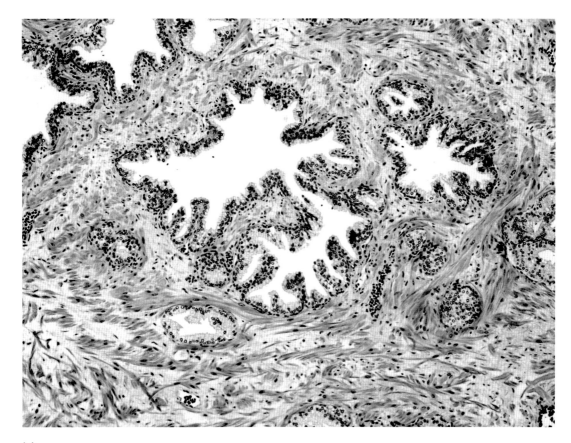

(a)

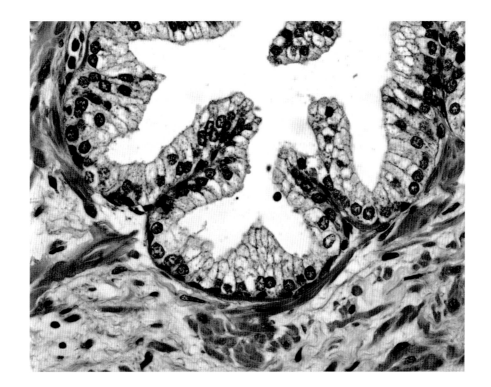

(b)

3

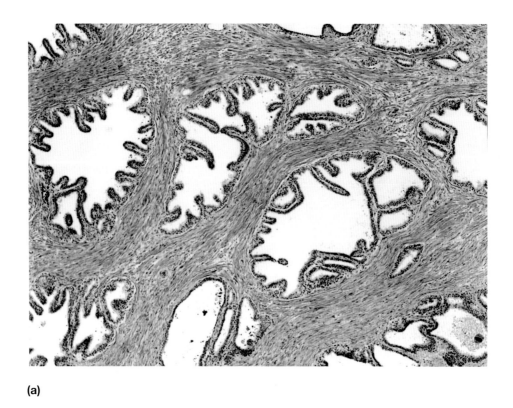

(a)

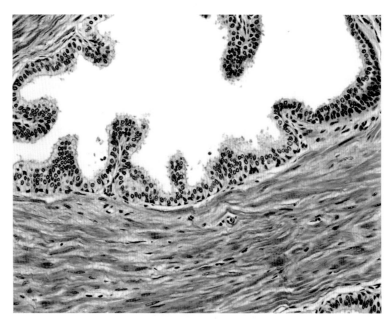

(b)

Figure 1.4 Normal central zone **(a)**, consisting of large acini with complex intraluminal ridges, papillary infoldings and epithelial arches set in a stroma of compact smooth muscle. The epithelium **(b)** varies from cuboidal to columnar.

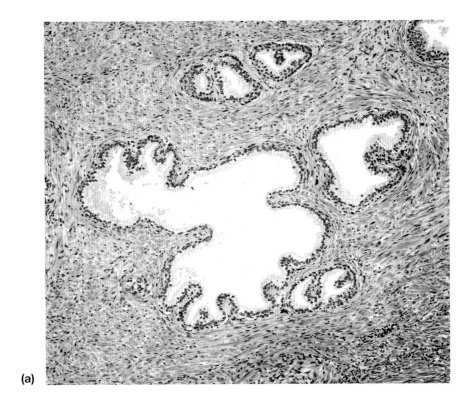

(a)

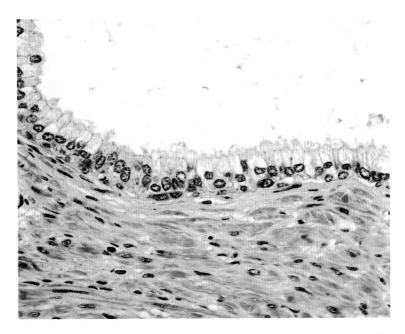

(b)

Figure 1.5 Normal transition zone **(a)**, consisting of simple acini and a compact stroma. The epithelium **(b)** is cuboidal or low columnar, with apical cytoplasmic blebs.

Table 1.1 Glandular zones of the human prostate: histological features

	Central zone	*Transition zone*	*Peripheral zone*
Volume of normal prostates (%)	25	5	70
Anatomic landmarks			
Intraprostatic relationships	Ejaculatory ducts	Surrounds proximal prostatic urethra	Distal prostatic urethra
Adjacent structures	Seminal vesicles	Bladder neck	Rectum
Urethral orifices of ducts	Verumontanum, adjacent to ejaculatory ducts	Posterolateral wall of proximal prostatic urethra at its distal end	Posterolateral wall of distal prostatic urethra
Distinctive histological features			
Epithelium	Complex, large polygonal glands with intraluminal ridges	Simple, small rounded glands	Simple, small rounded glands
Stroma	Compact	Compact	Loose
Biochemical differences			
Production of pepsinogen II	Yes	No	No
Production of tissue plasminogen activator	Yes	No	No
Lectin binding patterns			
LCA, Con-A, WGA, PNA-N, RCA-1	Yes	–	Yes
UEA-1, S-WGA, PNA	Yes	–	No
DBA, SBA, BS-I	No	–	No
Proposed embryonic origin	Wolffian duct	Urogenital sinus	Urogenital sinus

LCA = *Lens culinaris*; Con A = *Concanavalia ensiformis*; WGA = *Triticum vulgaris* (wheat germ); PNA-N = *Arachis hypogaea* (peanut) with neuraminidase predigestion; RCA-I = *Ricinus communis*; UEA-I = *Ulex europaeus*; S-WGA = succinyl-WGA; PNA = *Arachis hypogaea* (peanut); DBA = *Dolchus biflorus*; SBA = *Glycine max* (soybean); BS-I = *Bandeirea simplicifolia*; – = not evaluated.

the peripheral zone (Figure 1.5). The central zone and peripheral zone are often referred to together as the outer prostate or 'non-transition zone', whereas the transition zone and anterior fibromuscular stroma are often referred to as the inner prostate.

1.1.3 Normal epithelium of the prostate

The epithelium of the prostate is composed of three principal cell types: secretory cells, basal cells and neuroendocrine cells. The secretory luminal cells are cuboidal to columnar, with pale to clear cytoplasm. Despite having the lowest proliferative activity, these terminally differentiated cells produce prostate-specific antigen (PSA), prostatic acid phosphatase (PAP), acidic mucin and other secretory products.

The basal cells of the prostate form a flattened attenuated layer of inconspicuous elongate cells at the periphery of the glands surmounting the basement membrane (Figure 1.6).

These cells possess the highest proliferative activity of the prostatic epithelium, albeit low, and are thought to act as stem or 'reserve' cells that repopulate the secretory cell layer (Bonkhoff, Stein and Remberger, 1994). Basal cells apparently retain the ability to undergo metaplasia, including squamous differentiation in

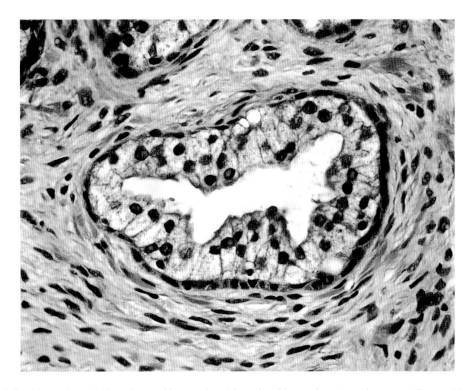

Figure 1.6   Normal prostatic acinus with prominent basal cell layer due to nuclear crowding and hyperchromasia. The basal cell layer is usually inconspicuous.

the setting of infarction and myoepithelial differentiation in sclerosing adenosis. Epidermal growth factor receptors have been identified in basal cells but not in secretory cells, suggesting that these cells play a role in growth regulation (Maygarden, Strom and Ware, 1992; Mellon *et al.*, 1992). Basal cells are selectively labeled with antibodies to high-molecular-weight keratins such as clone 34βE12 (keratin 903), a property which is exploited immunohistochemically in separating benign acinar processes such as atrophy (which retains a basal cell layer) from adenocarcinoma (which lacks a basal cell layer) (Figure 1.7).

Basal cells contain little or no PSA, PAP or mucin. The normal prostatic epithelium frequently displays foci of basal cell proliferation that are too small to warrant the diagnosis of basal cell hyperplasia (Chapter 4). Prostatic basal cells do not possess myoepithelial differentiation, unlike basal cells in the breast,

salivary glands, pancreas and other sites.

The neuroendocrine cells are the least common cell type of the prostatic epithelium, and are usually not identified in routine hematoxylin-and-eosin-stained sections except for rare cells with large eosinophilic granules (Adlakha and Bostwick, 1994; Di Sant' Agnese, 1995). Although their function is unknown, neuroendocrine cells probably have an endocrine–paracrine regulatory role in growth and development, similar to neuroendocrine cells in other organs, and contain multiple neuropeptides that can modulate cell growth and proliferation (Aprikian *et al.*, 1993; Bonkhoff *et al.*, 1991; Di Sant' Agnese, 1992, 1995; Di Sant' Agnese and Cockett, 1994; Di Sant' Agnese, 1995; Abrahamsson *et al.*, 1987). Androgen deprivation therapy does not appear to influence the number or distribution of neuroendocrine cells in the normal or neoplastic prostate (Aprikian *et al.*, 1993) Neuroendocrine cells

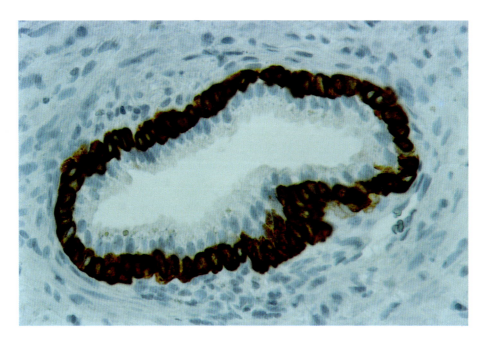

Figure 1.7 Intense cytoplasmic immunoreactivity in basal cells creates a continuous circumferential layer at the periphery of a benign prostatic acinus. Antikeratin 34ßE12 immunohistochemical stain.

coexpress PSA (Aprikian *et al.*, 1993) and androgen receptors (Abrahamsson *et al.*, 1993), suggesting a common cell of origin for epithelial cells and neuroendocrine cells in the prostate. Neuroendocrine cells are in greatest number near the verumontanum, suggesting a role in luminal constriction and dilatation. Serotonin and chromogranin are the best immunohistochemical markers of neuroendocrine cells in formalin-fixed sections of the prostate (Figures 1.8 and 1.9) (Adlakha and Bostwick, 1994; Abrahamsson *et al.*, 1987; Di Sant' Agnese, 1995).

Melanin-like (Fontana–Masson-positive) and lipofuscin-like (Ziehl–Neelsen-positive, S-100-protein-negative) pigment is frequently found in scattered foci in the normal and hyperplastic prostate (Figures 1.10–1.12).

It consists of granular yellow pigment within the epithelium or stroma, and is usually scant, although variable in amount (Brennick *et al.*, 1994). This pigment probably represents 'wear and tear' or 'old age' pigment resulting from endogenous cellular byproducts of the prostate epithelium. It is present in all zones of the prostate, and is randomly distributed.

1.1.4 Capsule

The capsule of the prostate consists of an inner layer of smooth muscle and an outer covering of collagen, with marked variability in the relative amounts in different areas. At the apex, the acinar elements become sparse and the capsule becomes ill-defined, composed of a mixture of

Figure 1.8 Neuroendocrine cells. **(a)** When present in normal prostatic epithelium, they are infrequent and variable in shape. **(b)** The cells in prostatic adenocarcinoma display dark cytoplasmic reaction product which fills the cytoplasm of scattered cells, obscuring the nuclei. Immunohistochemical stains for serotonin **(a)** and chromogranin **(b)**.

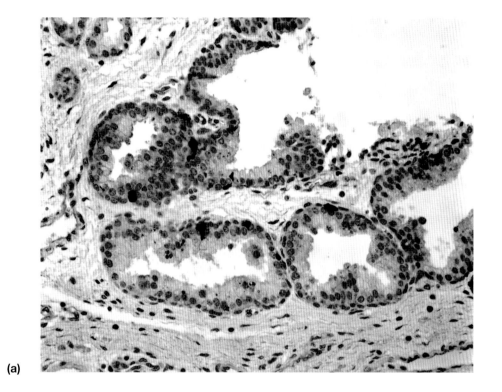

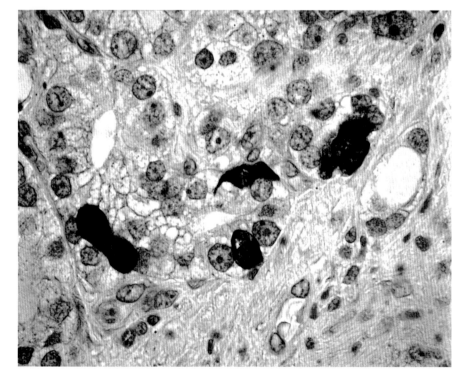

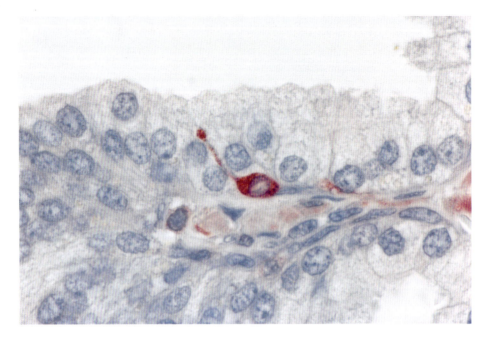

Figure 1.9 Neuroendocrine cell of the benign prostatic epithelium. Note the delicate slender cytoplasmic projections. Antiserotonin immunohistochemical stain.

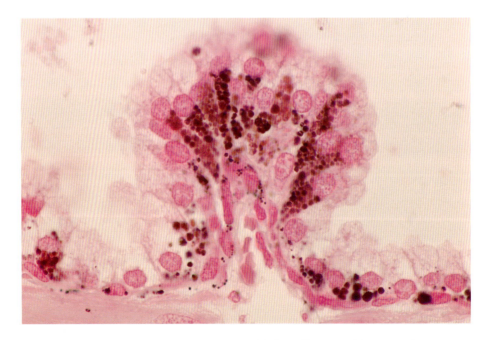

Figure 1.10 Melanin-like pigment in benign prostatic epithelium. Fontana—Masson stain.

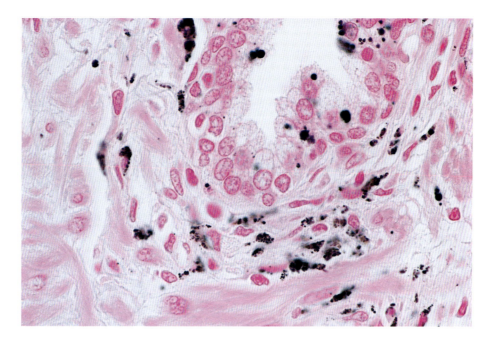

Figure 1.11 Melanin-like pigment in the periacinar prostatic stroma ('melanosis'). Fontana—Masson stain.

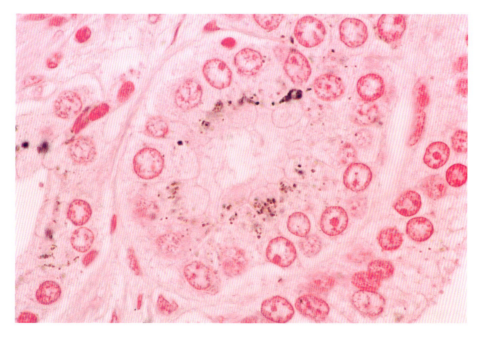

Figure 1.12 Melanin-like pigment in prostatic adenocarcinoma. This is an unusual finding, and is scant in amount. Fontana—Masson stain.

fibrous connective tissue, smooth muscle and striated muscle. As a result, the prostatic capsule cannot be regarded as a well-defined anatomic structure with constant features (Ayala *et al.*, 1989). In biopsy and surgical specimens, the capsule at the apex and bladder base is difficult to identify; consequently, it is often not possible to determine the presence of extraprostatic extension of cancer at these sites.

1.1.5 Nerve supply

The nerve supply of the prostate is furnished by paired neurovascular bundles that run along the posterolateral edge of the prostate from apex to base. Surgical sparing of these structures during radical prostatectomy may preserve sexual potency (Walsh, Lepor and Eggleston, 1983). Autonomic ganglia are clustered near the neurovascular bundles, sending out small nerve trunks which arborize over the surface of the prostate, penetrating through the capsule and branching to form an extensive network of nerve twigs within the prostate, which are often in intimate contact with the walls of ducts and acini. Caution is warranted in interpretation of perineural space invasion as an absolute criterion for the diagnosis of cancer, as this can be seen rarely in benign glands.

1.1.6 Blood supply

The blood supply of the prostate is furnished by one of the branches of the internal iliac artery. Veins drain directly into the prostatic plexus and an extensive arborizing network is present in the capsule. The venous drainage empties into the internal iliac vein. Lymphatics from the prostate drain mainly into the internal iliac lymph nodes, with lesser drainage into the external iliac and sacral lymph nodes.

1.2 SEMINAL VESICLES AND EJACULATORY DUCTS

The seminal vesicles arise during the 13th week of development as outpouchings of the lower mesonephric ducts. They are bounded by the prostate distally, the base of the bladder anteriorly and Denonvilliers fascia and the rectum posteriorly. Their anatomic distribution in this region is variable and they are occasionally found within the capsule of the prostate gland. The seminal vesicles may be palpable on digital rectal examination, and, when intimately associated with the prostate, may be mistaken for prostatic nodularity or induration. Up to 20% of prostate biopsies for nodularity contain fragments of seminal vesicle epithelium, a potential source of diagnostic confusion. In adults, the seminal vesicles measure about 6 cm in length and 2 cm in width, although there is wide variation in size and shape.

The mucosa displays complex papillary folds and irregular convoluted lumens, and the lining consists of a non-ciliated pseudostratified tall columnar epithelium.

The cells are predominately secretory, with microvesicular lipid droplets and characteristic lipofuscin pigment granules. The pigment is golden-brown and refractile, increasing in amount with age. These cells express androgen receptors like the prostatic epithelium, but not PSA or PAP. Secretory products include glycoproteins, fructose, prostaglandins and ascorbic acid. Up to 85% of the seminal fluid (normally 2–5 ml) originates in the seminal vesicles. The muscular wall consists of a thick circumferential coat of smooth muscle and is thought to serve a contractile function. The ducts of the seminal vesicles merge with the vas deferens on each side to form the ejaculatory ducts, and then enter the central zone of the prostate and converge prior to termination at the verumontanum and prostatic urethra (Figure 1.13).

The seminal vesicles begin to shrink in the seventh decade. The tall columnar cells lining the mucosa in young men are slowly replaced by flattened cuboidal cells, comprising 50% of the epithelium in men in the fifth decade of life and 2% in octogenarians. With advancing age, the stroma of the seminal vesicles becomes hyalinized and fibrotic.

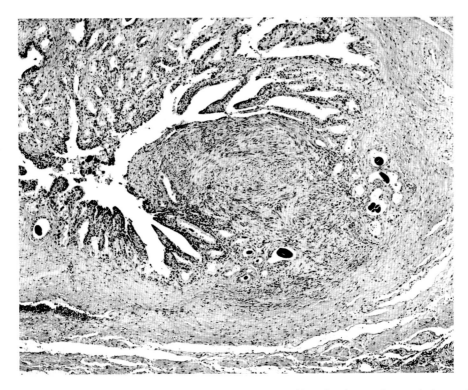

Figure 1.13 Ejaculatory duct near origin in the seminal vesicles. Note focal smooth muscle hyperplasia distorting lumen.

The flattening of the epithelium is accompanied by striking nuclear abnormalities, and highly atypical cells are present in about 75% of seminal vesicles in older men (Figure 1.15) (Arias-Stella and Takano-Moron, 1958; Kuo and Gomez, 1981; Mesonero and Oertel, 1991).

These cells have large irregular hyperchromatic nuclei with coarse chromatin and prominent nucleoli. Multinucleated cells are also present, as well as giant ring-shaped nuclei with large intranuclear cytoplasmic inclusions (Figure 1.14). These nuclear abnormalities are probably degenerative changes reflecting hormonal influences, and are not observed before age 20. When encountered in needle biopsies, such 'pseudomalignant' cytological atypia may lead to a mistaken diagnosis of prostatic carcinoma. Mitotic figures are absent. Difficulty may also be encountered in cytological

evaluation of fluids obtained by prostatic massage because seminal vesicular cells are frequently shed into the lumen. The distinctive lipofuscin-like pigment aids in their recognition (Koivuniemi and Tyrkku, 1976; Droese and Voeth, 1976; Mesonero and Oertel, 1991). Cells in prostatic aspirates derived from the seminal vesicles and ejaculatory ducts are often cytologically indistinguishable.

DNA content analysis reveals aneuploidy in 6.7% of seminal vesicles (Arber and Speights, 1991). Consequently, DNA analysis of prostate cancer specimens may yield false-positive results if contaminated by seminal vesicle tissue. It is uncertain why there is such a low level of aneuploidy in an organ with frequent and substantial cytological atypia.

Seminal vesicular cells are found as contaminants of cervical smears in 10% of specimens with spermatozoa, and may be diagnostically

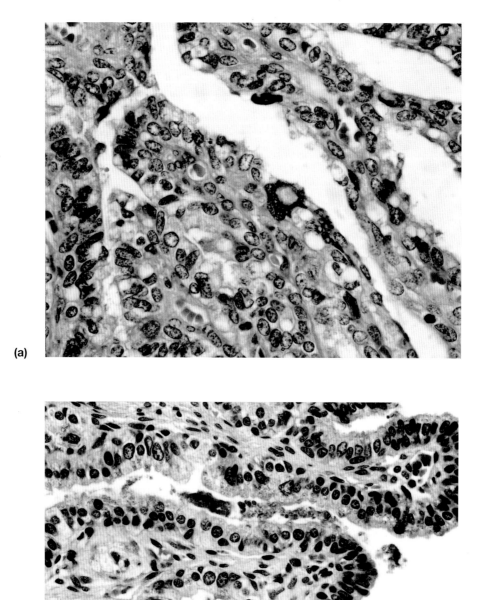

(a)

(b)

Figure 1.14　Seminal vesicle **(a)** and ejaculatory duct **(b)** epithelium have similar degree of severe cytological atypia, with occasional bizare giant cells.

confusing (Meisels and Ayotte, 1976). These cells contain foamy cytoplasm, scant pigment, vesicular hyperchromatic nuclei, sieve-like chromatin pattern and mild anisokaryosis.

Small 15–20 mm eosinophilic hyaline bodies, referred to as stromal hyaline bodies, are sometimes observed within the muscular wall of the seminal vesicles, vas deferens and prostate (Kuo and Gomez, 1958; Madara, Haggitt and Federman, 1978; Kovi, Jackson and Akberzie, 1979). These round to oval structures result from degeneration of smooth muscle fibers, and transition forms can be seen. Stromal hyaline bodies stain with Masson's trichrome and PAS, but do not stain with PTAH, methyl green pyronine, Feulgen, alcian blue at pH 2.5 or Congo red.

1.3 COWPER GLANDS

Cowper glands are small, paired bulbomembranous urethral glands which may be mistaken for prostatic carcinoma in biopsy specimens. These glands are composed of lobules of closely packed uniform acini lined by cytologically benign cells with abundant apical mucinous cytoplasm (Figure 1.15). Nuclei are inconspicuous. Carcinoma of Cowper glands is very rare, and is characterized by frank anaplasia of tumor cells.

1.4 IMMUNOHISTOCHEMISTRY

The most important immunohistochemical markers in prostate pathology are PSA, PAP and high-molecular-weight keratin 34βE12. Androgen receptors are a promising but unproven biomarker which has only become practical in recent years with the advent of microwave antigen retrieval. Other growth factors, oncogene products and cytoplasmic and membrane proteins are discussed in Chapter 16.

1.4.1 Prostate-specific antigen (PSA)

Immunohistochemical expression of PSA is useful for distinguishing high-grade prostate

cancer and urothelial carcinoma, colonic carcinoma, granulomatous prostatitis and lymphoma (Nadji et al., 1981; Stein et al., 1982; Sinha et al., 1986; Keillor and Aterman, 1987; Ordonez, Ro and Ayala, 1990; Brawn et al., 1994; Cote and Taylor, 1994; Bostwick, 1994a). PSA also facilitates identification of site of tumor origin in metastatic adenocarcinoma. A list of extraprostatic tissues and tumors that reportedly express PSA immunoreactivity is shown in Table 1.2 (Tepper et al., 1984; Pollen and Dreiling, 1984; Nowels, Kent and Rinsho, 1988; Golz and Schubert, 1989; Kamoshida and Tsutsumi, 1990; Spencer, Brodin and Ignatoff, 1990; Frazier et al., 1992; van Krieken, 1993; Cote and Taylor, 1994; Bostwick, 1994a; Elgamal et al., 1994; Sleater, Ford and Beers, 1994).

PSA can be detected in frozen sections, paraffin-embedded sections, cell smears and cytological preparations of normal and neoplastic prostatic epithelium (Figure 1.16).

Staining is invariably heterogeneous. Microwave antigen retrieval is usually not necessary, even in tissues that have been immersed in formalin for years. Formalin fixation is optimal for localization of PSA, and variation in staining intensity is only partially due to fixation and embedding effects (Sinha et al., 1986). Immunoreactivity is preserved in decalcified specimens, and may be enhanced.

1.4.2 Prostatic acid phosphatase (PAP)

Prostatic acid phosphatase (PAP) is a valuable immunohistochemical marker for identifying prostate cancer when used in combination with stains for PSA (Lowe and Trauzzi, 1993). Hammond et al. found that the intensity of PAP immunoreactivity correlated with patient survival, probably because of greater androgen responsiveness in immunoreactive cancers (Hammond et al., 1989). A list of extraprostatic tissues and tumors that reportedly express PAP immunoreactivity is shown in Table 1.3 (Choe et al., 1978; Shaw et al., 1981; Pollen and Dreiling, 1984; Tepper et al., 1984; Epstein, Kuhajda and Lieberman, 1986; Kimura and

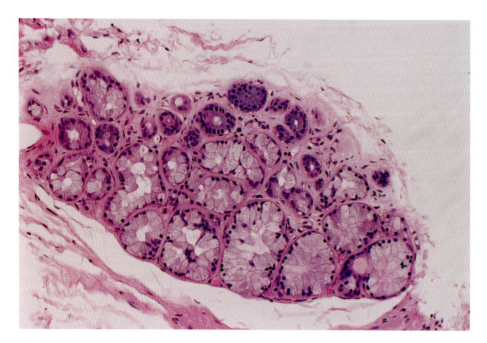

Figure 1.15 Cowper gland. This biopsy specimen contained a small, circumscribed, lobulated aggregate of benign uniform acini with abundant mucinous cytoplasm and small, dark basal nuclei.

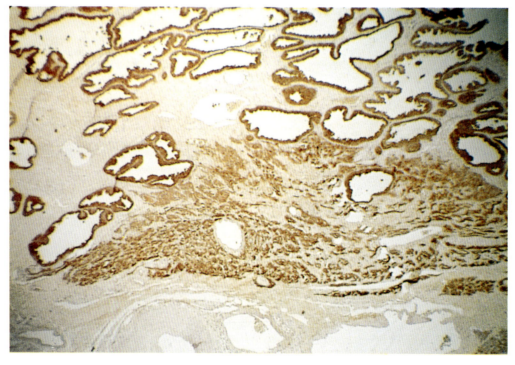

Figure 1.16 PSA immunoreactivity highlights adenocarcinoma along the capsule at the edge of the prostate; benign acini are also staining. Anti-PSA immunohistochemical stain.

Table 1.2 Immunoreactivity of prostate-specific antigen (PSA) in extraprostatic tissues and tumors (*Caveat*: In many of these tissues and tumors staining may be patchy, weak or equivocal. Many of these reports have not been confirmed or validated. Also, contemporary antibodies to PSA may have different specificity and sensitivity from those used in some of these studies.)

Extraprostatic tissues
  Urethra, periurethral glands, male and female
  Bladder, cystitis cystica and glandularis
  Urachal remnants
  Neutrophils
  Anus, anal glands (male only)

Extraprostatic tumors
  Mature teratoma
  Urethra, periurethral gland adenocarcinoma
    (female)
  Bladder, villous adenoma and adenocarcinoma
  Penis, extramammary Paget's disease
  Salivary gland, pleomorphic adenoma (male
    only)
  Salivary gland, carcinoma (male only)

Table 1.3 Immunoreactivity of prostatic acid phosphatase (PAP) in extraprostatic tissues and tumors (*Caveat*: in many of these tissues and tumors staining may be patchy, weak or equivocal. Many of these reports have not been confirmed or validated. Also, contemporary antibodies to PAP may have different specificity and sensitivity from those used in some of these studies.)

Extraprostatic cells and tissues
  Urethra, periurethral glands, male and female
  Bladder, cystitis cystica and glandularis
  Pancreas, islet cells
  Kidney, renal tubules
  Neutrophils
  Colon, neuroendocrine cells
  Anus, anal glands (male only)
  Stomach, parietal cells
  Liver, hepatocytes
  Breast, ductal epithelial cells

Extraprostatic tumors
  Bladder, adenocarcinoma
  Anus, cloagenic carcinoma
  Rectum carcinoid
  Other gastrointestinal carcinoids
  Pancreas, islet cell tumour
  Mature teratoma
  Breast, ductal carcinoma
  Salivary gland, pleomorphic adenoma (male
    only)
  Salivary gland, carcinoma (male only)

Sasano, 1986; Sobin *et al.*, 1986; Nowels, Kent and Rinsho, 1988; Kamoshida and Tsutsumi, 1990; Azumi, Traweek and Battifora, 1991; Fernandez *et al.*, 1992; van Krieken, 1993; Bostwick, 1994a; Cote and Taylor, 1994).

Serum PAP is less useful than PSA because of inherent problems in accuracy of measurement, including the requirement for special handling due to enzyme instability, diurnal fluctuation, variation resulting from prostatic digital examination and biopsy, and cross-reactivity with non-prostatic serum acid phosphatase produced by liver, bone, kidney, and blood cells. At present, serum PAP has little or no clinical utility.

1.4.3 Keratin 34βE12 (keratin 903; high-molecular-weight keratin)

Basal-cell-specific anti-keratin 34βE12 stains virtually all the normal basal cells of the prostate; there is no staining in the secretory and stromal cells. Basal cell layer disruption is present in 56% of cases of high-grade PIN,

more commonly in glands adjacent to invasive carcinoma than in distant glands. The amount of disruption increases with increasing grades of PIN, with loss of more than one-third of the basal cell layer in 52% of foci of high-grade PIN (Figure 1.17).

Early carcinoma occurs at sites of acinar outpouching and basal cell layer disruption (Bostwick and Brawer, 1987). Prostate cancer cells do not react with this antibody, although it may stain other cancers. Basal cell layer disruption also occurs in inflamed acini, atypical adenomatous hyperplasia and postatrophic hyperplasia (Brawer *et al.*, 1985; Bostwick and Brawer, 1987; Nagle *et al.*, 1987, 1991; Guinan *et al.*, 1989; Hedrick and Epstein, 1989; O'Malley, Grignon and Shum, 1990; Srigley *et al.*, 1990; Shah *et al.*, 1991; Okada *et al.*, 1992; Cheville and Bostwick, 1995).

Despite the clinical utility of high-molecular-weight keratin, caution is urged in interpretation because of the need to rely on negative results to separate adenocarcinoma from its mimics. Numerous confounding factors can interfere with staining, including poor tissue preservation and fixation and lack of enzyme predigestion.

1.4.4 Androgen receptors

Androgen receptors are present within androgen-responsive and androgen-unresponsive cells in prostatic adenocarcinoma. These receptors are widely distributed in the nuclei of the basal cell layer of the normal prostate, hyperplasia (Bonkhoff and Remberger, 1993), and localized and metastatic prostatic carcinoma (Sadi and Barrack, 1993; Ruizevald de Winter *et al.*, 1994). The percentage of cancer cells with androgen receptors is not predictive of time to progression after androgen-deprivation therapy (Sadi, Walsh and Barrack, 1991); however, there is greater heterogeneity of receptor immunoreactivity in adenocarcinoma which responds poorly to therapy (Sadi and Barrack, 1993). Androgen receptor expression in small cell carcinoma appears to predict poor outcome (Ferguson *et al.*, 1995). Androgen receptor gene mutations are present in up to 100% of cases of metastatic hormone-refractory prostate cancer (Taplin *et al.*, 1995). At present, there is no established role for androgen receptor assays in diagnosis and treatment of prostate cancer, although this is under active investigation.

1.5 PROSTATE SAMPLING TECHNIQUES

1.5.1 Needle biopsy

The introduction of the automatic, spring-driven 18-gauge core biopsy gun in the late 1980s began a new era in the sampling of the prostate for histological diagnosis. The 18-gauge needle offered important advantages over the older 14-gauge needle. The rate of post-biopsy infection declined from 7-39% to 0.81%, and hemorrhage with urinary clot retention fell from 3.2% to less than 1% (Bostwick, 1994b). The false-negative rate declined from 11–25% to 11% and the quality of the tissue sample improved, usually with little or no compression artifact at the edges of the specimen. The 18-gauge needle also allowed sextant biopsies (six cores, usually including three from each side at the apex, midportion and base) and seminal vesicle biopsies with minimal discomfort (Terris, McNeal and Stamey, 1992; Hammerer, Huland and Sparenberg, 1992; Stamey *et al.*, 1993). The main disadvantage of the 18-gauge needle is that it provides less than half as much tissue per needle core for pathological examination as the traditional 14-gauge biopsy. A greater number of biopsies in recent years contain less than 10% cancer due to the success of early detection efforts in identifying smaller tumors at earlier stages. Frequently, we encounter small suspicious foci in biopsies from asymptomatic young men who have no palpable abnormality and only slight elevation of serum PSA concentration; this issue is discussed in Chapter 6.

Inking the needle biopsy is useful for identifying the tissue cores in paraffin blocks, but this is infrequently performed. There is variation between laboratories in the number of serial sections obtained from prostate tissue blocks for routine examination; we routinely obtain at least three sections on each of two slides, yielding a minimum of six sections. It may be useful to have three slides cut routinely, submitting slides 1 and 3 for hematoxylin and eosin stain and retaining slide 2 for special studies such as immunohistochemistry for keratin 34βE12 or digital image analysis for DNA ploidy analysis. In our experience, recutting the block for additional levels is useful in about half of cases, with usually no more than four additional slides before the tissue specimen is exhausted.

1.5.2 Fine needle aspiration

Fine needle aspiration remains popular for cytological examination of the prostate in parts

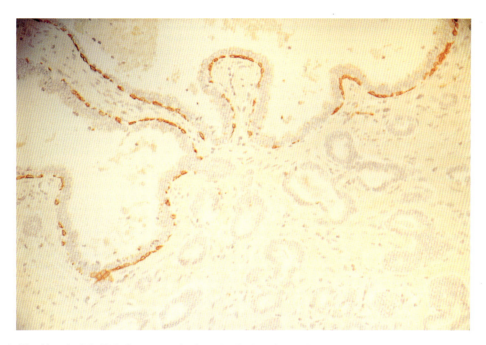

Figure 1.17 Keratin 34βE12 decorates the basal cells forming a discontinuous layer beneath the flat pattern of high-grade PIN (left and top); adenocarcinoma displays no immunoreactivity (center, right and bottom). Anti-keratin 34βE12 immunohistochemical stain.

of Europe and around the world, but interest in this method in the United States has dropped precipitously because of the ease of acquisition and interpretation of the 18-gauge needle core biopsy. Both techniques have similar sensitivity in the diagnosis of prostatic adenocarcinoma, and both are limited by small sample size; they are best considered as complementary techniques (Stilmant *et al.*, 1989; Maksem *et al.*, 1990; Maksem, 1995, 1996, 1997). Complications of fine needle aspiration occur in less than 2% of patients and are similar to those with needle core biopsy, including epididymitis, transient hematuria, hematospermia, fever and sepsis.

Fine needle aspiration produces clusters and small sheets of epithelial cells without stroma (Maksem, 1997) (Figure 1.18).

This enrichment for epithelium allows evaluation of single cells and the architectural relationship between cells. Benign and hyperplastic prostatic epithelium consist of orderly sheets of cells with distinct margins, creating a honeycomb-like pattern. Benign nuclei are uniform with finely granular chromatin and indistinct nucleoli; basal cells are often present at the edge. Prostatic carcinoma is distinguished from benign epithelium by increased cellularity, loss of cell adhesion, variation in nuclear size and shape, and nucleolar enlargement.

1.5.3 Transurethral resection (TURP)

The region of the prostate sampled by transurethral resection and needle biopsy tend to be different (McNeal *et al.*, 1988a). Transurethral resection specimens usually consist of tissue from the transition zone, urethra, periurethral area, bladder neck and anterior fibromuscular stroma (Table 1.4).

Studies of radical prostatectomies performed after transurethral resection show that the resection does not usually include tissue from the central or peripheral zone, and not all of the transition zone is removed. Most needle biopsy specimens consist only of tissue from

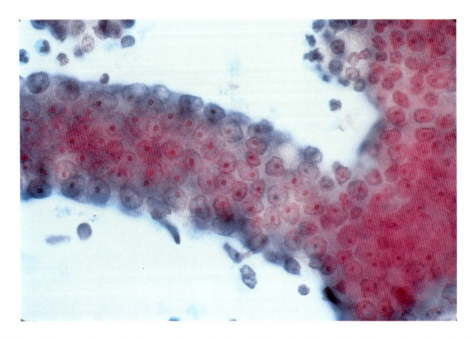

Figure 1.18 Adenocarcinoma in fine needle aspiration. Note cohesive cells with prominent nucleolomegaly. (Source: case courtesy of Dr John Maksem, Des Moines, IA.)

the peripheral zone, seldom including the central or transition zones.

Well-differentiated adenocarcinoma found incidentally in transurethral resection chips has usually arisen in the transition zone (McNeal *et al.*, 1988b). These tumors are frequently small and may be completely resected by transurethral resection. Poorly differentiated adenocarcinoma in transurethral resection chips usually represents part of a larger tumor that has invaded the transition zone from the peripheral zone.

The optimal number of chips to submit for histological evaluation from a transurethral resection specimen remains controversial, with some experts advocating complete submission even with large specimens that would require many cassettes (Rohr, 1987; Murphy *et al.*, 1986; Eble and Tejada, 1986; Vollmer, 1986). The Cancer Committee of the College of American Pathologists recommends a minimum of six cassettes for the first 30 g of tissue and one cassette for every 10 g thereafter (Henson, Hutter and Farrow, 1994).

1.5.4 Tissue artifacts

Cautery artifact is frequently extensive in transurethral resection specimens and often limits interpretation, particularly at the edges of the chips. The epithelium usually shows more damage than the stroma, with separation from the basement membrane, cellular disruption, loss of integrity of nuclear membranes and homogenization of the chromatin, creating featureless dark nuclei. In severely affected chips, coagulation necrosis is present, including tissue devitalization with loss of cell membranes and indistinct smeared chromatin.

Delayed fixation and air-drying commonly result in separation of the epithelium and the underlying basement membrane, as well as chromatin smearing and smudging (Figure 1.19).

This artifactual change is more prominent in malignant than benign acini, but both may be affected. Cell clusters floating in empty lumens may be mistaken for microvascular invasion.

Table 1.4 Glandular zones of the prostate: implications for disease

	Central zone	Transition zone	Peripheral zone
Tissue sampling techniques			
Transurethral resection	Poor	Good	Poor
Needle biopsy	Variable	Poor	Good
Involvement with pathological processes			
Atrophy	Infrequent	Variable	Frequent
Nodular hyperplasia	Rare	Frequent	Rare
Prostatitis	Infrequent	Variable	Frequent
Carcinoma (% of prostate cancers)	Infrequent (5)	Frequent (25)	Frequent (70)

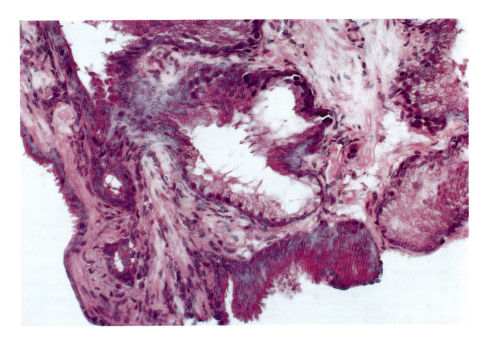

Figure 1.19 Artifactual drying of prostatic biopsy with chromatin smearing; this specimen is insufficient for diagnosis.

Degenerating lymphocytes and stromal myocytes may show vacuolization that mimics signet-ring-cell carcinoma (Alguacil-Garcia, 1986). In difficult cases, immunohistochemical stains are useful, with immunoreactivity for leukocyte common antigen in lymphocytes and smooth muscle actin in myocytes; both are negative for keratin AE1/AE3, PSA, and PAP.

REFERENCES

Abrahamsson, P. A., Wadstrom, L. B., Alumets, J. *et al.* (1987) Peptide-hormone- and serotonin-immunoreactive tumour cells in carcinoma of the prostate. *Pathol. Res. Pract.*, **182**, 298–307.

Abrahamsson, P. A., Ptak, A., Nakada, S. Y. *et al.* (1993) Immunohistochemical localization of the androgen receptors in neuroendocrine cells in human prostatic tissue and prostatic carcinoma. *Mod. Pathol.*, **6**, 54A.

Adlakha, H. and Bostwick, D. G. (1994) Paneth cell-like change in prostatic adenocarcinoma represents neuroendocrine differentiation: report of 30 cases. *Hum. Pathol.*, **25**, 135–139.

Alguacil-Garcia, A. (1986) Artifactual changes mimicking signet ring cell carcinoma in transurethral prostatectomy specimens. *Am. J. Surg. Pathol.*, **10**, 795–800.

Aprikian, A. G., Cordon-Cardo, C., Fair, W. R. *et al.* (1993) Characterization of neuroendocrine differentiation in human benign prostate and prostatic adenocarcinoma. *Cancer*, **71**, 3952–3965.

Arber, D. A. and Speights, V. O. (1991) Aneuploidy in benign seminal vesicle epithelium: an example of the paradox of ploidy studies. *Mod. Pathol.*, **4**, 687–689.

Arias-Stella, J. and Takano-Moron, J. (1958) Atypical epithelial changes in the seminal vesicle. *Arch. Pathol.*, **66**, 761–766.

Ayala, A. G., Ro, J. Y., Babaian, R. *et al.* (1989) The prostatic capsule: does it exist? Its importance in the staging and treatment of prostatic carcinoma. *Am. J. Surg. Pathol.*, **13**, 21–30.

Azumi, N., Traweek, S. T. and Battifora, H. (1991) Prostatic acid phosphatase in carcinoid tumors: immunohistochemical and immunoblot studies. *Am. J. Surg. Pathol.*, **15**, 787–790.

Bonkhoff, H. and Remberger, K. (1993) Widespread distribution of nuclear androgen receptors in the basal cell layer of the normal and hyperplastic human prostate. *Virchows Archiv Pathol. Anat.*, **422**, 35–38.

Bonkhoff, H., Stein, V. and Remberger, K. (1994) Multidirectional differentiation in the normal, hyperplastic, and neoplastic human prostate: simultaneous demonstration of cell-specific epithelial markers. *Hum. Pathol.*, **25**, 42–46.

Bonkhoff, H., Wernert, N., Dhom, G. *et al.* (1991) Relation of endocrine-paracrine cells to cell proliferation in normal, hyperplastic and neoplastic human prostate. *Prostate*, **19**, 91–98.

Bostwick, D. G. (1994a) Prostate-specific antigen. Current role in diagnostic pathology of prostate cancer. *Am. J. Clin. Pathol.*, **102**(Suppl 1), S31–S37.

Bostwick, D. G. (1994b) Gleason grading of prostatic needle biopsies: correlation with grade in 316 matched prostatectomies. *Am. J. Surg. Pathol.*, **18**, 796–803.

Bostwick, D. G. and Brawer, M. K. (1987) Prostatic intra-epithelial neoplasia and early invasion in prostatic cancer. *Cancer*, **59**, 788–794.

Brawer, M. K., Peehl, D. M., Stamey, T. A. and Bostwick, D. G. (1985) Keratin immunoreactivity in the benign and neoplastic human prostate. *Cancer Res.*, **45**, 3663–3667.

Brawn, P., Johnson, E. H., Foster, D. M. *et al.* (1994) Characteristics of prostatic infarcts and their effects of serum prostate-specific antigen and prostatic acid phosphatase. *Urology*, **44**, 71–75.

Brennick, J. B., O'Connell, J. X., Dickersin, G. R. *et al.* (1994) Lipofuscin pigmentation (so-called 'melanosis') of the prostate. *Am. J. Surg. Pathol.*, **18**, 446–454.

Cheville, J. C. and Bostwick, D. G. (1995) Post-atrophic hyperplasia of the prostate. *Am. J. Surg. Pathol.*, **19**, 1068–1076.

Choe, B. K., Pontes, E. J., Rose, N. R. *et al.* (1978) Expression of human prostatic acid phosphatase in a pancreatic islet cell carcinoma. *Invest. Urol.*, **15**, 312–316.

Cote, R. J. and Taylor, C. R. (1994) Prostate, bladder, and kidney, in *Immunomicroscopy: A Diagnostic Tool for the Surgical Pathologist*, 2nd edn, (eds C. R. Taylor and R. J. Cote), W. B. Saunders, Philadelphia, PA, pp. 256–276.

Di Sant' Agnese, P. A. (1992) Neuroendocrine differentiation in carcinoma of the prostate. Diagnostic, prognostic, and therapeutic implications. *Cancer*, **70**, 254–268.

Di Sant' Agnese, P. A. (1995) Neuroendocrine differentiation in prostatic carcinoma. Recent findings and new concepts. *Cancer*, **75**, 1850–1859.

Di Sant' Agnese, P. A. and Cockett, A. T. (1994) The prostatic endocrine-paracrine (neuroendocrine) regulatory system and neuroendocrine differentiation in prostatic carcinoma: a review and future directions in basic research. *J. Urol.*, **152**, 1927–1931.

Droese, M. and Voeth, C. (1976) Cytologic features of seminal vesicle epithelium in aspiration biopsy smears of the prostate. *Acta Cytologica*, **20**, 120–125.

Eble, J. N. and Tejada, E. (1986) Cost implications of sampling strategies for prostatic transurethral resection specimens: analysis of 549 cases. *Am. J. Clin. Pathol.*, **85**, 382.

Elgamal, A., van de Voorde, W., van Poppel *et al.* (1994) Immunohistochemical localization of prostate-specific markers within the accessory male sex glands of Cowper, Littre, and Morgagni. *Urology*, **434**, 84-90.

Epstein, J. I., Kuhajda, F. P. and Lieberman, P. H. (1986) Prostate-specific acid phosphastase immunoreactivity in adenocarcinomas of the urinary bladder. *Hum. Pathol.*, **17**, 939–945.

Ferguson, J. K., Sebo, T. A., Husmann, D. A. *et al.* (1995) Androgen receptor expression predicts survival in small cell carcinoma of the prostate. *J. Urol.*, **153**, 483A.

Fernandez, P. L., Gomez, M., Caballero, T. *et al.* (1992) Prostatic acid phosphatase in cloacogenic carcinoma. *Am. J. Surg. Pathol.*, **16**, 526–531.

Frazier, H. A., Humphrey, P. A., Burchette, J. L. *et al.* (1992) Immunoreactive prostate specific antigen in male periurethral glands. *J. Urol.*, **147**, 246–250.

Golz, R. and Schubert, G. E. (1989) Prostate specific antigen: immunoreactivity in urachal remnants. *J. Urol.*, **141**, 1480–1484.

Guinan, P., Shaw, M., Targonski, P. *et al.* (1989) Evaluation of cytokeratin markers to differentiate between benign and malignant prostatic tissue. *J. Surg. Oncol.*, **42**, 175–180.

Hammerer, P., Huland, H. and Sparenberg, S. (1992) Digital rectal examination, imaging, and systematic-sextant biopsy in identifying operable lymph node-negative prostatic carcinoma. *Eur. Urol.*, **22**, 281-287.

Hammond, M. E., Sause, W. T., Martz, K. L. *et al.* (1989) Correlation of prostate-specific acid phosphatase and prostate-specific antigen immunocytochemistry with survival in prostate carcinoma. *Cancer*, **63**, 461–466.

Hedrick, L. and Epstein, J. I. (1989) Use of keratin 903 as adjunct in the diagnosis of prostate carcinoma. *Am. J. Surg. Pathol.*, **13**, 389–396.

Henson, D. E., Hutter, R. V. P. and Farrow, G. M. (1994) Practice protocol for the examination of specimens removed from patients with carcinoma of the prostate gland. A publication of the Cancer Committee, College of American Pathologists. *Arch. Pathol. Lab. Med.*, **118**, 779–783.

Kamoshida, S. and Tsutsumi, Y. (1990) Extraprostatic localization of prostatic acid phosphatase and prostate specific antigen: distribution in cloacogenic glandular epithelium and sex-dependent expression in human anal gland. *Hum. Pathol.*, **21**, 1108–1115.

Keillor, J. S. and Aterman, K. (1987) The response of poorly differentiated prostatic tumors to staining for prostate specific antigen and prostatic acid phosphatase: a comparative study. *J. Urol.*, **137**, 894–898.

Kimura, N. and Sasano, N. (1986) Prostate-specific acid phosphatase in carcinoid tumors. *Virchows Arch. Pathol. Anat. Histol.*, **410**, 247–252.

Koivuniemi, A. and Tyrkku, J. (1976) Seminal vesicle epithelium in fine-needle aspiration biopsies of the prostate as a pitfall in the cytologic diagnosis of carcinoma. *Acta Cytologica*, **20**, 116–119.

Kovi, J., Jackson, M. A. and Akberzie, M. E. (1979) Unusual smooth muscle change in the prostate. *Arch. Pathol. Lab. Med.*, **103**, 204–205.

Kuo, P. M. and Gomez, L. G. (1981) Monstrous epithelial cells in human epididymis and seminal vesicles. A pseudomalignant change. *Am. J. Surg. Pathol.*, **5**, 483–490.

Lowe, F. C. and Trauzzi, S. J. (1993) Prostatic acid phosphatase in 1993: its limited clinical utility. *Urol. Clin. N. Am.*, **20**, 589–596.

McNeal, J. E. and Bostwick, D. G. (1990) Anatomy of the prostate: implications for disease, in *Pathology of the Prostate*, (ed. D. G. Bostwick), Churchill Livingstone, New York, pp. 1–14.

McNeal, J. E., Price, H., Redwine, E. A. *et al.* (1988a) Stage A versus stage B adenocarcinoma of the prostate: morphologic comparison and biologic significance. *J. Urol.*, **139**, 61–68.

McNeal, J. E., Redwine, E. A., Freiha, F. S. and Stamey, T. A. (1988b) Zonal distribution of prostatic adenocarcinoma. Correlation with histologic pattern and direction of spread. *Am. J. Surg. Pathol.*, **12**, 897–906.

Madara, J. L., Haggitt, R. C. and Federman, M. (1978) Intranuclear inclusions of the human vas deferens. *Arch. Pathol. Lab. Med.*, **102**, 648–650.

Maksem, J. A. (1995) Performance and processing of prostate aspiration biopsies: a strategy to ensure optimum cellularity and fixation. *J. Urol. Pathol.*, **3**, 347–354.

Maksem, J. (1996) Fine needle aspiration of the prostate gland used to detect a clinically significant asymptomatic cancer in the setting of benign prostatic enlargement. *Pathol. Case Reviews*, (in press).

Maksem, J. (1997) Fine needle aspiration of the prostate, in *Pathology of the Prostate*, (eds C. Foster and D. G. Bostwick), W. B. Saunders, Philadelphia, PA.

Maksem, J. A., Galang, C. F., Johenning, P. W. *et al.* (1990) Aspiration biopsy cytology of the prostate, in *Pathology of the Prostate*, (ed. D. G. Bostwick), Churchill Livingstone, New York, pp. 161–191.

Maygarden, S. J., Strom, S. and Ware, J. L. (1992) Localization of epidermal growth factor receptor by immunohistochemical methods in human prostatic carcinoma, prostatic intraepithelial neoplasia, and benign hyperplasia. *Arch. Pathol. Lab. Med.*, **1216**, 269–273.

Meisels, A. and Ayotte, D. (1976) Cells from the seminal vesicles: contaminants of the V-C-E smear. *Acta Cytologica*, **20**, 211–219.

Mellon, K., Thompson, S., Charlton, R. G. *et al.* (1992) p53, c-erbB-2 and the epidermal growth factor receptor in the benign and malignant prostate. *J. Urol.*, **147**, 496–499.

Mesonero, C. E. and Oertel, Y. C. (1991) Cells from ejaculatory ducts and seminal vesicles and diagnostic difficulties in prostatic aspirates. *Mod. Pathol.*, **4**, 723–726.

Murphy, W. M., Dean, P. J., Brasfield, J. A. *et al.* (1986) Incidental carcinoma of the prostate. How much sampling is adequate? *Am. J. Surg. Pathol.*, **10**, 170–176.

Nadji, M., Tabei, S. Z., Castro, A. *et al.* (1981) Prostatic-specific antigen: an immunohistologic marker for prostatic neoplasms. *Cancer*, **48**, 1229–1232.

Nagle, R. B., Ahmann, F. R., McDaniel, K. M. *et al.* (1987) Cytokeratin characterization of human prostatic carcinoma and its derived cell lines. *Cancer Res.*, **47**, 281-286.

Nagle, R. B., Brawer, M. K., Kittelson, J. *et al.* (1991) Phenotypic relationships of prostatic intraepithelial neoplasia to invasive prostatic carcinoma. *Am. J. Pathol.*, **138**, 119–128.

Nowels, K., Kent, E. and Rinsho, K. (1988) Prostate specific antigen and acid phosphatase-reactive cells in cystitis cystica and glandularis. *Arch. Pathol. Lab. Med.*, **112**, 734–738.

Okada, H., Tsubura, A., Okamura, A. *et al.* (1992) Keratin profiles in normal/hyperplastic prostates and prostate carcinoma. *Virchows Arch. Pathol. Anat.*, **421**, 157–161.

O'Malley, F. P., Grignon, D. J. and Shum, D. T. (1990) Usefulness of immunoperoxidase staining with high-molecular-weight cytokeratin in the differential diagnosis of small-acinar lesions of the prostate gland. *Virchows Arch. Pathol. Anat.*, **417**, 191–196.

Ordonez, N. G., Ro, J. Y. and Ayala, A. G. (1990) Application of immunocytochemistry in pathology, in *Pathology of the Prostate*, (ed. D. G. Bostwick), Churchill Livingstone, New York, pp. 137–160.

Pollen, J. J. and Dreiling, A. (1984) Immunohistochemical identification of prostatic acid phosphatase and prostate specific antigen in female periurethral glands. *Urology*, **23**, 303–307.

Rohr, L. R. (1987) Incidental adenocarcinoma in transurethral resection of the prostate. Partial versus complete microscopic examination. *Am. J. Surg. Pathol.*, **11**, 53–58.

Ruizevald de Winter, J. A., Janssen, P. J. A., Sleddens, H. M. E. B. *et al.* (1994) Androgen receptor status in localized and locally progressive hormone refractory human prostate cancer. *Am. J. Pathol.*, **144**, 735–746.

Sadi, M. V. and Barrack, E. R. (1993) Image analysis of androgen receptor immunostaining in metastatic prostate cancer. *Cancer*, **71**, 2574–2580.

Sadi, M. V., Walsh, P. C. and Barrack, E. R. (1991) Immunohistochemical study of androgen receptors in metastatic prostate cancer. Comparison of receptor content and response to hormonal therapy. *Cancer*, **67**, 3057–3064.

Shah, I. A., Schlageter, M. O., Stinnett, P. and Lechago, J. (1991) Cytokeratin immunohistochemistry as a diagnostic tool for distinguishing malignant from benign epithelial lesions of the prostate. *Mod. Pathol.*, **4**, 220–224.

Shaw, L. M., Yang, N., Brooks, J. J. *et al.* (1981) Immunochemical evaluation of the organ specificity of prostatic acid phosphatase. *Clin. Chem.*, **27**, 1505–1510.

Sinha, A. A., Hagen, K. A., Sibley, R. K. *et al.* (1986) Analysis of fixation effects on immunohistochemical localization of prostatic specific antigen in human prostate. *J. Urol.*, **136**, 722–727.

Sleater, J. P., Ford, M. J. and Beers, B. B. (1994) Extramammary Paget's disease associated with prostate adenocarcinoma. *Hum. Pathol.*, **25**, 615–617.

Sobin, L. H., Hjermstad, B. M., Sesterhenn, I. A. *et al.* (1986) Prostatic acid phosphatase activity in carcinoid tumors. *Cancer*, **58**, 136–143.

Spencer, J. R., Brodin, A. G. and Ignatoff, J. M. (1990) Clear cell adenocarcinoma of the urethra: evidence for origin within paraurethral ducts. *J. Urol.*, **143**, 122–125.

Srigley, J. R., Dardick, I., Hartwick, R. W. J. and Klotz, L. (1990) Basal epithelial cells of human prostate gland are not myoepithelial cells. A comparative immunohistochemical and ultrastructural study with the human salivary gland. *Am. J. Pathol.*, **136**, 957–966.

Stamey, T. A., Freiha, F. S., McNeal, J. E. *et al.* (1993) Localized prostate cancer. Relationship of tumor volume to clinical significance for treatment of prostate cancer. *Cancer*, **71**, 933–938.

Stein, B. S., Vangore, S., Peterson, R. O. *et al.* (1982) Immunoperoxidase localization of prostate-specific antigen. *Am. J. Surg. Pathol.*, **6**, 553–558.

Stilmant, M. M., Freedlund, M. C., De La Morenas, A. et. *al.* (1989) Expanded role for fine needle aspiration of the prostate. A study of 335 specimens. *Cancer*, **63**, 583–589.

Taplin, M.-E., Bubley, G. J., Shuster, T. D. *et al.* (1995) Mutation of the androgen-receptor gene in metastatic androgen-independent prostate cancer. *N. Engl. J. Med.*, **332**, 1393–1398.

Tepper, S. L., Jagirdar, J., Heath, D. *et al.* (1984) Homology between the female paraurethral (Skene's glands) and the prostate. *Arch. Pathol. Lab. Med.*, **108**, 423–427.

Terris, M. K., McNeal, J. E. and Stamey, T. A. (1992) Detection of clinically significant prostate cancer by transrectal ultrasound-guided systematic biopsies. *J. Urol.*, **148**, 829–832.

van Krieken, J. H. J. M. (1993) Prostate marker immunoreactivity in salivary gland neoplasms. A rare pitfall in immunohistochemistry. *Am. J. Surg. Pathol.*, **17**, 410–414.

Vollmer, R. T. (1986) Prostate cancer and chip specimens: Complete versus partial sampling. *Hum. Pathol.*, **17**, 285–290.

Walsh, P. C., Lepor, H. and Eggleston, J. C. (1983) Radical prostatectomy with preservation of sexual function: anatomical and pathological considerations. *Prostate*, **4**, 473–485.

2

INFLAMMATION

Patchy mild acute and chronic inflammation is present in most adult prostates, and is probably a normal finding (Blumenfeld, Tucci and Narayan, 1992). When the inflammation is severe, extensive, or clinically apparent, the term 'prostatitis' is warranted. There is a wide spectrum of prostatitis, many varieties of which are rare and poorly understood (Lopez-Plaza and Bostwick, 1990). Stamey considers prostatitis to be '[a] wastebasket of clinical ignorance' owing to significant variations in terminology, diagnostic criteria and treatment (Stamey, 1980).

2.1 ACUTE BACTERIAL PROSTATITIS

Patients with acute bacterial prostatitis present with sudden onset of fever, chills, irritative voiding symptoms and pain in the lower back, rectum and perineum. The prostate is swollen, firm, tender and warm. Microscopically, there are sheets of neutrophils surrounding prostatic glands, often with marked tissue destruction and cellular debris (Figure 2.1).

The stroma is edematous and hemorrhagic, and microabscesses may be present. Diagnosis is based upon culture of urine and expressed prostatic secretions; biopsy is contraindicated because of the potential for sepsis. Most cases

of acute prostatitis are caused by bacteria responsible for other urinary tract infections, including *Escherichia coli* (80% of infections), other Enterobacteriaceae, *Pseudomonas*, *Serratia*, *Klebsiella* (10–15%) and enterococci (5–10%). Gonococcal prostatitis due to *Neisseria gonorrheae* was common in the preantibiotic era but is rare today. Most cases of acute prostatitis respond to antibiotics.

Abscess is a rare complication, usually occurring in immunocompromised patients such as those with AIDS. Transrectal ultrasonography is a valuable method for preoperative diagnosis. Many patients with abscesses are treated by transurethral resection and antibiotics.

2.2 CHRONIC PROSTATITIS

Chronic bacterial prostatitis is a common cause of relapsing urinary tract infection, and is usually caused by *E. coli*. Clinical diagnosis is difficult, often requiring multiple urine cultures obtained after prostatic massage. Treatment is also vexing due to the inability of most intravenous antibiotics to enter the prostate and prostatic fluids when the organ is overrun with a chronic inflammatory infiltrate (Figure 2.2).

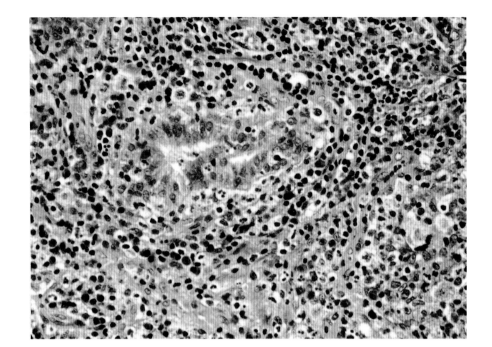

(a)

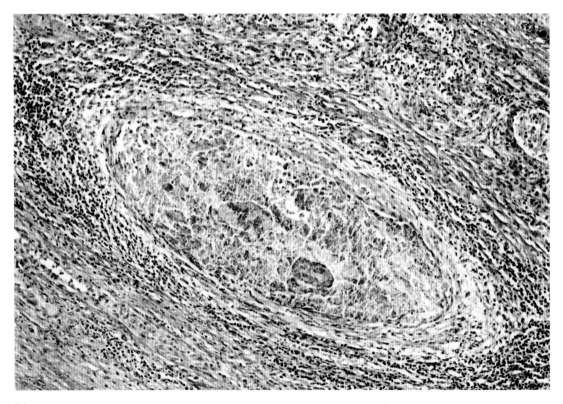

(b)

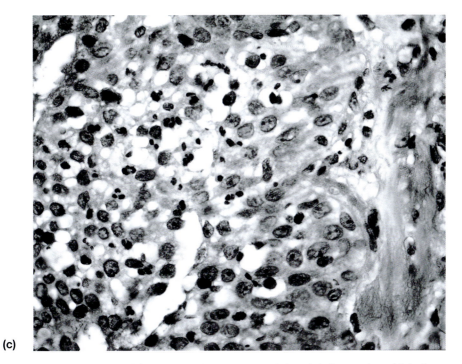

(c)

Figure 2.1 Acute inflammation. **(a)** There is a dense acute and chronic inflammation which obscures the acinar epithelium. **(b)** Constipated acinus with circumferential acute and chronic inflammation. **(c)** In this focus, the epithelium is proliferative and metaplastic, with scattered neutrophils.

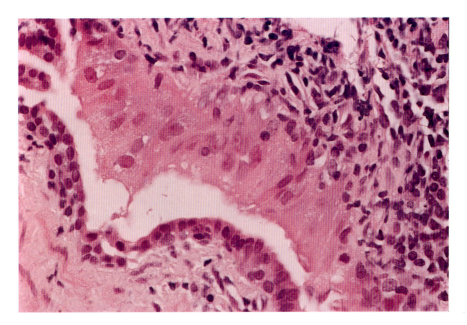

Figure 2.2 Inflammatory atypia in the setting of chronic inflammation. Note the metaplastic change which is adjacent to the inflammation. This was misinterpreted as high-grade PIN.

Also, prostatic calculi may contain bacteria embedded in the mineral matrix, and this serves as a nidus of recurring infection. The secretory products of the inflamed prostate are alkaline, with low levels of zinc, citric acid, spermine, cholesterol, antibacterial factors and certain enzymes.

Chronic abacterial prostatitis is more common than bacterial prostatitis, and rarely follows infection elsewhere in the urinary tract. Patients often complain of painful ejaculation. Cultures of urine and expressed prostatic secretions are negative. The etiological agent is unknown, but *Chlamydia, Ureaplasma* and *Trichomonas* have been proposed. This form of prostatitis has a prolonged indolent course with relapses and remissions. There appears to be no relationship between chronic prostatitis and the pathogenesis of benign prostatic hyperplasia (Helpap, 1994).

2.3 GRANULOMATOUS PROSTATITIS

Granulomatous prostatitis is a group of morphologically distinct forms of chronic prostatitis, the pathogenesis of which often cannot be determined. Causes include infection, tissue disruption following biopsy, BCG therapy, and others listed in Table 2.1 (Stamey, 1980; Stillwell, Engen and Farrow, 1987; Epstein and Hutchins, 1984; Lopez-Plaza and Bostwick, 1990).

The majority of patients have a prior history of urinary tract infection. The prostate is hard, fixed, and nodular, and cancer is usually suspected clinically. Urinalysis often shows pyuria and hematuria. Granulomatous prostatitis is probably caused by blockage of prostatic ducts and stasis of secretions, regardless of its etiology. The epithelium is destroyed and cellular debris, bacterial toxins and prostatic secretions including corpora amylacea, sperm and semen escape into the stroma, eliciting an intense localized inflammatory response (Figures 2.2–2.4).

This process is similar to intraprostatic sperm granuloma formation. Tissue eosinophilia may be prominent in prostates infested

with parasites, systemic allergic or auto-immune disease, iatrogenic post-TURP prostatitis or non-specific granulomatous prostatitis.

2.3.1 Granulomatous infections

Infectious granulomatous prostatitis is rare, and may be caused by bacteria, fungi, parasites, and viruses (Figure 2.5; Table 2.1).

Mycobacterium tuberculosis infection of the prostate only occurs after pulmonary infection or miliary dissemination. Small 1–2 mm caseating granulomas coalesce within the prostatic parenchyma, forming yellow nodules and streaks. Caseation and cavitation can be extensive. Brucellosis can mimic tuberculosis clinically and pathologically. Mycotic infections of the prostate are rare and invariably follow fungemia. Most of the deep mycoses induce necrotizing and non-necrotizing granulomas and fibrosis; *Candida albicans* is usually only associated with acute inflammation. Granulomas caused by *Schistosoma haematobium* are frequently found in the prostate as well as the bladder and seminal vesicles in endemic areas such as Egypt. The organisms lodge in vesicular and pelvic venous plexuses as the final habitat. The adult female schistosome migrates into the submucosa of the urinary bladder and prostatic stroma where she lays eggs that induce granuloma formation and fibrosis. Adenocarcinoma (Ma and Srigley, 1995) and squamous cell carcinoma (Adnani, 1985) of the prostate are rarely associated with schistosomiasis (Ma and Srigley, 1995). Herpes zoster infection may be associated with granulomatous prostatitis.

2.3.2 Postsurgical granulomatous prostatitis

Postsurgical granulomatous prostatitis can be identified years after transurethral resection of the prostate due to cauterization and surgical disruption of tissues (Figures 2.6 and 2.7) (Mies, Balogh and Stadecker, 1984; Koplovic,

Table 2.1 Classification of granulomatous prostatitis

I. *Infectious*
   A. Bacterial
      1. Tuberculosis
      2. Brucellosis
      3. Syphilis
   B. Fungal
      1. Coccidioidomycosis
      2. Cryptococcosis
      3. Blastomycosis
      4. Histoplasmosis
      5. Paracoccidiodomycosis
   C. Parasitic
      1. Schistosomiasis
      2. *Echinococcus*
      3. *Enterobius*
      4. *Linguatula*
   D. Viral
      1. Herpes zoster

II. *Iatrogenic*
   A. Postsurgical
   B. Postradiation
   C. BCG-associated
   D. Teflon-associated

III. *Malakoplakia*

IV. *Systemic granulomatous disease*
   A. Allergic ('eosinophilic')
   B. Sarcoidosis
   C. Rheumatoid
   D. Autoimmune/vascular
      1. Wegener's granulomatosis
      2. Polyarteritis nodosa
      3. Benign lymphocytic angiitis and granulomatosis (BLAG)
      4. Churg–Strauss vasculitis

V. *Idiopathic ('non-specific')*

Rivkind and Sherman, 1984). The granulomas are characteristically circumscribed and rimmed by palisading histiocytes with central fibrinoid necrosis. Multinucleated giant cells are frequently present. The striking histological resemblance of postsurgical granulomatous prostatitis to rheumatoid nodule suggests a hypersensitivity reaction or cell-mediated immune response. Tissue eosinophilia is present in many cases. Treatment is unnecessary for postsurgical prostatitis.

2.3.3 BCG-induced granulomatous prostatitis

Bacille Calmette–Guérin (BCG)-induced granulomatous prostatitis occurs in virtually all patients treated with intravesicular BCG immunotherapy for superficial urothelial carcinoma of the bladder (Oates *et al.*, 1988). The granulomas are characteristically discrete, with or without necrosis, and often contain numerous acid-fast bacilli. No therapy is required.

2.3.4 Teflon-induced granulomatous prostatitis

Periurethral and submucosal bladder injections of Teflon (polytetrafluoroethylene) have been used in the past for treatment of urinary incontinence. This foreign substance may migrate into the prostate and other sites, inducing a florid granulomatous response (Mahizia *et al.*, 1984; Politano, 1992; McKinney, Gaffet and Gillenwater, 1994; Orozco and Peters, 1995). Teflon in the prostate is basophilic, simulating neoplastic mucin dissecting through the prostatic stroma. Orozco and Peters recently described two cases of Teflon-induced granulomatous prostatitis in needle biopsies mimicking adenocarcinoma that occurred in patients 10 years after bladder injection (Orozco and Peters, 1995). Teflon tends to be more basophilic than mucin and appears filamentous and birefringent. The adjacent prostatic epithelium is rarely intact, and there are scattered or prominent multinucleated cells and other features of granulomatous prostatitis.

2.3.5 Malakoplakia

Malakoplakia is a granulomatous disease associated with defective intracellular lysosomal digestion of bacteria. It occasionally occurs in the prostate (Lopez-Plaza and Bostwick, 1990), presenting as a diffuse, indurated

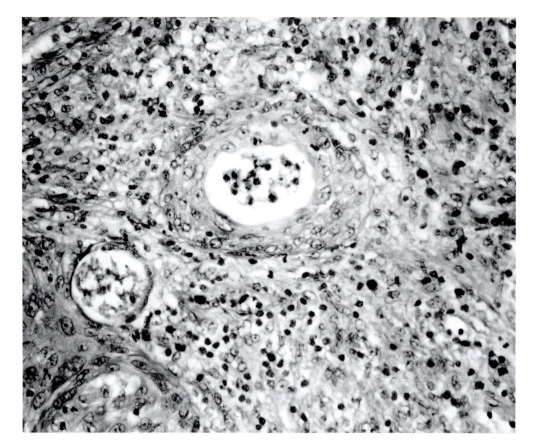

Figure 2.3 Necrotizing granulomatous prostatitis. The inflamed metaplastic epithelium merges with the cellular stroma.

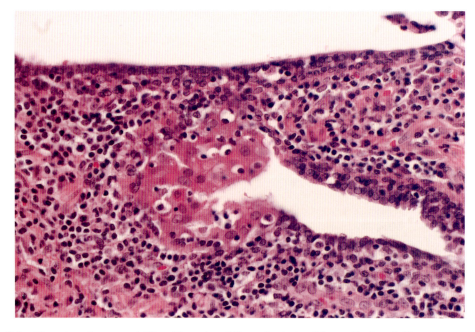

Figure 2.4 Granulomatous prostatitis with eosinophilic metaplasia of the epithelium (left).

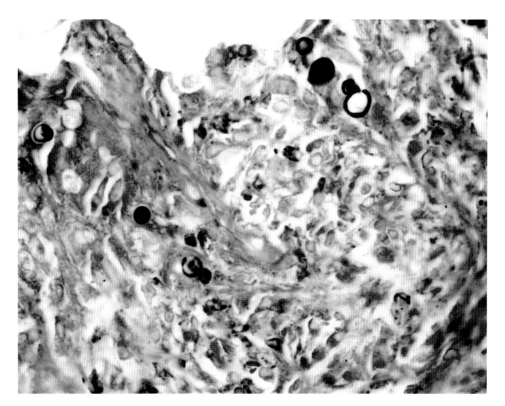

Figure 2.5 Blastomycosis of the prostate. Silver-stained fungal spores are present within areas of necrotizing granulomatous inflammation. Gomori's methenamine silver stain.

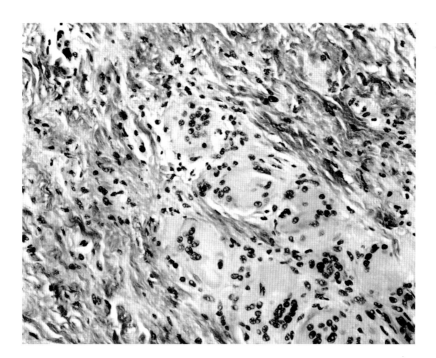

Figure 2.6 Granulomatous prostatitis following TURP, characterized by aggregates of multinucleated giant cells.

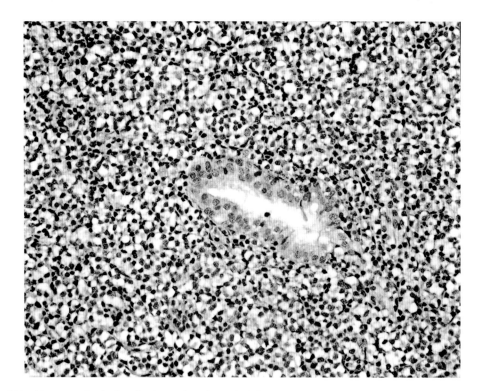

Figure 2.7 Non-neoplastic focally dense lymphocytic inflammation surrounding benign acinus. This was an incidental finding in a TURP specimen.

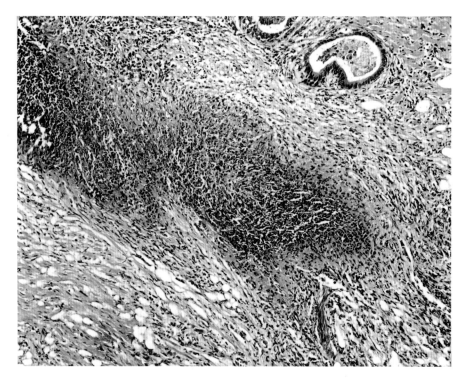

Figure 2.8 Wegener's granulomatosis with serpiginous necrosis rimmed by histiocytes mimicking post-TURP granulomatous prostatitis. This middle-aged man was subsequently found to have lung and kidney involvement.

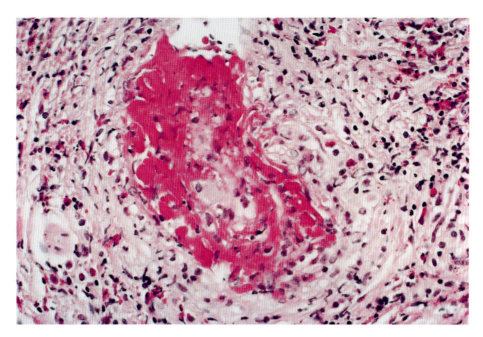

Figure 2.9 Churg–Strauss vasculitis with fibrin deposition. This prostate biopsy was the first evidence of systemic vasculitis.

mass clinically suggestive of prostatic carcinoma. *E. coli* is commonly isolated from urine cultures. Microscopically, the prostate is effaced by sheets of macrophages admixed with lymphocytes and plasma cells. Intracellular and extracellular Michaelis–Gutmann bodies are identified, appearing as sharply demarcated spherical structures with concentric 'owl's eyes' measuring 5–10 μm in diameter. PAS stain is useful in identifying non-mineralized forms and von Kossa stain for mineralized forms.

2.3.6 Allergic (eosinophilic) granulomatous prostatitis

Allergic granulomatous prostatitis is a component of Churg–Strauss syndrome. It should be diagnosed only in a patient with history of asthma or allergy with peripheral eosinophilia and systemic lesions. Histologically, it consists of granulomatous prostatitis with infiltrates of eosinophils, fibrinoid necrosis and vasculitis

(Epstein and Hutchins, 1984; Stillwell, Engen and Farrow, 1987). Treatment is steroids.

2.3.7 Wegener's granulomatosis

Prostatic involvement occurs in up to 7.4% of men with Wegener's granulomatosis, usually causing urinary obstruction, infection, hematuria and acute retention. The prostate is diffusely enlarged and often indurated. Urinalysis reveals microhematuria, red cell casts and proteinuria, features indicating renal involvement. The erythrocyte sedimentation rate is frequently elevated. The prostatic urethral mucosa is ragged and friable, and biopsy reveals necrotizing granulomatous inflammation with vasculitis (Figure 2.8).

Stellate and geographic granulomas are present, rimmed by palisading histiocytes and occasional multinucleated giant cells. Vasculitis involves small arteries and veins. Special stains for organisms are negative. Symptomatic prostatic involvement usually responds

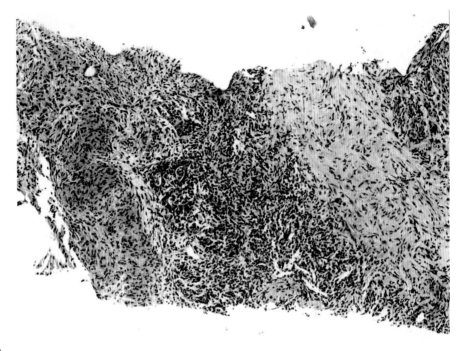

(a)

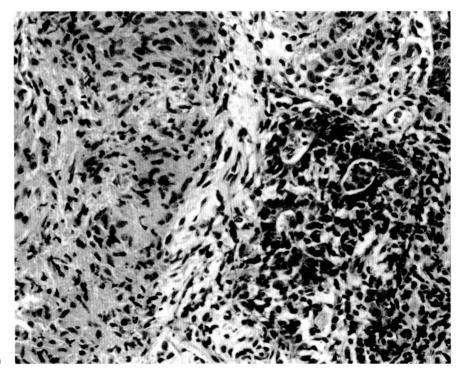

(b)

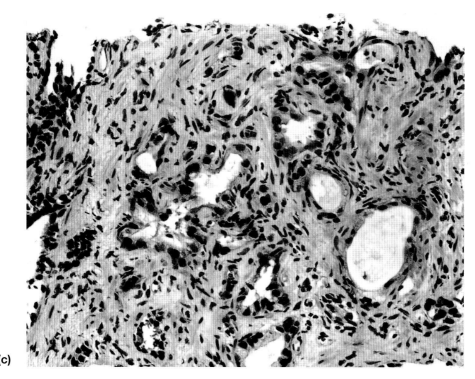

(c)

Figure 2.10 Idiopathic granulomatous prostatitis misinterpreted as poorly differentiated adenocarcinoma. At low magnification **(a)**, there is a dense cellular infiltrate. At high magnification **(b)**, the syncytial aggregate of histiocytes (left) stands in contrast with the chronic inflammation (right). Elsewhere in the biopsy core **(c)**, there is marked acinar distortion, anisonucleosis and nuclear hyperchromasia. These atypical reactive changes may mimic adenocarcinoma.

to chemotherapy, similar to pulmonary and renal involvement; TURP may also be helpful.

2.3.8 Other rare forms of granulomatous prostatitis

Other rare forms of granulomatous prostatitis include sarcoidosis, rheumatoid nodule, polyarteritis nodosa and silicone-induced prostatitis (Figure 2.9). Giant cell arteritis also rarely occurs in the prostate, sometimes without systemic involvement (Bretal-Laranga *et al.*, 1995; Lopez-Beltran, 1996).

2.3.9 Idiopathic prostatitis

Idiopathic (non-specific) granulomatous prostatitis ('of unknown cause') comprises the

majority of cases of granulomatous prostatitis (69%). The granulomas are usually non-caseating and associated with parenchymal loss and marked fibrosis. Classification of eosinophilic and non-eosinophilic types is probably of no clinical value. It is important to recognize the wide variety of inciting agents of granulomatous prostatitis and the histological clues that allow distinction of these different entities, but most cases elude definitive classification (Figure 2.10).

Induration may persist on physical examination for years even when there are no specific clinical symptoms. Up to 10% of patients with idiopathic granulomatous prostatitis do not respond to conservative management, developing severe urethral obstruction that requires TURP. However, transurethral resection is

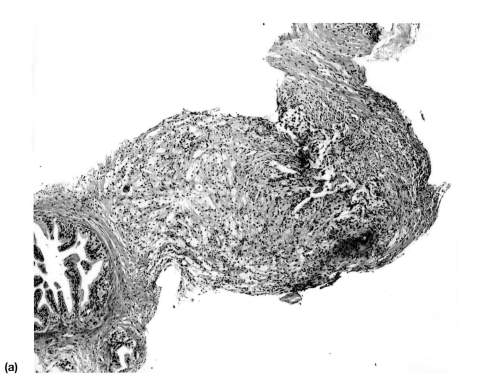

(a)

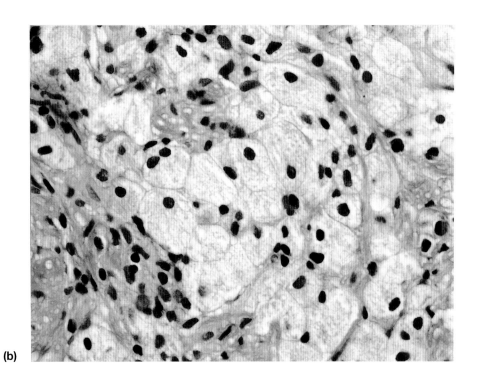

(b)

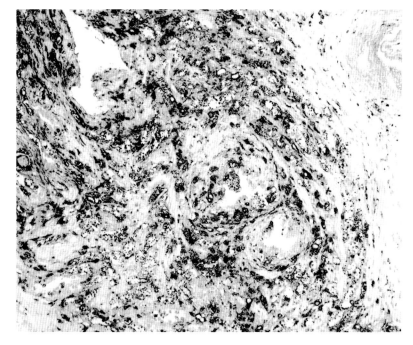

(c)

Figure 2.11 Xanthoma. **(a)** The needle core contains a collection of cells with clear cytoplasm misinterpreted as hypernephroid pattern of Gleason grade 4 adenocarcinoma. **(b)** The foamy histiocytes have small round to oval hyperchromatic nuclei. **(c)** There is intense cytoplasmic immunoreactivity for monocyte–macrophage marker KP-1. Immunohistochemical stain for KP-1.

Table 2.2 Clear cell proliferations of the prostate: differential diagnosis

Benign
  Atypical adenomatous hyperplasia with clear cell change
  Basal cell hyperplasia with clear cell change
  Cowper glands
  Mucinous metaplasia
  Paraganglia
  Storage disease
  Stromal nodular hyperplasia with myxoid matrix
  Xanthogranulomatous prostatitis
  Xanthoma

Malignant
  Clear cell adenocarcinoma of the prostate
    Transition zone cancer with clear cell pattern
    Status-postandrogen ablation ('nucleolus-poor' clear cell carcinoma)
    Mucinous carcinoma
    Signet-ring-cell carcinoma
  Epithelioid leiomyoma and leiomyosarcoma
  Secondary malignancies
    Clear cell carcinoma of the bladder
    Metastatic renal cell carcinoma, clear cell pattern
    Lymphoma with artifactual signet-ring cell-like pattern

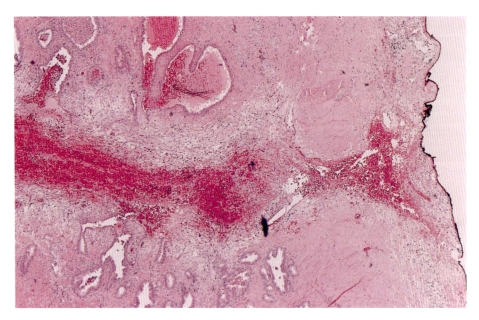

Figure 2.12 Line of hemorrhage denotes the needle track beneath the prostatic capsule on the right. This radical prostatectomy was obtained 2 weeks after sextant 18-gauge needle biopsies.

unsuccessful in up to 50% of cases, with some patients requiring multiple procedures.

2.3.10 Xanthoma

Xanthoma is a rare form of idiopathic granulomatous prostatitis that consists of a localized collection of cholesterol-laden histiocytes; it may also be seen in patients with hyperlipidemia (Figure 2.11) (Sebo *et al.*, 1994).

Xanthoma occurs in older men and is usually an incidental finding in patients undergoing transurethral resection or needle biopsy, although it may appear as a palpable nodule. Rare cases contain areas of typical granulomatous prostatitis, and the term xanthogranulomatous prostatitis is appropriate in such cases. Distinction from clear cell carcinoma ('hypernephroid' pattern) may be difficult and immunohistochemical stains for PSA and PAP often assist with this diagnostic concern (Table 2.2) (Presti and Weidner, 1991).

2.4 AIDS-RELATED PROSTATITIS

Patients infected with human immunodeficiency virus (HIV) are susceptible to opportunistic infections, including prostatitis, due in part to abnormalities of T- and B-lymphocyte function. Infectious prostatitis occurs in 14% of patients with acquired immunodeficiency syndrome (AIDS) and 3% with AIDS-related complex (ARC) or asymptomatic HIV infection. Prostatitis in these patients may be due to a variety of pathogens, including *E. coli*, *Klebsiella*, *Enterobacter*, *Serratia*, *Pseudomonas*, *Haemophilus parainfluenzae*, *Cryptococcus neoformans* and *Mycobacterium tuberculosis* (Selzman, Bennert and Kursh, 1994).

Patients with AIDS-related prostatitis may be asymptomatic or present with acute prostatitis, chronic prostatitis or abscess. Relapses are common despite prolonged antibiotic therapy.

2.5 PATHOLOGICAL CHANGES FOLLOWING NEEDLE BIOPSY

Contemporary transrectal 18-gauge needle biopsy of the prostate induces a predictable inflammatory response along a very narrow track (Bostwick, Vonk and Picado, 1994). The biopsy track consists of a partially collapsed cavity, often filled with red blood cells, rimmed by mixed acute and chronic inflammation, including lymphocytes, macrophages and occasional eosinophils (Figure 2.12).

There is a variable amount of hemosiderin pigment, granulation tissue and fibrosis, usually limited to the edge of the cavity. Venous thrombosis and foreign-body giant cell reaction are seen infrequently. Although tumor cells are frequently enmeshed within fibrous connective tissue, they are not seen within the cavity following 18-gauge biopsy (Bostwick, Vonk and Picado, 1994). Conversely, tumor is occasionally identified in the track following the wider 14-gauge biopsy, particularly with perineal biopsy (Greenstein *et al.*, 1989; Moul *et al.*, 1989; Zablow, 1989; Baech, Gote and Raahave, 1990; Haddad, 1990; Ryan and Peeling, 1990; Bastacky, Walsh and Epstein, 1991; Blight,1992).

Biopsy tracks in prostatectomies obtained 4–6 weeks after biopsy show fewer red blood cells and less acute inflammation than in those obtained earlier, but no other histological differences are noted. There is no evidence of florid granulomatous prostatitis or fibrinoid necrosis, which is often seen after transurethral resection. Biopsies involving benign prostatic tissue and cancer are histologically similar.

REFERENCES

Adnani, A. L. (1985) Schistosomiasis, metaplasia and squamous cell carcinoma of the prostate: histogenesis of the squamous cancer cells determined by localization of specific markers. *Neoplasma*, **32**, 613–622.

Baech, J., Gote, H. and Raahave, D. (1990) Perineal seeding of prostatic carcinoma after Trucut biopsy. *Urol. Int.*, **45**, 370–371.

Bastacky, S. S., Walsh, P. C. and Epstein, J. I. (1991) Needle biopsy associated tumor tracking of adenocarcinoma of the prostate. *J. Urol.*, **145**, 1003–1007.

Blight, E. M. Jr (1992) Seeding of prostate adenocarcinoma following transrectal needle biopsy. *Urology*, **39**, 297–298.

Blumenfeld, W., Tucci, S. and Narayan, P. (1992) Incidental lymphocytic prostatitis. Selective involvement with nonmalignant glands. *Am. J. Surg. Pathol.*, **16**, 975–981.

Bostwick, D. G., Vonk, J. and Picado, A. (1994) Pathologic changes in the prostate following contemporary 18-gauge needle biopsy: no apparent risk of local cancer seeding. *J. Urol. Pathol.*, **2**, 203–212.

Bretal-Laranga, M., Insua-Vilarino, S., Blanco-Rodriguez, J. *et al.* (1995) Giant cell arteritis limited to the prostate. *J. Rheumatol.*, **22**, 566–568.

Epstein, J. I. and Hutchins, G. M. (1984) Granulomatous prostatitis: distinction among allergic, non-specific, and posttransurethral resection lesions. *Hum. Pathol.*, **15**, 818–825.

Greenstein, A., Merimsky, E., Baratz, M. and Braf, Z. (1989) Late appearance of perineal implantation of prostatic carcinoma after perineal needle biopsy. *Urology*, **33**, 59–60.

Haddad, F. S. (1990) Risk factors for perineal seeding of prostate cancer after needle biopsy. *J. Urol.*, **143**, 587–588.

Helpap, B. (1994) Histological and immunohistochemical study of chronic prostatic inflammation with and without benign prostatic hyperplasia. *J. Urol. Pathol.*, **2**, 49–64.

Koplovic, J., Rivkind, A. and Sherman, Y. (1984) Granulomatous prostatitis with vasculitis. A sequel of transurethral prostatic resection. *Arch. Pathol. Lab. Med.*, **108**, 732–733.

Lopez-Beltran, A. (1996) Giant cell arteritis of the prostate. *Pathol. Case Rev.*, (in press).

Lopez-Plaza, I. and Bostwick, D. G. (1990) Prostatitis, in *Pathology of the Prostate*, (ed. D. G. Bostwick), Churchill Livingstone, New York.

Ma, T. K. F. and Srigley, J. R. (1975) Adenocarcinoma of prostate and schistosomiasis: a rare association. *Histopathology* **27**, 187–189.

McKinney, C. D., Gaffey, M. J. and Gillenwater, J. Y. (1994) Bladder outlet obstruction after multiple periurethral polytetrafluoroethylene injections. *J. Urol.*, **153**, 149–151.

Mahizia, A. A., Reiman, H. H., Myers, R. P. *et al.* (1984) Migration and granulomatous reaction after periurethral injection of polytef (Teflon). *J. A. M. A.*, **215**, 3277–3281.

Mies, C., Balogh, K. and Stadecker, M. (1984) Palisading prostate granulomas following surgery. *Am. J. Surg. Pathol.*, **8**, 217–221.

Moul, J. W., Miles, B. J., Skoog, S. J. and McLeod, D. G. (1989) Risk factors for perineal seeding of prostate cancer after needle biopsy. *J. Urol.*, **142**, 86–88.

Oates, R. D., Stilmant, M. M., Fredlund, M. C. *et al.* (1988) Granulomatous prostatitis following bacillus Calmette–Guèrin immunotherapy of bladder cancer. *J. Urol.*, **140**, 751–754.

Orozco, R. E. and Peters, R. L. (1995) Teflon granuloma of the prostate mimicking adenocarcinoma. Report of two cases. *J. Urol. Pathol.*, **3**, 365–368.

Politano, V. A. (1992) Transurethral polytef injection for post-prostatectomy urinary incontinence. *Br. J. Urol.*, **69**, 26–28.

Presti, B. and Weidner, N. (1991) Granulomatous prostatitis and poorly differentiated adenocarcinoma. Their distinction with the use of immunohistochemical methods. *Am. J. Clin. Pathol.*, **95**, 330–334.

Ryan, P. G. and Peeling, W. B. (1990) Perineal prostatic tumour seeding after 'Tru-Cut' needle biopsy: Case report and review of the literature. *Eur. Urol.*, **17**, 189–192.

Sebo, T. J., Bostwick, D. G., Farrow, G. M. *et al.* (1994) Prostatic xanthoma: a mimic of prostatic adenocarcinoma. *Hum. Pathol.*, **25**, 386–389.

Selzman, A. A., Bennert, K. W. and Kursh, E. D. (1994) Cryptococcal prostatitis causing urinary retention in an AIDS patient: a case report. *J. Urol. Pathol.*, **2**, 251–254.

Stamey, T. A. (1980) Urinary infections in males, in *Pathogenesis and Treatment of Urinary Tract Infections*, (ed. T. A. Stamey), Williams & Wilkins, Baltimore, MD, p. 1.

Stillwell, T. J., Engen, D. E. and Farrow, G. M. (1987) The clinical spectrum of granulomatous prostatitis: a report of 200 cases. *J. Urol.*, **138**, 320–323.

Zablow, A. I. (1989) Implantation of prostatic cancer after perineal needle biopsy. *Urology*, **33**, 449–451.

3

Non-neoplastic Metaplasia

The prostatic epithelium has an interesting but limited repertoire of responses to injury. These responses include a variety of metaplastic and proliferative lesions which may mimic adenocarcinoma (Table 3.1).

3.1 SQUAMOUS METAPLASIA

Squamous metaplasia results from a variety of insults to the prostate, including acute inflammation, infarction, radiation therapy and androgen deprivation therapy. The changes may be focal or diffuse, appearing as intraductal syncytial aggregates of flattened cells with abundant eosinophilic cytoplasm or cohesive aggregates of glycogen-rich clear cells with shrunken hyperchromatic nuclei (Figure 3.1). Keratinization is unusual except at the edge of infarcts or areas of acute inflammation. Squamous metaplasia commonly involves the prostatic urethra in patients with indwelling catheter.

3.2 MUCINOUS METAPLASIA

Mucinous metaplasia refers to clusters of tall columnar cells or goblet cells which are infrequently observed in the prostatic acinar epithelium (Figure 3.2) (Grignon and O'Malley, 1993).

This finding is invariably microscopic, and can also be seen in the urothelium of large

Table 3.1 Metaplastic changes of the prostate

Diagnosis	Features
Squamous metaplasia	Intraductal aggregates of flattened cells with eosinophilic cytoplasm, usually at edge of infarcts
Mucinous metaplasia	Mucin-producing columnar or goblet cells in the prostatic epithelium or urothelium
Neuroendocrine cells with eosinophilic granules	Isolated cells or small cell clusters with prominent eosinophilic cytoplasmic granules (usually seen as part of tumor)
Urothelial metaplasia	Urothelium within ducts and acini of the prostate; difficult to identify because of variable location of the normal transition–columnar junction
Nephrogenic metaplasia	Inflamed papillary mass of cystic or solid tubules in the urethra; rare

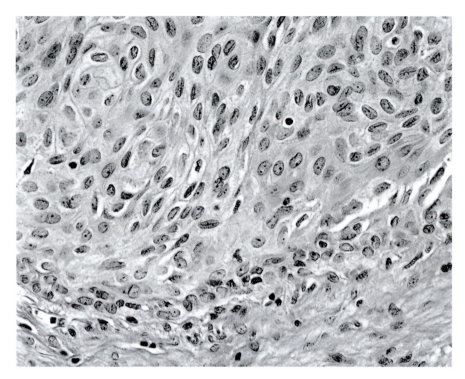

Figure 3.1 Squamous metaplasia. This syncytial aggregate of basal cells is whorled, with distinct cell borders. Note oval to elongate nuclei with central linear grooves (right).

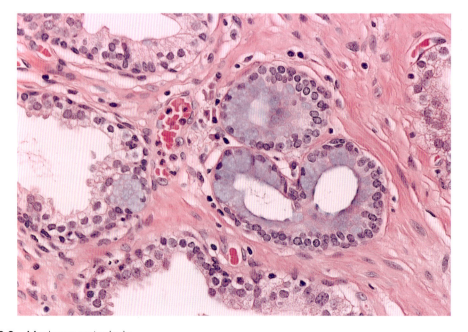

Figure 3.2 Mucinous metaplasia.

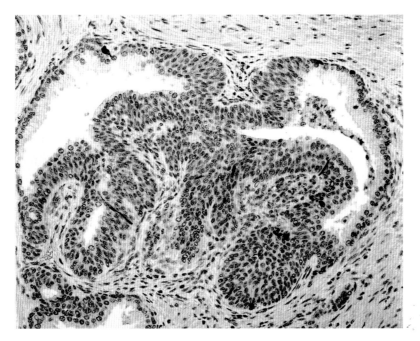

Figure 3.3 Urothelial metaplasia. This focus of thickened urothelium was found deep within the prostate in a radical prostatectomy specimen. Note the presence of columnar epithelium indicating the junction with the urothelium. Occasional neuroendocrine cells show dark reaction production (Immunohistochemical stain for serotonin).

periurethral prostatic ducts, foci of urothelial metaplasia, atrophy, nodular hyperplasia, basal cell hyperplasia and postatrophic hyperplasia. The cells contain acid mucin which stains with Mayer's mucicarmine, alcian blue (pH 2.7) and PAS following diastase predigestion; luminal secretions with similar staining are usually present. There is no immunoreactivity in mucinous metaplasia for PSA and PAP.

The differential diagnosis of mucinous metaplasia includes Cowper glands and adenocarcinoma. Unlike Cowper glands, mucinous metaplasia is usually focal within a small number of acini, lacking complete involvement of a lobular aggregate of acini.

3.3 NEUROENDOCRINE CELLS WITH EOSINOPHILIC GRANULES

Neuroendocrine cells with eosinophilic granules (NCEG; Paneth-cell-like change; PCLC)

are considered a distinct form of neuroendocrine differentiation in the prostatic epithelium, and may represent a normal finding rather than metaplasia (Haratake, Akio and Kenji, 1987; Frydman *et al.*, 1992; Weaver *et al.*, 1992; Weaver, Fadi and Abdul-Karim Srigley, 1992; Adlakha and Bostwick, 1994). This condition is characterized by isolated cells or small groups of cells with prominent eosinophilic cytoplasmic granules, present by routine hematoxylin-and-eosin-stained sections in 10% of serially sectioned radical prostatectomies. It is usually present focally, but is occasionally prominent and multifocal. NCEG are also present in isolated tumor cells or in continuous groups of cells, sometimes replacing an entire acinus. The distribution of NCEG is always patchy, and can be found in usual acinar carcinoma as well as cribriform, papillary and mucinous areas. The nuclei of NCEG are vesicular with prominent nucleoli, similar to other tumor cells. Luminal mucin is more common in cancer with NCEG than in cancer

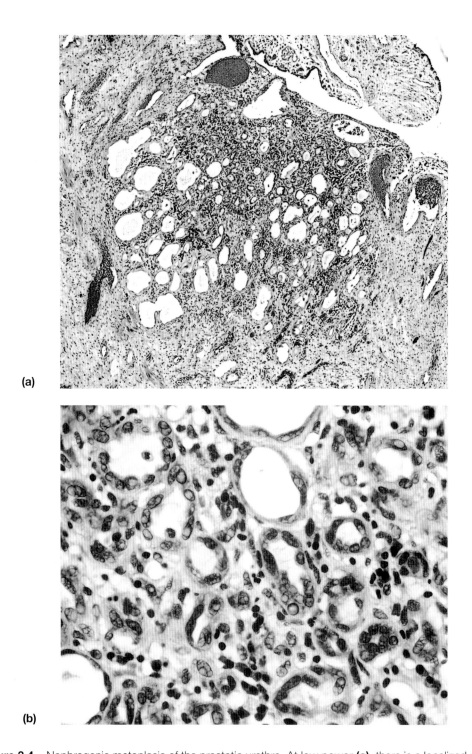

Figure 3.4 Nephrogenic metaplasia of the prostatic urethra. At low power **(a)**, there is a localized proliferation of irregular tubular structures immediately beneath the urethral epithelium (top right). At high magnification **(b)**, the small tubules are lined by flattened or hobnail cells. The stroma is chronically inflamed.

without NCEG. NCEG invariably display intense cytoplasmic immunoreactivity for chromogranin, neuron-specific enolase and serotonin. Many of these cells also express prostate-specific antigen and prostatic acid phosphatase. Lysozyme is negative.

NCEG are not associated with any factors predictive of aggressive behavior of prostate cancer, including tumor stage, serum PSA concentration and tumor grade, suggesting that this pattern of neuroendocrine differentiation is not indicative of poor prognosis (Adlakha and Bostwick, 1994).

NCEG account for only a small percentage of cells with neuroendocrine differentiation in benign prostatic acini and adenocarcinoma. Most neuroendocrine cells have small granules which are not apparent on hematoxylin-and-eosin-stained sections.

3.4 UROTHELIAL METAPLASIA (TRANSITIONAL METAPLASIA)

Urothelial metaplasia consists of urothelium within ducts and acini of the prostate beyond the normal transitional–columnar junction, arising apparently as a result of metaplastic change (Figure 3.3).

This junction is variable in location, creating difficulty in distinguishing metaplasia from normal urothelium in fragmented specimens such as transurethral resections and needle biopsies. Consequently, the diagnosis of metaplasia may be overused. Urothelial metaplasia is benign and easily distinguished from PIN by its characteristic architectural and cytological features.

3.5 NEPHROGENIC METAPLASIA (NEPHROGENIC ADENOMA)

Nephrogenic metaplasia most often occurs in adult patients in the urinary bladder, renal pelvis, ureter and urethra; prostatic urethral involvement is rare and extension

into the prostatic parenchyma may create diagnostic confusion with adenocarcinoma (Figure 3.4).

It usually follows instrumentation, urethral catheterization, infection, or calculi. Patients present with lower urinary tract symptoms, including hematuria, dysuria, obstruction and urethral mass (Martin and Santa Cruz, 1981; Carcamo Valor et al., 1992; Young, 1992; Malpica et al., 1994). Although the term nephrogenic adenoma is commonly used, it is a misnomer: this process is thought to be a reactive and metaplastic response to chronic inflammation or instrumentation and is not neoplastic.

Nephrogenic metaplasia appears as an exophytic papillary mass of cystic and solid tubules protruding from the urethral mucosa. The tubules may extend into the underlying prostate as a proliferation of small round to oval tubules, sometimes filled with colloid-like material. The lining consists of flattened or simple cuboidal cells, often with a distinctive hobnail appearance. Nuclei display finely granular uniform chromatin with inconspicuous nucleoli; occasional prominent nucleoli are observed. There is frequently chronic inflammation and edema of the stroma, but no desmoplasia is present.

The tubules contain scant or moderate mucin which is positive with alcian blue and PAS stains. The basement membrane is accentuated with PAS stain. Epithelial membrane antigen is positive in the tubular epithelial cells, and high-molecular-weight keratin 34βE12 stains many of the basal cells. PSA, PAP, and CEA are negative (Malpica et al., 1994).

REFERENCES

Adlakha, H. and Bostwick, D. G. (1994) Paneth cell-like change in prostatic adenocarcinoma represents neuroendocrine differentiation: report of 30 cases. *Hum. Pathol.*, **25**, 135–139.

Carcamo Valor, P. I., San Millan Arruti, J. P., Cozar Olmo, J. M. et al. (1992) Nephrogenic adenoma of the upper and lower urinary tract. Apropos of 22 cases. *Arch. Esp. Urol.*, **45**, 423–427.

Frydman, C. P., Bleiweiss, I. J., Unger, P. D. *et al.* (1992) Paneth cell-like metaplasia of the prostate gland. *Arch. Pathol. Lab. Med.*, **116**, 274–276.

Grignon, D. J. and O'Malley, F. P. (1993) Mucinous metaplasia in the prostate gland. *Am. J. Surg. Pathol.*, **17**, 287–290.

Haratake, J., Akio, H. and Kenji, I. (1987) Argyrophilic adenocarcinoma of the prostate with paneth cell-like granules. *Acta Pathol. Jpn.*, **37**, 831–836.

Malpica, A., Ro, J. Y., Troncoso, P. *et al.* (1994) Nephrogenic adenoma of the prostate gland: a clinicopathologic and immunohistochemical study of eight cases. *Hum. Pathol.*, **25**, 390–395.

Martin, S. A. and Santa Cruz, D. J. (1981) Adenoma-toid metaplasia of prostatic urethra. *Am. J. Clin. Pathol.*, **75**, 185–189.

Weaver, M. G., Fadi, W. and Abdul-Karim Srigley, J. R. (1992) Paneth cell-like change and small cell carcinoma of the prostate. Two divergent forms of prostatic neuroendocrine differentiation. *Am. J. Surg. Pathol.*, **16**, 1013–1016.

Weaver, M. G., Fadi, W., Abdul-Karim Srigley, J. *et al.* (1992) Paneth cell-like change of the prostate gland: a histological immunohistochemical and electron microscopic study. *Am. J. Surg. Pathol.*, **16**, 62–68.

Young, R. H. (1992) Nephrogenic adenomas of the urethra involving the prostate gland: a report of two cases of a lesion that may be confused with prostatic adenocarcinoma. *Mod. Pathol.*, **5**, 617–620.

4

HYPERPLASIA AND NODULAR HYPERPLASIA

Enlargement of the prostate, also known as nodular hyperplasia or benign prostatic hyperplasia (BPH; benign prostatic enlargement – BPE; adenofibromyomatous hyperplasia – AFH), consists of overgrowth of the epithelium and fibromuscular tissue of the transition zone and periurethral area. Symptoms are caused by interference with muscular sphincteric function and by obstruction of urine flow through the prostatic urethra. These symptoms, referred to as lower urinary tract symptoms (LUTS), include urgency, difficulty in starting urination, diminished stream size and force, increased frequency, incomplete bladder emptying and nocturia.

4.1 USUAL ACINAR AND STROMAL HYPERPLASIA

Development of nodular hyperplasia includes three pathological changes: nodule formation, diffuse enlargement of the transition zone and periurethral tissue, and enlargement of nodules (McNeal, 1990). In men under 70 years of age, diffuse enlargement predominates; in older men, epithelial proliferation and expansile growth of existing nodules predominates, probably as the result of androgenic and other hormonal stimulation. The proportion of epithelium to stroma increases as symptoms become more severe (Shapiro et al., 1992).

Grossly, nodular hyperplasia consists of variably sized nodules that are soft or firm, rubbery and yellow-gray, and bulge from the cut surface upon transection (Figure 4.1).

If there is prominent epithelial hyperplasia in addition to stromal hyperplasia, the abundant luminal spaces create soft and grossly spongy nodules which ooze a pale/white watery fluid. If the nodular hyperplasia is predominantly fibromuscular, there may be diffuse enlargement or numerous trabeculations without prominent nodularity. Degenerative changes include calcification and infarction. Nodular hyperplasia usually involves the transition zone, but occasionally nodules arise from the periurethral tissue at the bladder neck. Protrusion of bladder neck nodules into the bladder lumen is referred to as median lobe hyperplasia (Figure 4.1).

Microscopically, nodular hyperplasia is composed of varying proportions of epithelium and stroma (fibrous connective tissue and smooth muscle). The most common are adenomyofibromatous nodules, which contain all elements (Figures 4.2 and 4.3).

The diagnosis of nodular hyperplasia is often used by pathologists in needle biopsy specimens when only normal benign

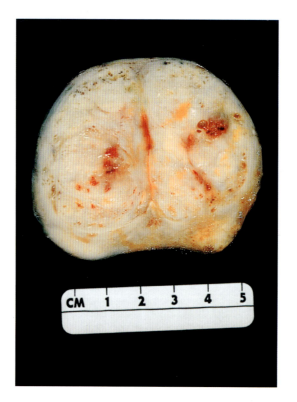

(a)

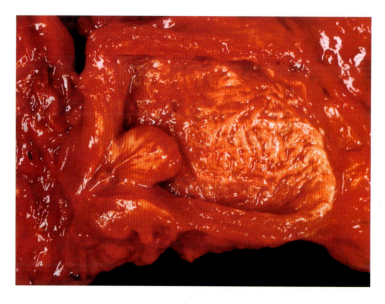

(b)

Figure 4.1 Nodular hyperplasia, gross appearance. **(a)** Transverse section of the prostate shows massive nodular hyperplasia with small foci of hemorrhagic infarction. A focus of adenocarcinoma forms an ill-defined mass in the peripheral zone at the lower right of the specimen. **(b)** Hyperplasia of the median lobe of the prostate has created an exophytic mass that protrudes into the bladder.

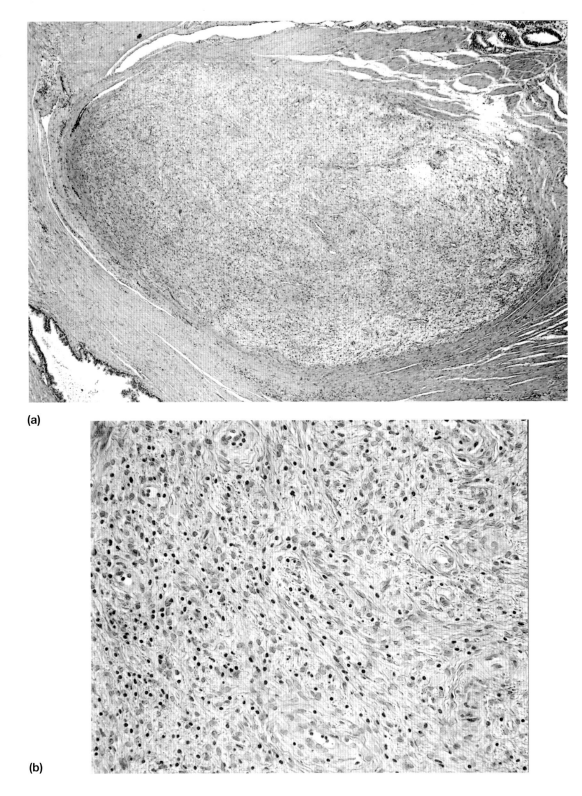

Figure 4.2 Pure stromal nodule of nodular hyperplasia. **(a)** This nodule is uniform and circumscribed. **(b)** The nodule consists of stromal fibroblasts with scattered lymphocytes.

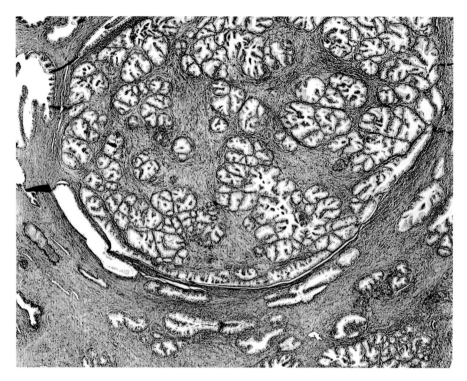

Figure 4.3 Mixed epithelial–stromal nodule of nodular hyperplasia. Note the dilated peripheral sinus which forms the boundary of the nodule with the transition zone stroma. This sinus often goes in and out of the plane of section, and may appear incomplete.

peripheral zone prostatic tissue is present. The transition zone is infrequently sampled by needle biopsies unless the urologist specifically targets this area or there is massive nodular hyperplasia which compresses the peripheral zone. We require the presence of at least part of a nodule for the diagnosis of nodular hyperplasia in needle biopsies. Narrow 18-gauge biopsies virtually never contain the entire nodule unless it is very small and fortuitously sampled. Casual use of the term 'nodular hyperplasia' for benign prostatic tissue may mislead the urologist into believing that a palpable nodule or hypoechoic focus of concern has been sampled and histologically evaluated; it is of clinical value for the pathologist to correlate the light-microscopic findings with the clinical impression. Variants of nodular hyperplasia are compared in Table 4.1.

Vascular insufficiency probably accounts for infarction of hyperplastic nodules, seen in up to 20% of resected cases. The center of the nodule undergoes hemorrhagic necrosis, often with reactive changes in the residual epithelium at the periphery, including squamous metaplasia and transitional cell metaplasia.

4.2 ATROPHY AND POSTATROPHIC HYPERPLASIA

Atrophy is a common microscopic finding, consisting of small distorted glands with flattened epithelium, hyperchromatic nuclei and stromal fibrosis. It is usually idiopathic, and the prevalence increases with advancing age. At low magnification, atrophy may be confused with adenocarcinoma due to prominent acinar architectural distortion. At high

Table 4.1 Histopathological variants of nodular hyperplasia

Variant	Microscopic features	Usual location
Atypical adenomatous hyperplasia	Localized proliferation of small acini in association with BPH nodule which architecturally mimics adenocarcinoma but lacks cytological features of malignancy	Transition zone
Basal cell hyperplasia	Proliferation of basal cells two or more cells in thickness; may have prominent nucleoli (atypical basal cell hyperplasia) or form a nodule (basal cell adenoma)	Transition zone
Cribriform hyperplasia	Acini with distinctive cribriform pattern, often with clear cytoplasm; easily mistaken for proliferative acini of the central zone	Transition zone
Hyperplasia of mesonephric remnants	Rare benign lobular proliferation of small acini with colloid-like material in the lumens; may mimic nephrogenic metaplasia focally; acini do not apparently express PSA or PAP	All zones (very rare)
Postatrophic hyperplasia	Atrophic acini with epithelial proliferative changes; easily mistaken for adenocarcinoma due to architectural distortion	All zones
Sclerosing adenosis	Circumscribed proliferation of small acini in a dense spindle cell stroma without significant atypia; usually solitary and microscopic	Transition zone
Stromal hyperplasia with atypical giant cells	Stromal nodules in the setting of BPH with increased cellularity and nuclear atypia	Transition zone
Verumontanum mucosal gland hyperplasia	Small benign acinar proliferation involving the verumontanum	Verumontanum

magnification, atrophy usually lacks significant nuclear and nucleolar enlargement except in cases of postatrophic hyperplasia. The nucleus-to-cytoplasmic ratio is high because of scant cytoplasm, and nuclei are dark.

Clusters of atrophic prostatic acini which display proliferative epithelial changes are referred to as postatrophic hyperplasia (PAH; postinflammatory hyperplasia; partial atrophy; postsclerotic hyperplasia) (Figure 4.4) (Franks, 1954; Cheville and Bostwick, 1995). PAH is at the extreme end of the morphological continuum of acinar atrophy which most closely mimics adenocarcinoma (Table 4.2).

This continuum varies from mild acinar irregularity, with a flattened layer of attenuated cells with scant cytoplasm, to that of PAH, in which the lining cells are low cuboidal with moderate cytoplasm. There is no sharp division in this continuum between atrophy and PAH, challenging the utility of PAH as a

distinct entity. However, the morphological similarity of PAH and carcinoma creates the potential for misdiagnosis, sometimes resulting in unnecessary prostatectomy (Cheville and Bostwick, 1995). To avoid this potentially tragic misinterpretation, the pathologist should have an understanding of this extreme morphological variant of atrophy. We believe that PAH is a diagnostic category for atrophic acini that most closely mimic adenocarcinoma, recognizing that this is merely a descriptive term.

PAH consists of a microscopic lobular cluster of five to 15 small acini with distorted contours reminiscent of atrophy. One or more larger dilated acini are usually present within these round to oval clusters, and the small acini appear to bud off of the dilated acinus, imparting a lobular appearance to the lesion. The small acini are lined by a layer of cuboidal secretory cells with mildly enlarged nuclei

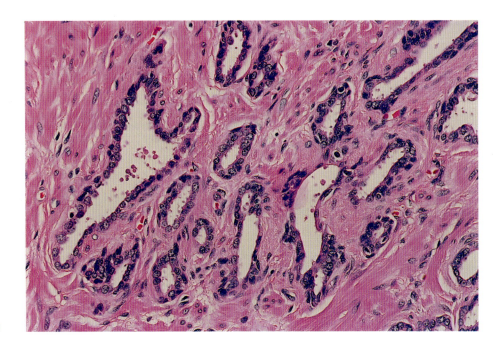

(a)

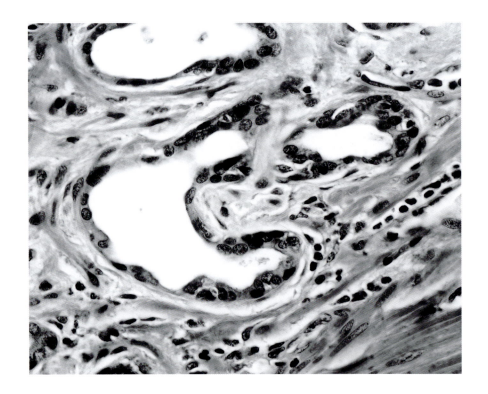

(b)

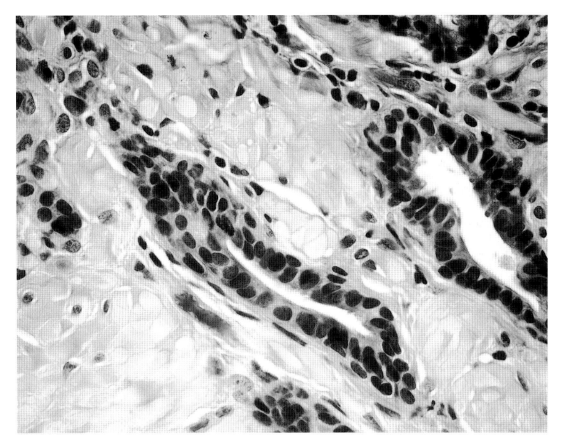

(c)

Figure 4.4 Postatrophic hyperplasia. **(a)** The acini are variable in size and shape, set in a fibrous stroma. Part of the epithelium is flattened, indicating atrophy, but other areas show low cuboidal epithelium, and luminal secretory blebs. **(b)** The epithelial lining is irregular, with hyperchromatic nuclei. **(c)** These elongate acini have enlarged nuclei with hyperchromasia. Nucleoli are inconspicuous.

with an increased nucleus-to-cytoplasmic ratio when compared with adjacent benign epithelial cells. The nuclei contain evenly distributed and finely granular chromatin, and nucleoli are usually small, although mildly enlarged basophilic nucleoli are focally present in 39% of cases. The cytoplasm is often basophilic or finely granular to clear, and luminal cytoplasmic apocrine-like blebs are present in 33% of cases. Luminal mucin is occasionally present in PAH. Corpora amylacea are present in 75% of cases of PAH, but crystalloids are rare.

The basal cell layer is usually present in PAH, but is often inconspicuous by routine light microscopy. Basal cell hyperplasia is rarely seen in foci of PAH. Immunohistochemical stains for high-molecular-weight keratin (antibody 34βE12) reveal a focally fragmented basal cell layer in some cases. Adjacent prostatic acini always show at least focal atrophy.

Stromal changes are always present in PAH, ranging from smooth muscle atrophy to dense sclerosis with compression of acini. In cases with sclerosis, the acinar lumens are

Table 4.2 Postatrophic hyperplasia versus low-grade carcinoma

	Postatrophic hyperplasia	*Low-grade adenocarcinoma*
Architecture		
Low power	Lobular small acinar proliferation, usually with central large dilated acini or acinus	May be lobular and circumscribed
Acinar contours	Irregular, 'atrophic'	May be rounded or smooth
Basal cell layer		
Light microscopy	Usually intact; may be inconspicuous	Absent
High-molecular-weight keratin (34βE12) immunoreactivity	Intact or fragmented	Absent
Stromal changes	Smooth muscle atrophy, often with dense periacinar sclerosis	With or without stromal sclerosis
Cytology		
Nuclei	Mild enlargement	Enlarged
Nucleoli	Usually inconspicuous	Usually prominent
Cytoplasm	Basophilic	Usually pale due to greater amount of cytoplasm
Basophilic mucin	Rare	May be present
Crystalloids	Rare	May be present
Adjacent acini	Often atrophic	Variable

compressed and showed marked distortion. Subtyping of PAH into lobular and postsclerotic subtypes is useful only to allow recognition of PAH and distinguish it from mimics such as low-grade adenocarcinoma, and we prefer not to subtype PAH. Also, PAH is often associated with patchy chronic inflammation; infrequently, dilated acini contain luminal neutrophils.

PAH is distinguished from carcinoma by its characteristic lobular architecture, intact or fragmented basal cell layer, inconspicuous or mildly enlarged nucleoli and adjacent acinar atrophy with stromal fibrosis or smooth muscle atrophy (Table 4.2). Low-grade adenocarcinoma is the most important differential diagnosis. PAH usually has a lobular pattern on low power, similar to Gleason pattern 2 and 3 adenocarcinoma. However, the lobular pattern in PAH is less distinct in cases with abundant stromal sclerosis, and there may be a pseudoinfiltrative growth pattern with fibrous entrapment of acini. Nucleolar changes are also useful in separating PAH and carcinoma, although some cases of low-grade carcinoma

have only scattered large nucleoli. Mildly enlarged nucleoli may be present in PAH, but only focally, and the majority of cells have small nucleoli. The separation of PAH from carcinoma is most difficult in needle biopsy specimens in which only a portion of the lesion is sampled, and awareness of this entity assists in this distinction.

4.3 STROMAL HYPERPLASIA WITH ATYPICAL GIANT CELLS

Stromal hyperplasia with atypia consists of stromal nodules in the transition zone with increased cellularity and nuclear atypia (Figures 4.5 and 4.6) (Leong, Vogt and Yu, 1988; Eble and Tejada, 1991).

These may appear as solid stromal nodules (often erroneously referred to as atypical leiomyoma) or with atypical cells interspersed with benign glands. Stromal nuclei are large, hyperchromatic and often multinucleated or vacuolated, with inconspicuous nucleoli (Figure 4.6(a)). There are no mitotic figures and

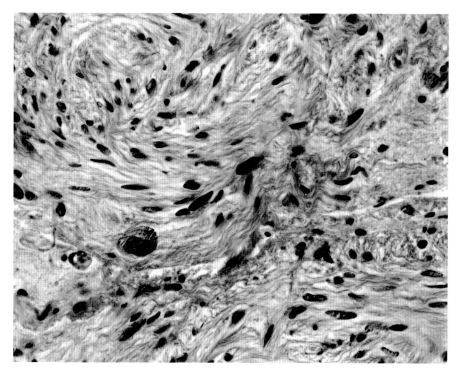

Figure 4.5 Stromal hyperplasia with atypical giant cells.

no necrosis. Stromal hyperplasia with atypia has no malignant potential, and the atypical cells are considered degenerative.

4.4 BASAL CELL HYPERPLASIA AND BASAL CELL PROLIFERATIONS

There are three patterns of benign basal cell hyperplasia, including typical basal cell hyperplasia, atypical basal cell hyperplasia and basal cell adenoma (Grignon *et al.*, 1988; Epstein and Armas, 1992; Deveraj and Bostwick, 1993) (Table 4.3). Neoplastic basal cell proliferations, referred to as adenoid basal cell tumor, adenoid cystic carcinoma, and basal cell carcinoma, are described in Chapter 8.

4.4.1 Basal cell hyperplasia

Basal cell hyperplasia consists of a proliferation of basal cells two or more cells in thickness at the periphery of prostatic acini (Figure 4.7) (Dermer, 1978; Cleary, Choi and Ayala, 1983; Grignon *et al.*, 1988; Deveraj and Bostwick, 1993).

It sometimes appears as small nests of cells surrounded by compressed stroma, often associated with chronic inflammation. The nests may be solid or cystically dilated, and are occasionally punctuated by irregular round luminal spaces, creating a cribriform pattern. Basal cell hyperplasia frequently involves only part of an acinus, and sometimes protrudes into the lumen, retaining the overlying secretory cell layer (Figure 4.8(a)); less commonly, there is symmetric duplication of the basal cell layer at the periphery of the acinus.

The proliferation may protrude into the acinar lumen, retaining the overlying secretory luminal epithelium. Symmetrical circumferential thickening of the basal cell layer is less frequent than eccentric thickening, and these changes do not result from tangential sectioning.

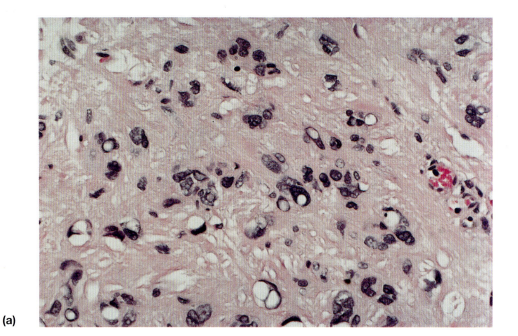

(a)

(b)

Figure 4.6 Stromal hyperplasia with atypical cells. **(a)** Symplastic changes of many of the myocytes, including nuclear and cytoplasmic vacuolization. **(b)** In another case, there is focal crowding of mycoytes with variation in nuclear size. No mitotic figures were observed in either of these cases despite exhaustive sectioning.

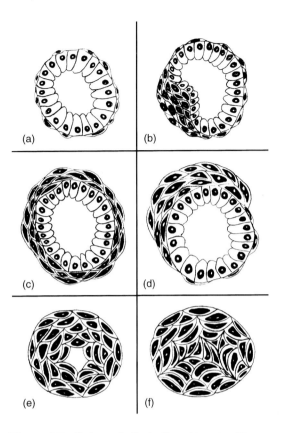

Figure 4.7 Schematic illustration of basal cell hyperplasia in the prostate. **(a)** Normal prostatic gland with thin peripheral layer of basal cells and overlying columnar secretory luminal cell layer. **(b)** Focal basal cell proliferation with mild distortion of the glandular luminal contour. **(c)** Symmetric circumferential proliferation of basal cells, at least 2 cells in thickness. **(d)** Eccentric focus of atypical basal cell hyperplasia with prominent nucleoli, eccentric pattern. **(e)** Basal cell hyperplasia with loss of secretory cell layer (note retention of glandular lumen); compare with **(f)** — 'solid' pattern of basal cell hyperplasia, with absence of lumen. (Source: reprinted with permission from Deveraj and Bostwick, 1993).

The basal cells in basal cell hyperplasia are enlarged, ovoid or round, and plump (epithelioid), with large, pale, ovoid nuclei, finely reticular chromatin and a moderate amount of cytoplasm. Nucleoli are usually inconspicuous (less than 1 μm in diameter) except in atypical BCH (see below).

Sclerosing basal cell hyperplasia is identical to typical basal cell hyperplasia except for the presence of delicate lace-like fibrosis or dense irregular sclerotic fibrosis and hyperplastic smooth muscle surrounding and distorting hyperplastic basal cell aggregates. It is not associated with carcinoma, but occasionally may be confused with malignancy.

Clear cell change is common in basal cell hyperplasia, often with a cribriform pattern; cribriform pattern without clear cell change is rare. Squamous metaplasia is infrequent, usually associated with infarction. Chronic inflammation is a common association, but is non-specific. Occasional nuclear grooves and nuclear 'bubble' artifact are observed. Focal calcification is evident in some cases, and may be present within the basal cell nests.

4.4.2 Atypical basal cell hyperplasia

Atypical basal cell hyperplasia is identical to basal cell hyperplasia except for the presence of large prominent nucleoli (Figure 4.8). The nucleoli are round to oval and lightly eosinophilic. There is chronic inflammation in the majority of cases, suggesting that nucleolomegaly is a reflection of reactive atypia. A morphological spectrum of nucleolar size is observed in basal cell proliferations, and only those with more than 10% of cells exhibiting prominent nucleoli are considered atypical (Deveraj and Bostwick, 1993). This lesion is significant because of the potential for misdiagnosis as adenocarcinoma.

4.4.3 Basal cell adenoma

Basal cell adenoma consists of one or more large round, usually solitary circumscribed nodules of acini with basal cell hyperplasia in the setting of nodular hyperplasia. The nodules contain uniformly spaced aggregates of hyperplastic basal cells which form small solid nests or cystically dilated acini. Condensed stroma is seen at the periphery,

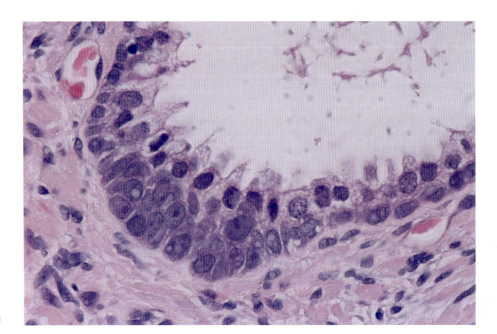

(a)

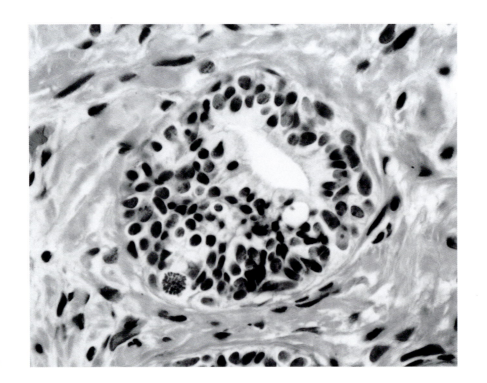

(b)

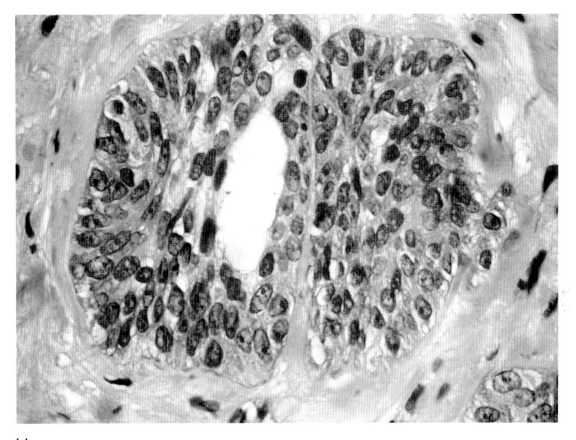

(c)

Figure 4.8 Atypical basal cell hyperplasia. **(a)** The basal cell nuclei are enlarged and round, with central enlarged nucleoli. Note the secretory cell layer at the surface, consisting of cells with pale finely vacuolated cytoplasm and darkly staining nuclei with irregular nuclear outlines. **(b)** In another case, the basal cell nuclei are slightly enlarged, with punctate dark nucleoli. **(c)** A third case of atypical basal cell hyperplasia, demonstrating variation in nuclear size and shape.

and often traverses the adenomatous nodules, creating incomplete lobulation in some cases. Stroma is normal or slightly increased in density and may be basophilic without myxoid change adjacent to cell nests.

The basal cells in basal cell adenoma are plump, with large nuclei, scant cytoplasm, and inconspicuous nucleoli, although large prominent nucleoli are rarely observed. Many cells are cuboidal or 'epithelioid', particularly near the center of the cell nests, and some contain clear cytoplasm. Prominent calcific debris is often present within acinar lumens.

Multiple basal cell adenomas are referred to as basal cell adenomatosis. Basal cell adenoma invariably arises in association with nodular hyperplasia, and appears to be a variant with no malignant potential.

4.4.4 Immunohistochemical findings

Basal cell hyperplasia (typical and atypical forms) displays intense cytoplasmic immunoreactivity in virtually all of the cells with high-molecular-weight keratin 34βE12 (Table 4.3).

Table 4.3 Basal cell proliferations of the prostate: diagnostic criteria and immunohistochemical profile (±, <5% of cells were positive) (Source: from Devaraj and Bostwick, 1993, with permission)

	Normal basal cell layer	Basal cell hyperplasia (BCH)	Atypical basal cell hyperplasia	Basal cell adenoma	Adenoid basal cell carcinoma
Architecture	Near-continuous single cell layer	Small cell nests (solid or cystic), usually in nodular hyperplasia, two cell layer minimum	Same as BCH	Round circumscribed nodule of BCH	Infiltrating 'adenoid cystic' pattern or basaloid pattern; myxoid stroma
Cytology	Small elongate cells, ovoid nuclei, scant cytoplasm	Large ovoid nuclei, indistinct nucleoli, scant cytoplasm, may have clear cytoplasm	Same as BCH, but with nucleolomegaly	Same as BCH, may have nucleolomegaly	Basaloid cells with large nuclei
Immunohistochemical findings					
Basal-cell-specific keratin 34βE12	+	+	+	+	+ (patchy)
Prostate-specific antigen	−	+ (patchy)	+ (patchy)	+ (focal)	±
Prostatic acid phosphatase	−	+ (patchy)	+ (patchy)	+ (focal)	±
Chromogranin	−	±	±	±	±
S-100 protein	−	±	±	±	−
Neuron-specific enolase	−	±	±	−	−

Immunoreactivity for PSA, PAP, chromogranin, S-100 protein and neuron-specific enolase is present in rare basal cells in the majority of cases.

4.4.5 Differential diagnosis

The differential diagnosis of basal cell proliferations includes a wide variety of benign and malignant lesions. Atypical adenomatous hyperplasia may be confused with basal cell hyperplasia, but does not usually have a prominent basal cell layer, and displays a fragmented keratin 34βE12-immunoreactive basal cell layer. Sclerosing adenosis may be difficult to separate from sclerosing basal cell hyperplasia and these lesions may coexist; however, sclerosing adenosis has no smooth muscle in the sclerotic stroma and displays myoepithelial differentiation (intense cytoplasmic immunoreactivity with keratin 34βE12, S-100 protein and muscle-specific actin, as well as ultrastructural evidence of cytoplasmic myofilaments).

Seminal vesicle and ejaculatory duct epithelium may also be confused with basal cell hyperplasia and adenoma, particularly in small specimens such as needle biopsies and rarely in transurethral resection specimens. The proliferation and stratification of lining cells with cytological atypia may resemble small foci of solid basal cell hyperplasia. The seminal vesicular epithelium is distinguished by the presence of secretory luminal cells, significant cytological atypia (particularly in the senile seminal vesicle) and distinctive abundant yellow to golden-brown lipochrome pigment.

The normal urothelium of the prostatic urethra and periurethral ducts resembles basal cell hyperplasia histologically and immunohistochemically. Also, transitional metaplasia may occur in the medium-sized and small ducts in the prostate, sometimes in association with inflammation and reactive atypia with mild nucleolomegaly.

Urethral polyp, although uncommon, may be confused with basal cell hyperplasia and adenoma, particularly in small cystoscopic specimens and needle biopsies. Urethral polyp includes proliferative papillary urethritis, ectopic prostatic tissue, nephrogenic metaplasia and inverted papilloma.

Prostatic intraepithelial neoplasia may be mistaken for atypical basal cell hyperplasia and is distinguished by the presence of cytological abnormalities in secretory luminal cells of medium-sized to large acini, intense cytoplasmic PSA and PAP immunoreactivity in the abnormal cells and an intact or fragmented keratin 34βE12-immunoreactive basal cell layer.

Well differentiated adenocarcinoma is distinguished from BCH by the presence of PSA- and PAP-immunoreactive luminal secretory cells with nucleolomegaly, frequent luminal crystalloids and absence of a keratin 34βE12-immunoreactive basal cell layer. Similar criteria allow separation of the cribriform variant of adenocarcinoma, adenoid cystic carcinoma, basal cell hyperplasia with or without clear cell change and clear cell cribriform hyperplasia.

4.5 CRIBRIFORM HYPERPLASIA

Cribriform hyperplasia, including clear cell cribriform hyperplasia, consists of a nodule of glands arranged in a distinctive cribriform pattern (Figures 4.9 and 4.10).

The cells from such glands usually have pale to clear cytoplasm and small uniform nuclei with inconspicuous nucleoli (Ayala *et al.*, 1986; Frauenhoffer *et al.*, 1991). The basal cell layer in cribriform hyperplasia may have enlarged nuclei, and this lesion should be distinguished from high-grade PIN and carcinoma by the lack of prominent nucleoli in acinar cells.

4.6 ATYPICAL ADENOMATOUS HYPERPLASIA

Atypical adenomatous hyperplasia (AAH; atypical hyperplasia; small acinar atypical hyperplasia; adenosis; atypical adenosis) is a

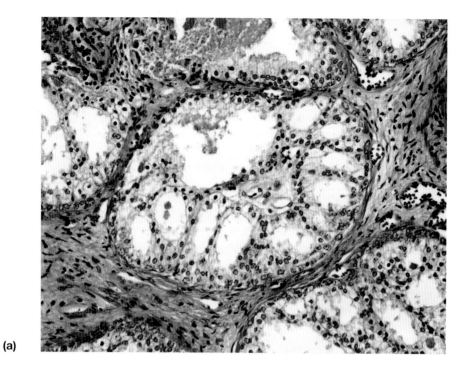

(a)

(b)

Figure 4.9 Clear cell cribriform hyperplasia. **(a)** At low magnification, the fenestrations are irregular in size and shape and are contained within expanded acini. **(b)** At high magnification, another case had a more solid proliferation of cells with pale, finely vacuolated cytoplasm, uniform nuclei with open chromatin pattern and small inconspicuous nucleoli.

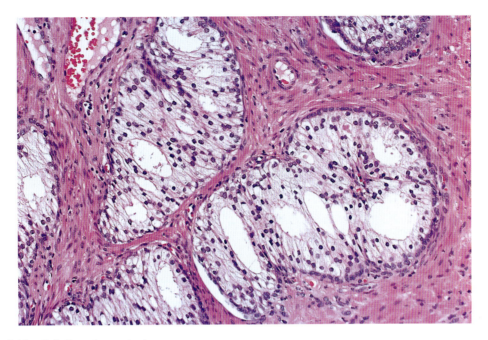

Figure 4.10 Cribriform hyperplasia.

localized proliferation of small acini within the prostate that may be mistaken for carcinoma (Figures 4.11–4.16) (Bostwick *et al.*, 1993, 1994; Bostwick and Qian, 1995).

Small acinar proliferations in the prostate form a morphological continuum ranging from benign proliferations with minimal architectural and cytological atypia to those in which the degree of atypia is such that they are easily recognized as well-differentiated adenocarcinoma. The proliferations are easily distinguished at widely spaced points of the spectrum; however, no abrupt change is apparent along the continuum. The greatest difficulty in distinguishing AAH from carcinoma is with lesions containing nucleoli intermediate in size between benign and malignant (Table 4.4; Figure 4.17).

To accommodate this borderline group, we recommend separating small acinar proliferations into AAH (probably benign) and atypical small acinar proliferation (possibly benign, but having some features of carcinoma). Importantly, lesions in the category of 'atypical small acinar proliferation' may have enlarged nucle-

oli, but they maintain a fragmented basal cell layer, similar to that seen in AAH. Furthermore, these lesions generate considerable discordance among observers. In view of the uncertainty of the nature of these lesions, some pathologists may prefer a more non-committal term such as 'atypical small acinar proliferation, not further classified.' Some authors use the term adenosis rather than AAH for these lesions.

Atypical adenomatous hyperplasia varies in incidence from 19.6% (transurethral resection specimens) to 24% (autopsy series in 20–40-year-old men) (Brawn *et al.*, 1989). It can be found throughout the prostate, but is usually present near the apex and in the transition zone and periurethral area (Bostwick and Qian, 1995).

4.6.1 Separation of AAH and cancer

AAH is distinguished from well-differentiated carcinoma by the following:

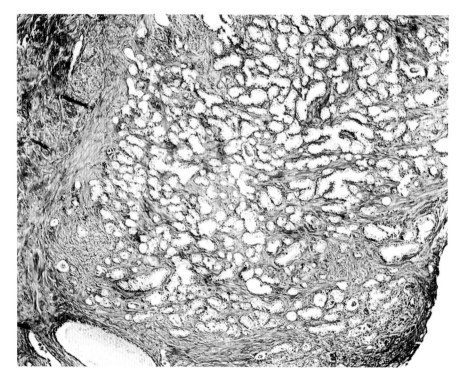

Figure 4.11 Atypical adenomatous hyperplasia. The small acinar proliferation shows variation in size, shape and spacing in a moderately cellular stroma.

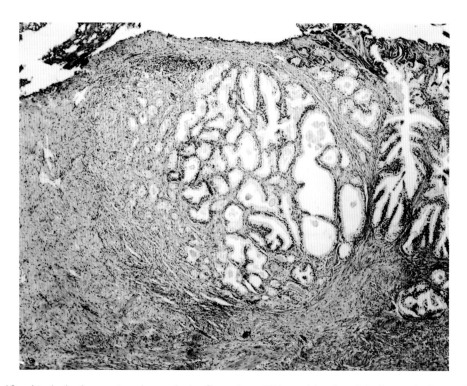

Figure 4.12 Atypical adenomatous hyperplasia. One edge of this nodule of nodular hyperplasia consists of a proliferation of small pale acini set in a cellular stroma.

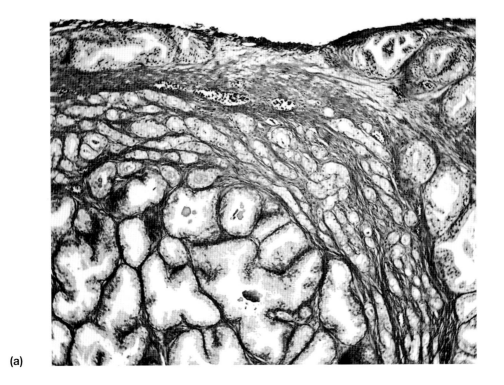

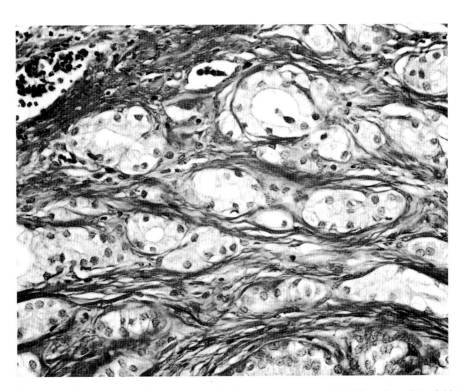

Figure 4.13 Atypical adenomatous hyperplasia. **(a)** Linear arrays of small acini hug the edge of this nodule of nodular hyperplasia, architecturally mimicking well-differentiated adenocarcinoma. **(b)** The acini lack cytological features of malignancy, without significant nuclear or nucleolar enlargement.

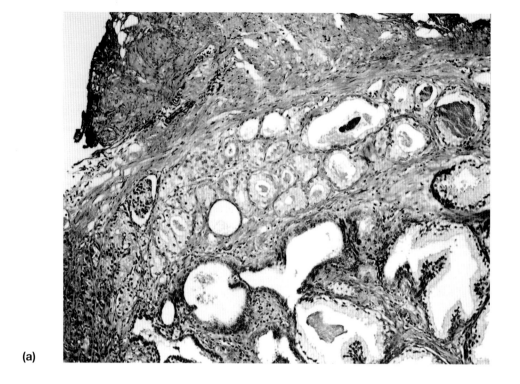

(a)

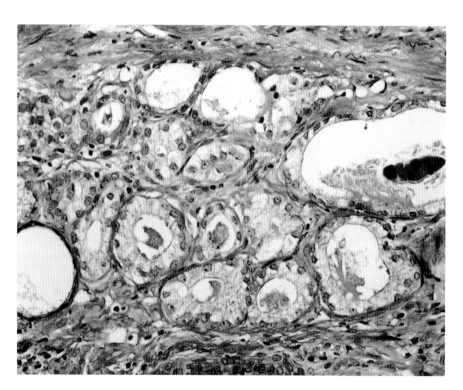

(b)

Figure 4.14 Atypical adenomatous hyperplasia. **(a)** At the edge of a hyperplastic nodule, there is a minute nest of small acini with pale cytoplasm. **(b)** At high magnification, the small acini contain uniform small nuclei and punctate nucleoli without signficant enlargement.

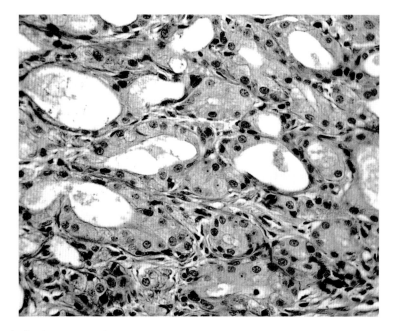

Figure 4.15 Atypical adenomatous hyperplasia. The closely packed cluster of acini contain small nuclei and minute punctate nucleoli.

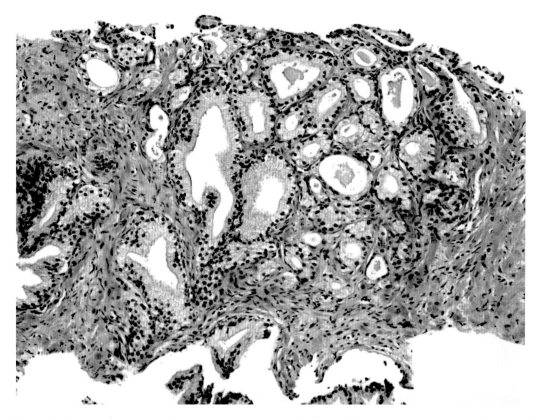

Figure 4.16 Atypical adenomatous hyperplasia on needle biopsy. Although very rare on needle biopsy, AAH is occasionally observed, consisting of a small acinar proliferation in intimate association with larger acini of nodular hyperplasia. We require that most or all of the focus is present on the biopsy to diagnose AAH in order to avoid underdiagnosis of adenocarcinoma.

Table 4.4 Atypical adenomatous hyperplasia versus well-differentiated adenocarcinoma

	Atypical adenomatous hyperplasia	*Carcinoma (Gleason grades 1 and 2)*
Architectural and associated features		
Low power	Circumscribed or limited infiltration	Circumscribed or limited infiltration
Lesion size	Variable	Variable
Gland size	Variable	Less variable
Gland shape	Variable	Less variable
Crystalloids	Infrequent (16%)	Frequent (75%)
Corpora amylacea	Frequent (32%)	Infrequent (13%)
Basophilic mucin	Infrequent	Frequent
Nuclear features		
Nuclear size variation	Less variable	Variable
Chromatin	Uniform/granular	Uniform or variable
Parachromatin clearing	Infrequent	Frequent
Nucleoli	Inconspicuous	Prominent
Nucleoli (largest)	2.5 µm (rare)	3.0 µm
Nucleoli (mean)	<1.0 µm	1.8 µm
Nucleoli >1 µm	18%	77%
Basal cell layer		
Hematoxylin and eosin stain	Inconspicuous	Absent
Antikeratin stain (high molecular weight)	Fragmented	Virtually absent

- inconspicuous nucleoli;
- fragmented basal cell layer;
- infrequent crystalloids (Table 4.4).

All measures of nucleolar size allow separation of AAH from adenocarcinoma, including mean nucleolar diameter, largest nucleolar diameter and percentage of nucleoli greater than 1 µm in diameter. There is apparently widespread acceptance of Gleason's criterion of nucleolar diameter greater than 1 µm for separating well-differentiated cancer (Gleason primary grades 1 and 2) from other proliferative lesions such as AAH (Gleason, 1985).

Despite the utility of these features, the absolute distinction between AAH and carcinoma is still difficult in some cases. Other morphological features are not useful in distinguishing AAH from adenocarcinoma, including lesion shape, circumscription, multifocality, average acinar size, variation in acinar size and shape, chromatin pattern, and the amount and tinctorial quality of the cytoplasm. AAH and cancer contain acidic mucin in the majority of cases (Epstein and Fynheer, 1992; Goldstein, Qian and Bostwick, 1995).

4.6.2 Immunohistochemistry of AAH

Immunohistochemistry is often useful in the diagnosis of AAH. The basal cell layer is characteristically discontinuous and fragmented in AAH, but absent in cancer, a feature that can be demonstrated in routine formalin-fixed sections with basal-cell-specific antikeratin 34βE12 (Figure 4.18).

4.6.3 Differential diagnosis

Histological mimics of AAH include nodular hyperplasia without atypia (Figure 4.19), simple lobular atrophy, postatrophic

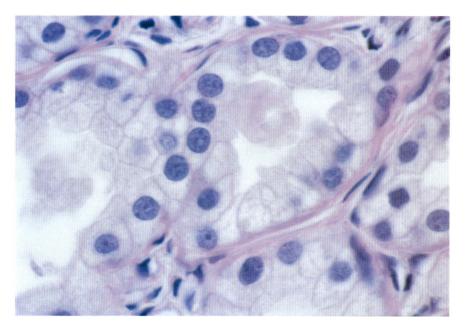

Figure 4.17 Atypical adenomatous hyperplasia. Note uniform round nuclei without prominent nucleoli.

hyperplasia, sclerosing atrophy, basal cell hyperplasia, atypical basal cell hyperplasia and metaplastic changes associated with radiation, infarction and prostatitis. Many mimics display architectural and cytological atypia, including nucleolomegaly, and caution is warranted in interpretation of scant specimens, cauterized or distorted specimens, and specimens submitted with incomplete patient history.

AAH is uncommonly associated with sclerosis, but further study is needed to determine the relationship to sclerosing adenosis. Sclerosing adenosis differs from AAH by displaying myoepithelial features of the basal cells and an exuberant stroma of fibroblasts and loose ground substance. AAH should also be distinguished from lobular atrophy and postatrophic hyperplasia. Simple atrophy consists of shrunken acini that demonstrate strong basal-cell-specific antikeratin immunoreactivity. Postatrophic hyperplasia may be difficult to separate from AAH since proliferating luminal cells with small amounts of clear cytoplasm may occur in an atrophic background. These

cells may demonstrate cytological atypia, sometimes with luminal mucin. Both may have a fragmented basal cell layer.

4.6.4 Clinical significance of AAH

There are three unanswered questions with AAH. First, does 'atypical small acinar proliferation of uncertain significance' represent underdiagnosed adenocarcinoma? Six of eight cases in our study created considerable diagnostic discord among the participants (Bostwick *et al.*, 1993). Critics could reasonably argue that the lack of concordance for this lesion indicates that it is not a distinct entity but merely a reflection of our uncertainty; also, the criteria for distinguishing this lesion from AAH and cancer may be difficult to apply in practice.

Second, does Gleason primary grade 1 adenocarcinoma represent overdiagnosed adenocarcinoma? These lesions are uncommon; most agree that Gleason primary grade 2 adenocarcinoma (infiltrating acini) is malignant,

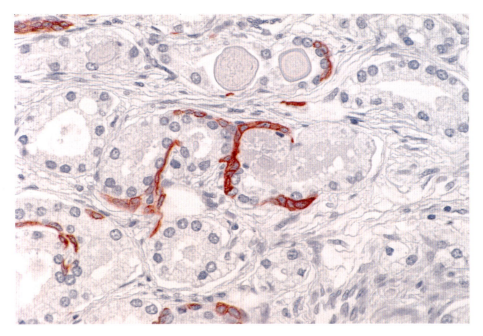

Figure 4.18 Keratin 34βE12 immunoreactivity in the fragmented basal cell layer of atypical adenomatous hyperplasia. Antikeratin 34βE12 immunohistochemical stain.

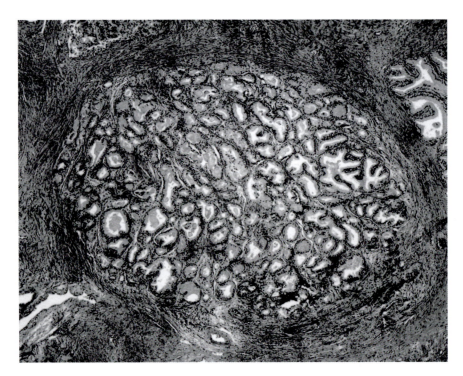

Figure 4.19 Adenomatous hyperplasia (non-atypical), also referred to as the small acinar pattern of nodular hyperplasia. Unlike atypical adenomatous hyperplasia, the small acinar proliferation of non-atypical adenomatous hyperplasia comprises the entire nodule.

but what is the true biological potential of the uniform circumscribed proliferation of Gleason primary grade 1 adenocarcinoma? Presently, we consider these to be malignant, following the suggestion of Gleason and others.

Third, is AAH a precursor of adenocarcinoma? AAH has been proposed as a premalignant lesion of the prostate because of the following:

- increased incidence in association with carcinoma (15% in 100 prostates without carcinoma at autopsy, and 31% in 100 prostates with cancer at autopsy);
- topographic relationship with small-acinar carcinoma;
- age peak incidence that precedes that of carcinoma;
- increasing AgNOR count;
- increased nuclear area and diameter;
- a proliferative cell index similar to that of small-acinar carcinoma but significantly higher than that of normal and hyperplastic prostatic epithelium;
- rare cases with genetic instability (Qian, Bostwick and Jenkins, 1995).

Some authors claim that the link between cancer and AAH is an epiphenomenon and that the data are insufficient to conclude that AAH is a premalignant lesion (Srigley, 1988; Epstein, 1994). It has also been suggested that AAH may be related to a subset of cancer that arises in the transition zone in association with benign prostatic hyperplasia (Helpap, 1980; Bostwick et al., 1992). Although the biological significance of AAH is uncertain, its light-microscopic appearance and immunophenotype allow it to be separated from carcinoma.

4.6.5 The pathologist's approach to AAH

When AAH is encountered in prostatic specimens, we believe that all tissue should be embedded and made available for examination; serial sections of suspicious foci may be useful. Needle biopsies rarely contain AAH,

and we require that most or all of the focus be present for diagnosis, recognizing the potential for sampling AAH-like areas in adenocarcinoma. The identification of AAH should not influence or dictate therapeutic decisions; however, the clinical importance of these lesions is not understood and close surveillance and follow-up appear to be indicated, particularly for cases considered as atypical small acinar proliferation of uncertain significance.

4.7 SCLEROSING ADENOSIS

Sclerosing adenosis of the prostate, originally described as adenomatoid or pseudoadenomatoid tumor, consists of a benign circumscribed proliferation of small acini set in a dense spindle cell stroma (Chen and Schiff, 1983; Hulman, 1989; Young and Clement, 1987; Sakamoto, Tsuneyoshi and Enjoji, 1991; Jones, Clement and Young, 1991; Collina et al., 1992; Grignon et al., 1992). It is an incidental finding in transurethral resection specimens for benign prostatic hyperplasia, present in about 2% of specimens; rare cases are associated with elevated serum PSA concentration. Sclerosing adenosis is usually solitary and microscopic, but may be multifocal and extensive.

4.7.1 Diagnostic criteria

The acini in sclerosing adenosis are predominantly well-formed and small to medium in size, but may form minute cellular nests or clusters with abortive lumens (Figure 4.20).

The cells lining the acini display a moderate amount of clear to eosinophilic cytoplasm, often with distinct cell margins. The basal cell layer may be focally prominent and hyperplastic, particularly in acini thickly rimmed by cellular stroma (Figures 4.20 and 4.21). In some areas, the acini merge with the exuberant stroma of fibroblasts and loose ground substance. There is usually no significant

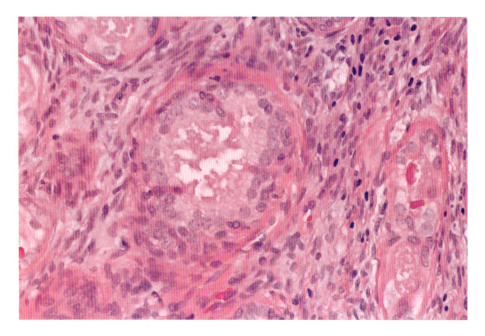

Figure 4.20   Sclerosing adenosis with benign acini set in a cellular stroma.

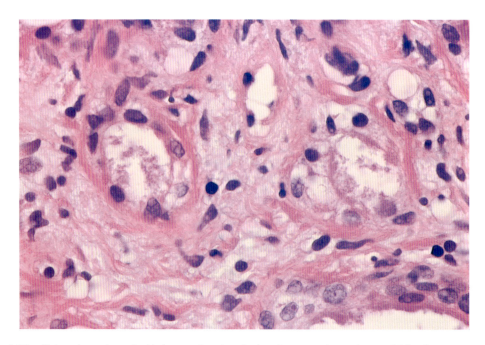

Figure 4.21   Sclerosing adenosis. Note prominent periacinar basement membrane thickening.

cytological atypia of the epithelial cells or stromal cells, but some cases may show moderate atypia.

4.7.2 Immunohistochemical and ultrastructural studies

The unique immunophenotype of sclerosing adenosis is a valuable diagnostic clue that distinguishes it from adenocarcinoma (Table 4.5). The basal cells show immunoreactivity for S-100 protein and muscle-specific actin, unlike normal prostatic epithelium or carcinoma (Srigley *et al.*, 1990); consequently, sclerosing adenosis is considered a form of metaplasia (Figure 4.22).

The basal cell layer is intact or fragmented and discontinuous in sclerosing adenosis as demonstrated with immunohistochemical stains for high-molecular-weight keratin 34βE12, compared with absence of staining in carcinoma. PSA and PAP are present within secretory luminal cells.

Ultrastructural studies demonstrate myoepithelial differentiation in sclerosing adenosis, with collections of thin filaments and dense bodies (Grignon *et al.*, 1992).

4.7.3 Differential diagnosis of sclerosing adenosis

Sclerosing adenosis should be distinguished from lobular atrophy and postatrophic hyperplasia. Both of these lesions tend to be lobulated. Simple atrophy consists of shrunken acini, whereas postatrophic hyperplasia contains proliferating luminal cells with small amounts of clear cytoplasm. The cells may demonstrate some degree of cytological atypia and luminal mucin may be identified. Other histological mimics of sclerosing adenosis include sclerosing atrophy, basal cell hyperplasia, atypical basal cell hyperplasia and metaplastic changes associated with radiation, infarction and prostatitis.

Table 4.5 Sclerosing adenosis versus adenocarcinoma

	Sclerosing adenosis	*Adenocarcinoma*
Architecture	Lobular small acinar proliferation; may form cell nests or clusters; prominent cellular stroma	May be lobular and circumscribed
Acini	Round and smooth; appear to merge with stroma due to pale staining	May be rounded or smooth
Basement membrane	Prominent thickening	Inconspicuous
Basal cell layer		
Light microscopy	Usually intact and often hyperplastic	Absent
High-molecular-weight keratin (34βE12) immunoreactivity	Intact or discontinuous	Absent
Stromal changes	Prominent cellular stroma without atypia	Without or without stromal sclerosis
Cytology		
Nuclei	Mild enlargement	Enlarged
Nucleoli	Usually inconspicuous	Usually prominent
Cytoplasm	Clear or eosinophilic	Usually pale due to greater amount of cytoplasm
Immunoreactivity		
S-100 protein	Yes (basal cells)	No
Actin	Yes (basal cells)	No

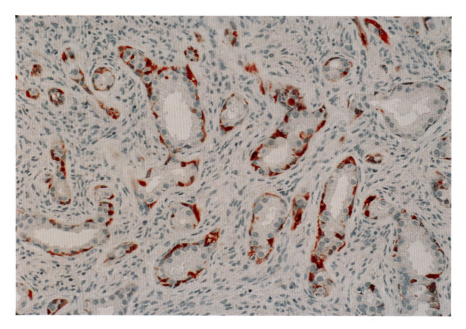

Figure 4.22 S-100 protein stain in sclerosing adenosis. There is prominent immunoreactivity in most of the basal cells.

AAH is occasionally associated with sclerosis, but lacks the dense periacinar hyalinized fibrosis sometimes seen in sclerosing adenosis. Immuno-histochemical studies reveal a fragmented and discontinuous basal cell layer in AAH, whereas sclerosing adenosis usually retains an intact basal cell layer. The myoepithelial differentiation of sclerosing adenosis is distinctive. Both lesions arise chiefly in the transition zone and are usually incidental findings in TURP specimens with nodular hyperplasia.

Sclerosing adenosis can be distinguished from adenocarcinoma by:

- distinctive fibroblastic stroma, which is rarely seen in carcinoma;
- benign cytology, with epithelial cells and stromal cells that lack prominent nucle-omegaly and nucleolomegaly usually seen in prostatic carcinoma;
- hyalinized periacinar stroma occasionally seen in sclerosing adenosis;
- intact basal cell layer;
- frequent association with nodular hyperplasia;

- immunophenotype of S-100 protein and actin immunoreactivity.

4.8 VERUMONTANUM MUCOSAL GLAND HYPERPLASIA

This is an uncommon form of small acinar hyperplasia that mimics well-differentiated adenocarcinoma (Gagucas, Brown and Wheeler, 1995) (Table 4.6).

It is invariably small, less than 1 mm, often multifocal and limited anatomically to the verumontanum, utricle, ejaculatory ducts and adjacent prostatic urethra and ducts. The acini are small and closely packed, with an intact basal cell layer, small uniform nuclei and inconspicuous nucleoli. The basal cells display immunoreactivity for high-molecular-weight keratin, and are S-100-protein-negative. This lesion is rare in needle biopsies and is almost never sampled in transurethral resections because of the sparing of the verumontanum by this procedure.

Table 4.6 Verumontanum mucosal gland hyperplasia (VMGH) versus adenocarcinoma

	VMGH	Adenocarcinoma
Location	Verumontanum	Anywhere in prostate
Size	Small (< 1 mm)	Any size
Architecture	Lobular small acinar proliferation; may be multifocal	May be lobular and circumscribed; usually multifocal
Basal cell layer		
Light microscopy	Usually intact; may be inconspicuous	Absent
High-molecular-weight keratin (34βE12) immunoreactivity	Usually intact	Absent
Stromal changes	With or without stromal sclerosis	With or without stromal sclerosis
Cytology		
Nuclei	Mild enlargement	Enlarged
Nucleoli	Usually inconspicuous	Usually prominent
Cytoplasm	Basophilic or clear on low power	Usually pale due to greater amount of cytoplasm
Basophilic mucin	Rare	May be present
Crystalloids	Rare	May be present

4.9 HYPERPLASIA OF MESONEPHRIC REMNANTS

Hyperplasia of mesonephric remnants in the prostate and periprostatic tissues is a rare and benign mimic of adenocarcinoma that is usually identified in TURP specimens (Table 4.7).

According to Gikas, Del Buono and Epstein, it shares many features with mesonephric hyperplasia of the female genital tract, including apparent infiltration of the stroma and neural spaces, lobular arrangement of small acini or solid nests lined by a single cell layer, prominent nucleoli and eosinophilic intratubular material. We encountered one case in which the lobular pattern was lost and the acini were infiltrative.

Two histopathological patterns have been described, both with a lobular pattern and cuboidal cell lining. One pattern consists of small acini that contain colloid-like material reminiscent of thyroid follicles. The lining consists of a single layer of cuboidal cells without significant cytological atypia. The second pattern consists of small acini or solid nests of cells with empty lumens, reminiscent of nephrogenic metaplasia. Acini may be atrophic or exhibit micropapillary projections lined by cuboidal cells. Prominent nucleoli are usually absent, but are present in rare cases, compounding the diagnostic confusion.

The diagnosis may be confirmed by cellular immunoreactivity for keratin 34βE12 and lack of immunoreactivity for PSA and PAP. One of the original cases was misdiagnosed as adenocarcinoma, resulting in unnecessary prostatectomy.

4.10 ASSOCIATION OF NODULAR HYPERPLASIA AND PROSTATE CANCER

There are a number of similarities between nodular hyperplasia and cancer (Bostwick *et al.*, 1992). Both display a parallel increase in prevalence with patient age according to autopsy studies, although cancer lags by 15–20 years. Both require androgens for growth and development, and both may respond to androgen deprivation treatment. Most cancers arise in patients with concomitant nodular hyperplasia, and cancer is found incidentally in a significant number (10%) of transurethral prostatectomy specimens. Nodular hyperplasia

Table 4.7 Mesonephric remnants versus adenocarcinoma

	Mesonephric remnants	*Adenocarcinoma*
Architecture	Lobular small acinar proliferation Two patterns: (1) Small acini with colloid-like material; (2) Small acini with empty lumens or solid nests	May be lobular and circumscribed
Acinar contours	May be rounded or smooth; may be atrophic or contain intraluminal micropapillary projections lined by cuboidal cells	May be rounded or smooth
Basal cell layer		
Light microscopy	Usually intact; may be inconspicuous	Absent
High-molecular-weight keratin (34βE12) immunoreactivity	Intact	Absent
Stromal changes	With or without stromal sclerosis	With or without stromal sclerosis
Cytology		
Nuclei	Mild enlargement	Enlarged
Nucleoli	Usually inconspicuous	Usually prominent
Cytoplasm	Basophilic or clear on low power	Usually pale due to greater amount of cytoplasm
Luminal contents	Often with colloid-like material	May have basophilic mucin
Immunoreactivity		
PSA	No	Yes
PAP	No	Yes

may be related to prostate cancer arising in the transition zone, perhaps in association with certain forms of hyperplasia.

REFERENCES

Ayala, A. G., Srigley, J. R., Ro, J. Y. *et al.* (1986) Clear cell cribriform hyperplasia of prostate. *Am. J. Surg. Pathol.*, **10**, 665–672.

Bostwick, D. G. and Qian, J. (1995) Atypical adenomatous hyperplasia of the prostate. Relationship with carcinoma in 217 whole-mount radical prostatectomies. *Am. J. Surg. Pathol.*, **19**, 506–518.

Bostwick, D. G., Cooner, W. H., Denis, L. *et al.* (1992) The association of benign prostatic hyperplasia and cancer of the prostate. *Cancer*, **70**, 291–301.

Bostwick, D. G., Srigley, J., Grignon, D. *et al.* (1993) Atypical adenomatous hyperplasia of the prostate: morphologic criteria for its distinction from well-differentiated carcinoma. *Hum. Pathol.*, **24**, 819–832.

Bostwick, D. G., Algaba, F., Amin, M. B. *et al.* (1994) Consensus statement on terminology: recommendation to use atypical adenomatous hyperplasia in place of adenosis of the prostate. *Am. J. Surg. Pathol.*, **18**, 1069–1070.

Brawn, P. N., Speights, V. O., Contin, J. U. *et al.* (1989) Atypical hyperplasia in prostates of 20 to 40 year old men. *J. Clin. Pathol.*, **42**, 383–386.

Chen, K. T. K. and Schiff, J. J. (1983) Adenomatoid prostatic tumor. *Urology*, **21**, 88–89.

Cheville, J. C. and Bostwick, D. G. (1995) Post-atrophic hyperplasia of the prostate. A histologic mimic of prostatic adenocarcinoma. *Am. J. Surg. Pathol.*, **19**, 1068–1076.

Cleary, K. R., Choi, H. Y. and Ayala, A. G. (1983) Basal cell hyperplasia of the prostate. *Am. J. Clin. Pathol.*, **80**, 850–854.

Collina, G., Botticelli, A. R., Martinelli, A. M. *et al.* (1992) Sclerosing adenosis of the prostate. Report of three cases with electron microscopy and immunohistochemical study. *Histopathology*, **20**, 505–510.

Dermer, G. B. (1978) Basal cell proliferation in benign prostatic hyperplasia. *Cancer*, **41**, 1857–1862.

Devaraj, L. T. and Bostwick, D. G. (1993) Atypical basal cell hyperplasia of the prostate: immuno-phenotypic profile and proposed classification of basal cell proliferations. *Am. J. Surg. Pathol.*, **17**, 645–659.

Eble, J. N. and Tejada, E. (1991) Prostatic stromal hyperplasia with bizarre nuclei. *Arch. Pathol. Lab. Med.*, **115**, 87–89.

Epstein, J. I. (1994) Adenosis vs. atypical adenomatous hyperplasia of the prostate (letter). *Am. J. Surg. Pathol.*, **18**, 1070–1071.

Epstein, J. I. and Armas, O. A. (1992) Atypical basal cell hyperplasia of the prostate. *Am. J. Surg. Pathol.*, **16**, 1205–1214.

Epstein, J. I. and Fynheer, J. (1992) Acidic mucin in the prostate: can it differentiate adenosis from adenocarcinoma? *Hum. Pathol.*, **23**, 1321–1325.

Franks, L. M. (1954) Atrophy and hyperplasia in prostate proper. *J. Pathol. Bact.*, **68**, 617–621.

Frauenhoffer, E. E., Ro, J. Y., El-Naggar, A. K. et. al. (1991) Clear cell cribriform hyperplasia of the prostate: immunohistochemical and flow cytometric study. *Am. J. Clin. Pathol.*, **95**, 446–453.

Gagucas, R. J., Brown, R. W. and Wheeler, T. M. (1995) Verumontanum mucosal gland hyperplasia. *Am. J. Surg. Pathol.*, **19**, 30–36.

Gikas, P. W., Del Buono, E. A. and Epstein, J. I. (1992) Florid hyperplasia of mesonephric remnants involving prostate and periprostatic tissue: possible confusion with adenocarcinoma. *Am. J. Surg. Pathol.*, **16**, 454–459.

Gleason, D. F. (1985) Atypical hyperplasia, benign hyperplasia, and well-differentiated adenocarcinoma of the prostate. *Am. J. Surg. Pathol.*, **9**, 53–67.

Goldstein, N. S., Qian, J. and Bostwick, D. G. (1995) Mucin expression in atypical adenomatous hyperplasia of the prostate. *Hum. Pathol.*, **26**, 887–891.

Grignon, D. J., Ro, J. Y., Ordonez, N. G., Ayala, A. G. and Cleary, K. R. (1988) Basal cell hyperplasia, adenoid basal cell tumor, and adenoid cystic carcinoma of the prostate gland: an immunohistochemical study. *Hum. Pathol.*, **19**, 1425–1433.

Grignon, D. J., Ro, J. Y., Srigley, J. R. et al. (1992) Sclerosing adenosis of the prostate gland. A lesion showing myoepithelial differentiation. *Am. J. Surg. Pathol.*, **16**, 383–391.

Helpap, B. (1980) The biological significance of atypical hyperplasia of the prostate. *Virchows Arch. Pathol. Histol.*, **387**, 307–317.

Hulman, G. (1989) 'Pseudoadenomatoid' tumor of prostate. *Histopathology*, **14**, 317–323.

Jones, E. C., Clement, P. B. and Young, R. H. (1991) Sclerosing adenosis of the prostate gland. A clinicopathologic and immunohistochemical study of 11 cases. *Am. J. Surg. Pathol.*, **15**, 1171–1180.

Leong, S. S., Vogt, P. F. and Yu, G. M. (1988) Atypical stroma with muscle hyperplasia of prostate. *Urology*, **31**, 163–167.

McNeal, J. E. (1990) The pathobiology of nodular hyperplasia, in *Pathology of the Prostate*, (ed. D. G. Bostwick), Churchill Livingstone, New York, pp. 31–36.

Qian, J., Bostwick, D. G. and Jenkins, R. B. (1995) Chromosomal anomalies in atypical adenomatous hyperplasia and carcinoma of the prostate using fluorescence in situ hybridization. *Urology*, **46**, 837–842.

Sakamoto, N., Tsuneyoshi, M. and Enjoji, M. (1991) Sclerosing adenosis of the prostate. Histopathologic and immunohistochemical analysis. *Am. J. Surg. Pathol.*, **15**, 660–667.

Shapiro, E., Becich, M. J., Hartanto, V. et al. (1992) The relative proportion of stromal and epithelial hyperplasia is related to the development of symptomatic benign prostatic hyperplasia. *J. Urol.*, **147**, 1293–1297.

Srigley, J. R. (1988) Small-acinar patterns in the prostate gland with emphasis on atypical adenomatous hyperplasia and small-acinar carcinoma. *Sem. Diag. Pathol.*, **5**, 254–257.

Srigley, J. R., Dardick, I. Hartwick, R. W. J. and Kotz, L. (1990) Basal epithelial cells of human prostate gland are not myoepithelial cells. A comparative immunohistochemical and ultrastructural study with human salivary gland. *Am. J. Surg. Pathol.*, **136**, 957–963.

Young, R. H. and Clement, P. B. (1987) Sclerosing adenosis of the prostate. *Arch. Pathol. Lab. Med.*, **11**, 363–366.

5

MISCELLANEOUS BENIGN LESIONS AND CYSTS

5.1 AMYLOIDOSIS

Localized amyloidosis is rarely present in the prostate or urethra, but is common in the seminal vesicles (senile seminal vesicle amyloidosis), observed at autopsy in 5–8% of men between 46 and 60 years of age, 13–23% between 61 and 75 years and 21–34% over 75 years (Pitkanen *et al.*, 1983; Seidman *et al.*, 1989; Khan *et al.*, 1992; Coyne and Kealy, 1993; Ramchandani *et al.*, 1993). It often extends bilaterally along the ejaculatory ducts, forming linear or massive nodular subepithelial deposits of amorphous eosinophilic fibrillar material (Figure 5.1). Basement membrane thickening is observed, and deposits may be seen within the vesicular lumens, occasionally causing significant luminal narrowing (Chapter 14).

Special stains which confirm the diagnosis of amyloid include:

- Congo red, which appears red by light microscopy with apple-green polarization birefringence;
- methylene blue, which reveals green polarization birefringence;
- crystal violet and toluidine blue, which impart a metachromatic appearance to the deposits;

- periodic-acid–Schiff (PAS) and sulfated alcian blue stains, which are weakly to moderately positive.

The composition of localized seminal vesicle and ejaculatory duct amyloid is histochemically unique (permanganate-sensitive, non-AA, non-B2M, non-pre-albumin type), apparently derived from secretory protein of the epithelium; amyloid at other sites is derived from light chains or serum amyloid protein.

5.2 PIGMENTED LESIONS

Descriptions of pigment within the prostate gland are limited chiefly to blue nevus and prostatic melanosis, both of which are uncommon benign lesions. In melanosis, the pigment is melanin-like, according to histochemical, ultrastructural and immunohistochemical findings (see Figures 1.10–1.12). Another distinctive type of pigment is more frequently encountered in the normal prostatic epithelium, consisting of delicate or coarse golden yellow-brown cytoplasmic granules which may be inconspicuous or rarely prominent (Figure 5.2). This pigment can cause diagnostic confusion with ejaculatory ductal and seminal

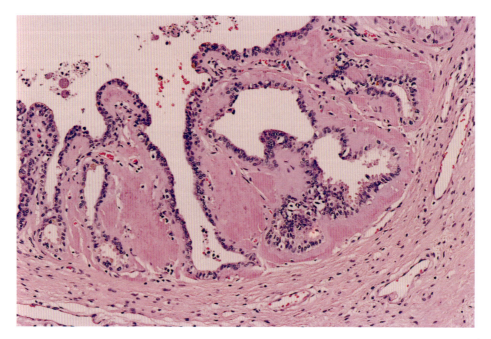

Figure 5.1   Amyloidosis of the ejaculatory ducts

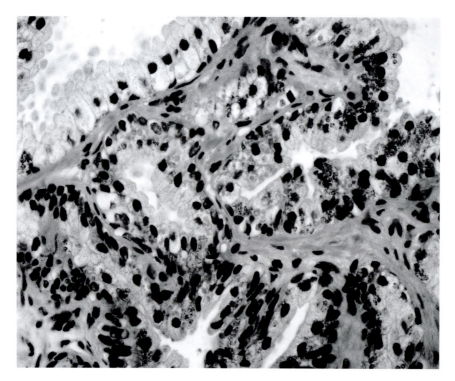

Figure 5.2   Prostatic epithelial pigmentation. Note granular pigment within the epithelium, reminiscent of that seen in the seminal vesicles.

vesicular epithelium, particularly when it is found in abundance or in limited or artifactually distorted biopsies and transurethral resection specimens.

5.2.1 Melanosis

The prostate contains two distinct types of pigment: the common melanin-like, lipofuscin-like pigment present in benign prostate epithelium (Guillian and Zelman, 1970; Seman, Gallager and Johnson, 1982), high-grade PIN (Bostwick *et al.*, 1993; Brennick *et al.*, 1994) and prostatic adenocarcinoma (Ro *et al.*, 1988; Rios and Wright, 1976; Aguilar, Gaffney and Finnerty, 1982); and melanin, which is rare and found only in prostatic melanocytic lesions such as blue nevus, melanosis and malignant melanoma. Melanin-like, lipofuscin-like pigment is common in the normal prostate, present in the epithelium in 89% of cases and in the stroma in 78% (D. G. Bostwick and M. A. Amin, unpublished observations). It is widely distributed, including the transition zone (67%), central zone (56%), peripheral zone (89%) and periurethral glands (56%). This pigment is most commonly seen in the basal portion of the secretory luminal cells, but is variable in location and amount. The reported incidence of this melanin-like, lipofuscin-like prostatic pigment in the normal prostate varies from 4% to 70% (Tannenbaum, 1974; Guillian and Zelman, 1970; Seman, Gallager and Johnson, 1982).

Pigment in the prostate has some resemblance to pigment in the seminal vesicular and ejaculatory ductal epithelium, particularly when it is present in abundance, and may cause diagnostic confusion in scant specimens such as needle biopsies or transurethral resection specimens which may contain foci with cytological atypia (Kuo and Gomez, 1981). However, the pigment granules tend to be less coarse and refractile, and have a unique histochemical profile that allows them to be distinguished from seminal vesicular tissue: melanin-like (Fontana–Masson-stain-positive and potassium-permanganate-bleaching-sensitive) and lipofuscin-like (prolonged

Ziehl–Neelsen-stain-positive and S-100-negative); unlike pigment in seminal vesicle epithelium which is not melanin-like (Fontana–Masson-stain-negative).

These findings suggest that this pigment is different from typical cutaneous melanin; the lipofuscin-like material ('wear and tear' or 'old age' pigment) is probably endogenous cellular byproducts of prostate epithelium rather than of melanocytic origin. Its only significance is to be aware of its distribution such that epithelium or stroma with pigment is not necessarily of seminal vesicle origin.

5.2.2 Blue nevus

In blue nevus, melanin pigment is contained within dendritic bipolar cells in the stroma, (Nigogosyan *et al.*, 1963; Jao *et al.*, 1971; Block, Weber and Schinella, 1971; Langley and Weitzner, 1974; Tannenbaum, 1974; Ro *et al.*, 1988) whereas in prostatic melanosis it is chiefly in the epithelium (Goldman, 1968; Gardner and Spitz, 1971; Rios and Wright, 1976; Aguilar, Gaffney and Finnerty, 1982). Premelanosomes and melanosomes are present ultrastructurally in the cells of prostatic blue nevus, indicating that they are melanocytic. Conversely, only stage IV melanosomes have been described in the epithelial cells. Immunohistochemistry revealed S-100 reactivity in the stromal cells in one case, confirming the ultrastructural findings (Ro *et al.*, 1988).

5.2.3 Melanoma

Malignant melanoma was the first reported pigmented lesion of the prostate (Berry and Reese, 1953), and, since that report in 1953, other cases have been reported (Simard, Rognon and Pilorce, 1964).

5.3 ENDOMETRIOSIS

A case of endometriosis was described in the prostate of a 78-year-old man with a long

Table 5.1 Prostatic cysts: differential diagnosis

Type of cyst	Location	Size	Sperm within
Prostatic cyst	Lateral	Variable	No
Seminal vesicle cyst	Lateral	Large	Yes
Diverticulum of ejaculatory duct or ampulla	Lateral	Variable	Yes
Müllerian duct cyst	Midline	Large	No

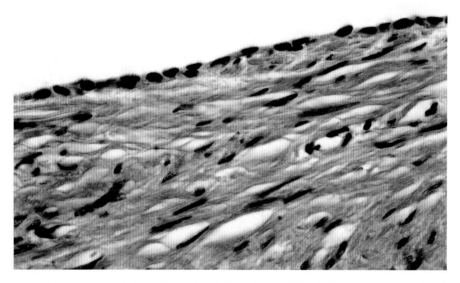

Figure 5.3 Ejaculatory duct cyst. A single layer of flattened epithelial cells lines the inner surface of this small 1 cm diameter cyst of the ejaculatory ducts near the verumontanum.

history of estrogen therapy for prostate cancer (Beckman *et al.*, 1985). It arose as a small, pale red mass proximal to the internal urethral orifice and extended into the prostate. This case and similar cases reported in the male bladder are invariably associated with hematuria and androgen deprivation therapy for prostatic adenocarcinoma.

5.4 PROSTATIC CYST

Giant multilocular prostatic cystadenoma is a large tumor composed of acini and cysts lined by prostatic-type epithelium set in a hypocellular fibrous stroma (Watanabe *et al.*, 1990; Maluf *et al.*, 1991; Levy, Gogate and Hampel, 1993; Lim *et al.*, 1993). This rare tumor arises in

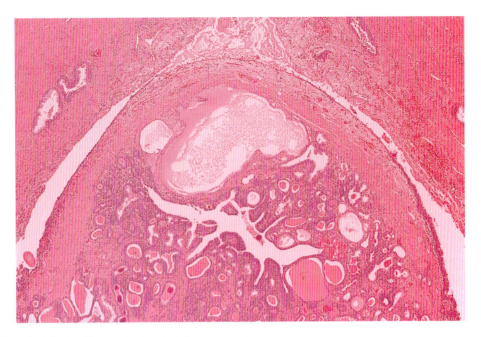

Figure 5.4   Incipient müllerian duct cyst at the verumontanum

men between the ages of 28 and 80 years as a large midline prostatic or extraprostatic mass causing urinary obstruction. The epithelial lining displays PSA immunoreactivity. Surgical excision is usually curative, although it may recur if incompletely excised. The differential diagnosis includes phyllodes tumor, multilocular peritoneal inclusion cyst, multicystic mesothelioma, müllerian duct cyst, seminal vesicle cyst, lymphangioma and hemangiopericytoma. The light-microscopic appearance of the cyst lining is useful in separating these lesions (Table 5.1).

Other benign unilocular cysts which may be sampled by biopsy include seminal vesicle cyst, ejaculatory duct cyst (Figure 5.3) (Elder and Mostwin, 1984; Mayersak, 1989; Pryor and Hendry, 1991) and müllerian duct cyst (Figure 5.4) (Gevenois *et al.*, 1990; Hendry and Pryor, 1992). Location is often useful, recognizing that seminal vesicle cyst is typically lateral whereas müllerian duct cyst is midline.

Echinococcal cyst is usually associated with prominent inflammation, and organisms are often demonstrable (DeKlotz, 1976).

5.5 EJACULATORY DUCT ADENOFIBROMA

A case of benign adenofibroma of the ejaculatory duct was recently reported (Mai and Walley, 1994). This incidental autopsy finding consisted of a small polypoid mass of epithelium and stroma which projected into a cystically dilated duct. Adenomatoid tumor of the ejaculatory duct has also been described (Fan and Johnson, 1985).

REFERENCES

Aguilar, M., Gaffney, E. F. and Finnerty, D. P. (1982) Prostatic melanosis with involvement of benign and malignant epithelium. *J. Urol.*, **128**, 825–827.

Beckman, E. N., Pintado, S. O., Leonard, G. L. and Sternberg, W. H. (1985) Endometriosis of the prostate. *Am. J. Surg. Pathol.*, **9**, 374–379.

Berry, N. E. and Reese, L. (1953) Malignant melanoma which had its first clinical manifestation in the prostate gland. *J. Urol.*, **69**, 286–290.

Block, N. L., Weber, D. and Schinella, R. (1972) Blue nevi and other melanotic lesions of the prostate: report of 3 cases and review of literature. *J. Urol.*, **107**, 85–87.

Bostwick, D. G. and Eble, J. N. (1996) *Urologic Surgical Pathology*, Mosby-Yearbook, St Louis, MO.

Bostwick, D. G., Amin, M. B., Dundore, P. *et al.* (1993) Architectural patterns of high grade prostatic intraepithelial neoplasia. *Hum. Pathol.*, **24**, 298–310.

Brennick, J. B., O'Connell, J. X., Dickersin, G. R. *et al.* (1994) Lipofuscin pigmentation (so-called 'melanosis') of the prostate. *Am. J. Surg. Pathol.*, **18**, 446–454.

Coyne, J. D. and Kealy, W. F. (1993) Seminal vesicle amyloidosis: morphological, histochemical and immunohistochemical observations. *Histopathology*, **22**, 173–176.

DeKlotz, R. J. (1976) Echinococcal cyst involving the prostate and seminal vesicles: a case report. *J. Urol.*, **115**, 116–117.

Elder, J. S. and Mostwin, J. L. (1984) Cyst of the ejaculatory duct/urogenital sinus. *J. Urol.*, **132**, 768–771.

Fan, K. and Johnson, D. F. (1985) Adenomatoid tumor of ejaculatory duct. *Urology* **25**, 653–654.

Gardner, W. A. and Spitz, W. U. (1971) Melanosis of the prostate gland. *Am. J. Clin. Pathol.*, **56**, 762–764.

Gevenois, P. A., Van Sinoy, M. L., Sintzoff, S. A. Jr *et al.* (1990) Cysts of the prostate and seminal vesicles: MR imaging findings in 11 cases. *Am. J. Roentgenol.*, **155**, 1021–1024.

Goldman, R. L. (1968) Melanogenic epithelium in the prostate gland. *Am. J. Clin. Pathol.*, **49**, 75–78.

Guillian, R. A. and Zelman, S. (1970) The incidence and probable origin of melanin in the prostate. *J. Urol.*, **104**, 151–153.

Hendry, W. F. and Pryor, J. P. (1992) Müllerian duct (prostatic utricle) cyst: diagnosis and treatment in subfertile males. *Br. J. Urol.*, **69**, 79–82.

Jao, W., Fretzin, D., Christ, M. L. and Prinz, L. M. (1971) Blue nevus of the prostate gland. *Arch. Path.*, **91**, 187–191.

Khan, S. M., Birch, P. J., Bass, P. S. *et al.* (1992) Localized amyloidosis of the lower genitourinary tract: a clinicopathological and immunohistochemical study of nine cases. *Histopathology*, **21**, 143–147.

Kuo, P. M. and Gomez, L. G. (1981) Monstrous epithelial cells in human epididymis and seminal vesicles. A pseudomalignant change. *Am. J. Surg. Pathol.*, **5**, 483–490.

Langley, J. W. and Weitzner, S. (1974) Blue nevus and melanosis of prostate. *J. Urol.*, **112**, 359–361.

Levy, D. A., Gogate, P. A. and Hampel, N. (1993) Giant multilocular prostatic cystadenoma: a rare clinical entity and review of the literature. *J. Urol.*, **150**, 1920–1922.

Lim, D. J., Hayden, R. T., Murad, T. *et al.* (1993) Multilocular prostatic cystadenoma presenting as a large complex pelvic cystic mass. *J. Urol.*, **149**, 856–859.

Mai, K. T. and Walley, V. M. (1994) Adenofibroma of the ejaculatory duct. *J. Urol. Pathol.*, **2**, 301–305.

Maluf, H. M., King, M. E., DeLuca, F. R. *et al.* (1991) Giant multilocular prostatic cystadenoma: a distinctive lesion of the retroperitoneum in men. A report of two cases. *Am. J. Surg. Pathol.*, **15**, 131–137.

Mayersak, J. S. (1989) Urogenital sinus–ejaculatory duct cyst: a case report with a proposed clinical classification and review of the literature. *J. Urol.*, **142**, 1330–1332.

Nigogosyan, G., De la Pava, S., Pickeren, J. W. and Woodruff, M. W. (1963) Blue nevus of prostate gland. *Cancer*, **16**, 1097–1099.

Pitkanen, P., Westermark, P., Cornwell, G. G. III *et al.* (1983) Amyloid of the seminal vesicles. A distinctive and common localized form of senile amyloidosis. *Am. J. Pathol.*, **110**, 64–69.

Pryor, J. P. and Hendry, W. F. (1991) Ejaculatory duct obstruction in subfertile males: analysis of 87 patients. *Fertil. Steril.*, **56**, 725–730.

Ramchandani, P., Schnall, M. D., LiVolsi, V. A. *et al.* (1993) Senile amyloidosis of the seminal vesicles mimicking metastatic spread of prostatic carcinoma on MR images. *Am. J. Roentgenol.*, **161**, 99–100.

Rios, C. N. and Wright, J. R. (1976) Melanosis of the prostate gland: report of a case with neoplastic epithelium involvement. *J. Urol.*, **115**, 616–617.

Ro, J. Y., Grignon, D. J., Ayala, A. G. *et al.* (1988) Blue nevus and melanosis of the prostate, electron-microscopic and immunohistochemical studies. *Am. J. Clin. Pathol.*, **90**, 530–535.

Seidman, J. D., Shmookler, B. M., Connolly, B. *et al.* (1989) Localized amyloidosis of seminal vesicles: report of three cases in surgically obtained material. *Mod. Pathol.*, **2**, 671–675.

Seman, G., Gallager, S. and Johnson, D. E. (1982) Melanin-like pigment in the human prostate. *Prostate*, **3**, 59–72.

Simard, C., Rognon, L. M. and Pilorce, G. (1964) Le problème du naevus bleu prostatique. *Ann. Anat. Pathol. (Paris)*, **9**, 469–474.

Tannenbaum, M. (1974) Differential diagnosis in uropathology. Melanotic lesions of prostate: blue nevus and prostatic epithelial melanosis. *Urology*, **5**, 617–621.

Watanabe, J., Konishi, T., Takeuchi, H. and Tomoyoshi, T. (1990) A case of giant prostatic cystadenoma. *Acta Urol. Jpn.*, **36**, 1077–1079.

6

PROSTATIC INTRAEPITHELIAL NEOPLASIA (PIN)

Prostatic intraepithelial neoplasia refers to the precancerous end of the morphological continuum of cellular proliferations within pre-existing prostatic ducts, ductules and acini. PIN is divided into two grades (low-grade and high-grade) to replace the previous three-grade system (PIN 1 is considered low-grade, and PIN 2 and 3 are considered high-grade) (Table 6.1) (McNeal and Bostwick, 1986; Bostwick, 1995a).

The continuum from low-grade PIN to high-grade PIN and early invasive cancer is characterized by basal cell layer disruption, progressive loss of markers of secretory differentiation and increasing nuclear and nucleolar abnormalities, proliferative activity, microvessel density, genetic instability and DNA content. Autopsy studies indicate that PIN precedes carcinoma by 10 years or more; low-grade PIN first emerges in men in the third decade of life (Sakr *et al.*, 1993).

6.1 DIAGNOSTIC FEATURES OF PIN

At low-power magnification, acini containing PIN usually appear hyperchromatic because of proliferation and crowding of the inner secretory cells. The acini are medium-sized or large, with smooth-sculpted rounded contours, similar to adjacent benign acini. PIN in biopsies usually involves single acini or small clusters of acini, but is occasionally more extensive.

At medium- and high-power magnification, crowding, heaping up and irregular spacing of the secretory cell layer of PIN is pronounced, in marked contrast with benign acini (Figures 6.1–6.6).

The presence of partial acinar involvement is particularly helpful. Overlapping nuclei are prominent and cell borders are usually inapparent. Along the luminal surface, the cells often display cytoplasmic blebs reminiscent of apocrine secretion.

In low-grade PIN, the epithelium lining ducts and acini are heaped up, crowded, and irregularly spaced, with marked variation in nuclear size (Figure 6.3; Table 6.1). Elongated hyperchromatic nuclei and small nucleoli are also present, but are not prominent. The diagnosis of PIN requires a combination of cytological and architectural features, and lesions displaying some but not all features are considered atypical but not neoplastic. Some pathologists prefer not to report low-grade PIN, recognizing the difficulty in separating this lesion from benign epithelium and reactive atypia.

High-grade PIN is considered the precursor of most cases of prostate cancer (McNeal *et al.*,

Table 6.1 Prostatic intraepithelial neoplasia (PIN): diagnostic criteria

	Low-grade PIN (formerly PIN 1)	High-grade PIN (formerly PIN 2 and 3)
Architecture	Epithelial cell crowding and stratification, with irregular spacing	Similar to low-grade PIN; more crowding and stratification; four patterns: tufting, micropapillary, cribriform and flat
Cytology		
Nuclei	Enlarged, with marked size variation	Enlarged; some size and shape variation
Chromatin	Normal	Increased density and clumping
Nucleoli	Rarely prominent	Occasionally to frequently large and prominent, similar to invasive carcinoma; sometimes multiple
Basal cell layer	Intact	May show some disruption
Basement membrane	Intact	Intact

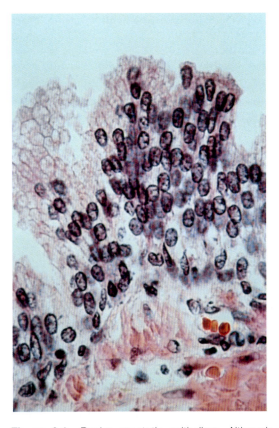

Figure 6.1 Benign prostatic epithelium. Although there is cell proliferation, spacing is uniform and nuclei are small without nucleolomegaly. Compare with Figures 6.2—6.6, showing PIN.

1991; Bostwick, 1995). This microscopic finding consists of a proliferation of epithelial cells with cytological changes mimicking cancer, including nuclear and nucleolar enlargement (Figures 6.2–6.7).

High-grade PIN resembles low-grade PIN, but nucleolomegaly, cell crowding and stratification are more pronounced and nuclear size is less variable because the majority of nuclei are enlarged. The presence of prominent nucleoli, often multiple, is typical of high-grade PIN and of great diagnostic utility (McNeal and Bostwick, 1986; Helpap, 1988; Montironi et al., 1990; De La Torre et al., 1993; Bostwick, 1995). In less severe foci of high-grade PIN (formerly PIN grade 2), greater variability in nuclear size is observed, but some markedly enlarged forms are present (Montironi et al., 1990). Nucleoli may be single or multiple, and are often eccentric and in contact with the chromatinic rim (Helpap, 1988).

The basal cell layer at the periphery is usually inconspicuous and may be difficult to appreciate by routine light microscopy; rarely, it is prominent at low power, partially or completely encircling acini containing PIN. Fragmentation of the basal cell layer is a distinctive finding in about half of acini with high-grade PIN, but often requires immunohistochemical studies with keratin 34βE12 for

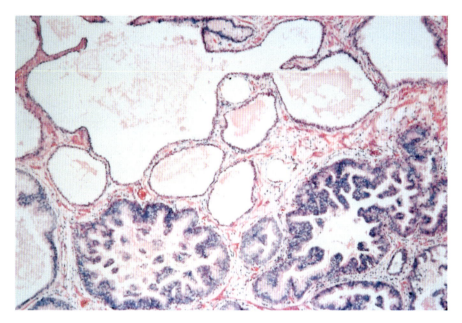

Figure 6.2 High-grade PIN. At low magnification, the hyperchromasia due to nuclear crowding is prominent (bottom) and stands in contrast with the adjacent benign acini (top).

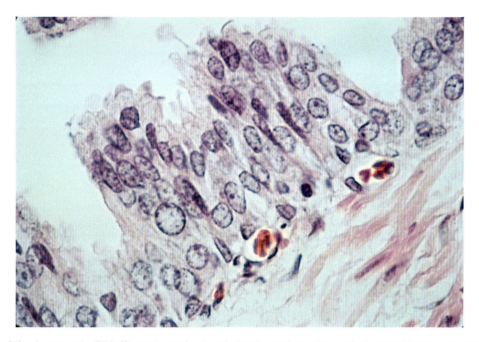

Figure 6.3 Low-grade PIN. There is marked variation in nuclear size and shape without nucleolomegaly. Compare with high-grade PIN in Figure 6.4.

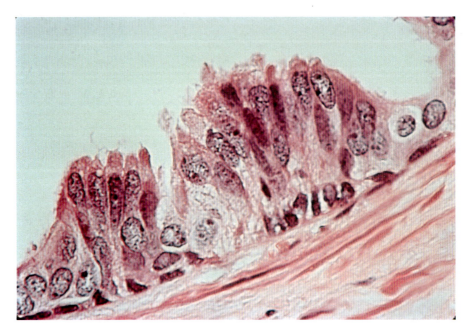

Figure 6.4   High-grade PIN. Nuclei are enlarged, with granular chromatin and nucleolomegaly.

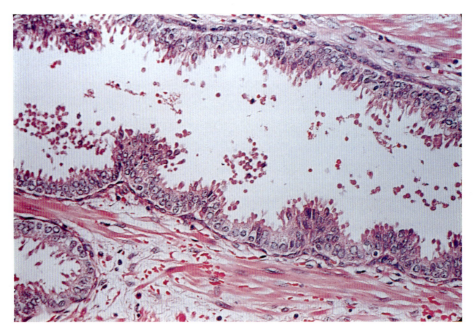

Figure 6.5   Tufting pattern of high-grade PIN. Small mounds of cells protrude into the lumen. This focus has a prominent basal cell layer at the periphery.

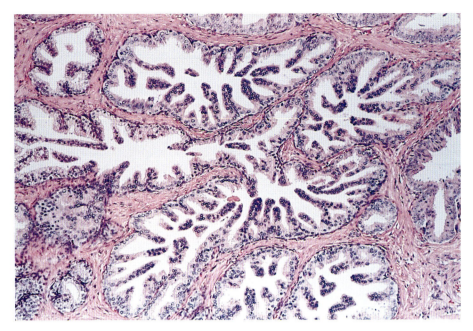

Figure 6.6 Micropapillary pattern of high-grade PIN. Elongate finger-like projections of epithelium protrude into the lumens.

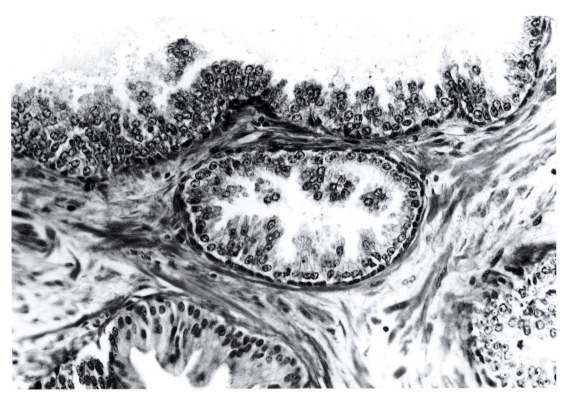

Figure 6.7 High-grade PIN involving multiple medium size and large acini. Note prominent basal cell layer. (Source: courtesy of Dr Magda Stilmant, Boston, MA.)

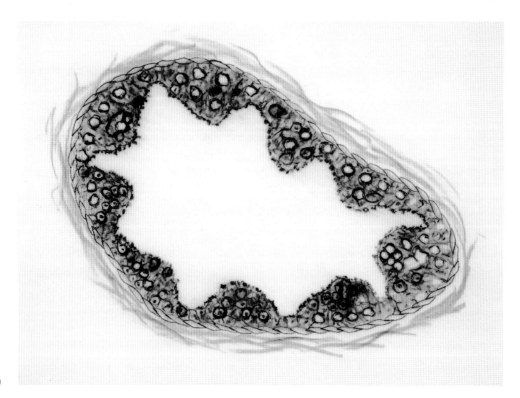

(a)

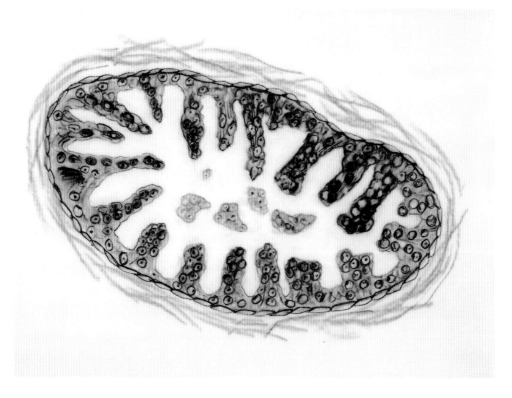

(b)

94

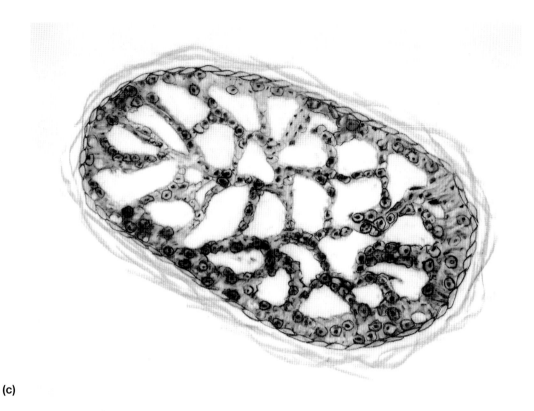

(c)

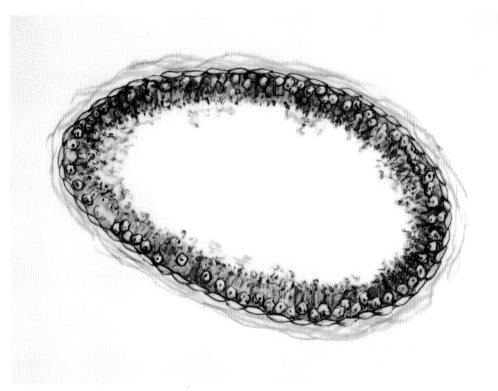

(d)

Figure 6.8 Architectural patterns of high-grade PIN. **(a)** Tufting pattern. **(b)** Micropapillary pattern. **(c)** Cribriform pattern. **(d)** Flat pattern. (Source: reproduced with permission from Bostwick *et al.* , 1993.)

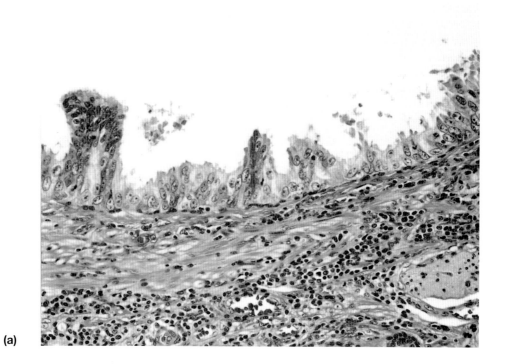

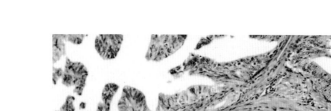

(a)

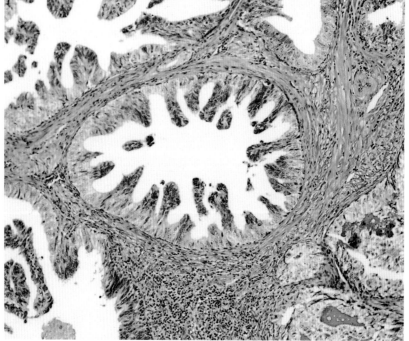

(b)

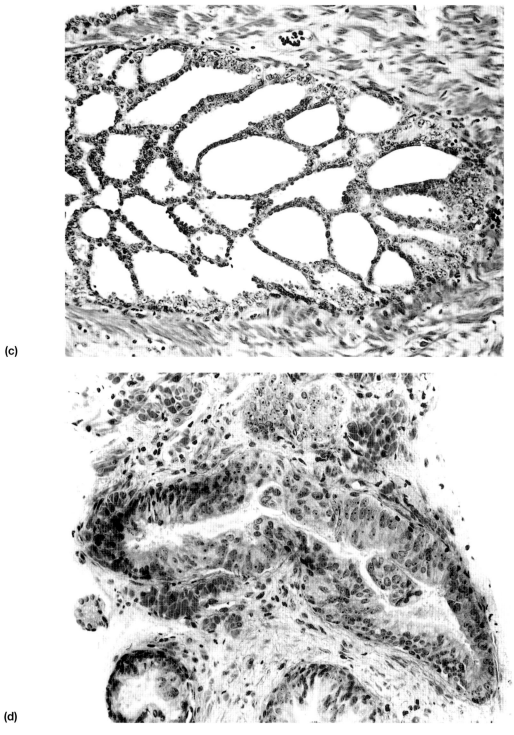

(c)

(d)

Figure 6.9 High-grade PIN. **(a)** Tufting pattern. **(b)** Micropapillary pattern. **(c)** Cribriform pattern. **(d)** Flat pattern. (Source: **(d)** courtesy of Dr Magda Stilmant, Boston, MA.)

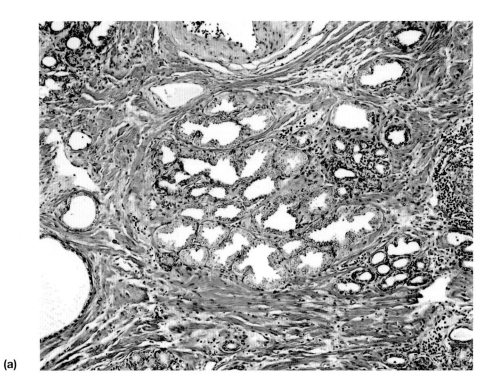

(a)

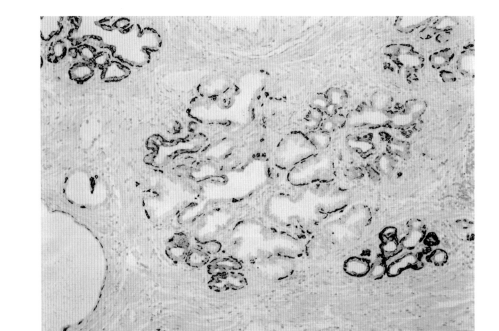

(b)

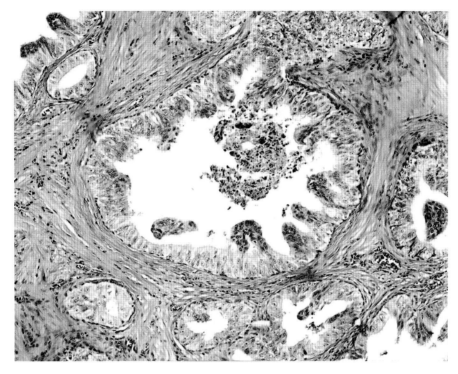

(c)

Figure 6.10 Unusual patterns of high-grade PIN. **(a)** Lobular pattern of high-grade PIN involving small acini; in our experience, this is very rare. Compare with **(b)**, showing fragmentation of the basal cell layer demonstrated with antikeratin 34ßE12 immunoreactivity. **(c)** Mixed micropapillary and tufted pattern with central necrosis; prostatic acini with prominent luminal necrosis usually represent adenocarcinoma.

identification (see Figure 1.19) (Bostwick and Brawer, 1987).

There are four main architectural patterns of high-grade PIN: tufting, micropapillary, cribriform and flat (Figures 6.5, 6.6, 6.8, 6.9) (Bostwick *et al.*, 1993).

The patterns often merge with each other, although fields with a single pattern may be present. PIN with solid luminal epithelial proliferation (solid pattern of PIN) and luminal necrosis (comedonecrosis pattern of PIN) is very rare in prostates from untreated patients (Figure 6.10). Familiarity with these patterns aids in recognition of PIN and avoids potential diagnostic pitfalls. Other than diagnostic utility, there is no known clinical significance to the different patterns.

PIN and cancer are almost always multifocal in the prostate (Qian, Wollan and Bostwick,

1996). PIN spreads through prostatic ducts in three different patterns, similarly to prostatic carcinoma. In the first pattern, neoplastic cells replace the normal luminal secretory epithelium, with preservation of the basal cell layer and basement membrane. Foci of high-grade PIN are usually indistinguishable from ductal spread of carcinoma by routine light microscopy. In the second pattern, there is direct invasion through the ductal or acinar wall, with disruption of the basal cell layer. In the third pattern, neoplastic cells invaginate between the basal cell layer and columnar secretory cell layer ('pagetoid spread'), a very rare finding. Early invasive carcinoma occurs at sites of acinar outpouching and basal cell disruption. A model of prostatic carcinogenesis has been proposed based on the morphological continuum of PIN and the multi-step

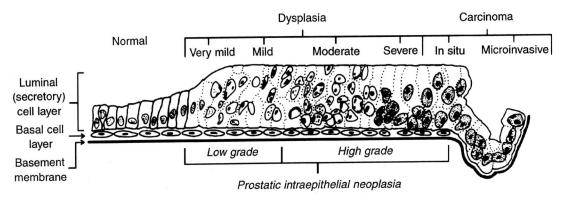

Figure 6.11 Morphological continuum from normal prostatic epithelium through increasing grades of PIN to early invasive carcinoma, according to the disease-continuum concept. Low-grade PIN (grade 1) corresponds to very mild to mild dysplasia. High-grade PIN (grades 2 and 3) corresponds to moderate to severe dysplasia and carcinoma *in situ*. The precursor state ends when malignant cells invade the stroma; this invasion occurs where the basal cell layer is disrupted. Notice that the dysplastic changes occur in the superficial (luminal) secretory cell layer, perhaps in response to luminal carcinogens. Disruption of the basal cell layer accompanies the architectural and cytological features of high-grade PIN and appears to be a necessary prerequisite for stromal invasion. The basement membrane is retained with high-grade PIN and early invasive carcinoma. (Source: modified with permission from Bostwick and Brawer, 1987).

theory of transformation (Figure 6.11) (Bostwick and Brawer, 1987).

6.2 PIN AFTER THERAPY

There is a marked decrease in the prevalence and extent of high-grade PIN in prostates after androgen deprivation therapy compared with prostates from untreated patients (Figure 6.12) (Ferguson *et al.*, 1994).

This decrease is accompanied by epithelial hyperplasia, cytoplasmic clearing and prominent acinar atrophy, with decreased ratio of acini to stroma. These findings indicate that the dysplastic prostatic epithelium is hormone-dependent. In the normal prostatic epithelium, luminal secretory cells are more sensitive to the absence of androgen than basal cells, and these results show that the cells of high-grade PIN share this androgen sensitivity. The loss of normal, hyperplastic and dysplastic epithelial cells with androgen deprivation is probably due to acceleration of programmed single cell death (apoptosis)

with subsequent exfoliation into acinar lumens (Montironi *et al.*, 1993a).

In our experience, PIN is difficult or impossible to recognize after radiation therapy (Bostwick, D. G., unpublished observations). The significant cytological changes following radiation overlap with many of those in PIN, and we avoid this diagnosis in such circumstances. Conversely, Arakawa *et al.* found that the incidence of high-grade PIN in salvage radical prostatectomies from patients with recurrent cancer was similar to that in non-irradiated prostates, although the extent of PIN measured in number of foci was less (Arakawa *et al.*, 1995).

6.3 CLINICAL SIGNIFICANCE OF PIN

The clinical significance of recognizing PIN is based on its strong association with prostatic carcinoma. High-grade PIN is encountered in up to16.5% of contemporary needle biopsies in urology office practice (Figure 6.13) (Bostwick, Qian and Frankel, 1995); by comparison, the

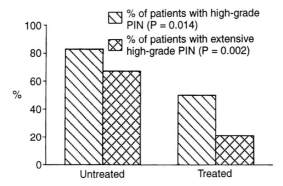

Figure 6.12 Histogram comparing the prevalence and extent of high-grade PIN following androgen deprivation in 24 treated and 24 untreated patients. Dark bars indicate prevalence; cross-hatched bars indicate extent in high power microscopic fields. (Source: reproduced with permission from Ferguson *et al.*, 1994.)

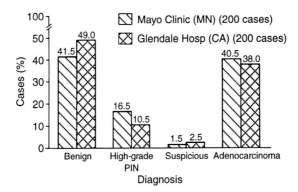

Figure 6.13 Comparative incidence of findings in 200 consecutive needle biopsies from the Mayo Clinic (MN) and Glendale Hospital (CA). There is no significant difference in the incidence of benign findings (including low-grade PIN), high-grade PIN, atypical small acinar proliferation suspicious for malignancy and adenocarcinoma between the two institutions (Source: data from Bostwick, Qian and Frankel, 1995.)

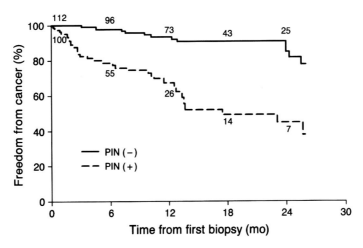

Figure 6.14 Freedom from cancer from time of first biopsy according to the presence or absence of high-grade PIN. (Source: reproduced with permission from Davidson *et al.*, 1995.)

American Cancer Society National Cancer Detection Project identified PIN and cancer in 17 (5.2%) and 58 (15.8%) of men over 50 years of age, respectively, from a series of 330 biopsies from men participating in an early detection project (Mettlin *et al.*, 1991).

High-grade PIN has a high predictive value as a marker for adenocarcinoma, and identification in biopsy specimens warrants further search for concurrent invasive carcinoma (Figure 6.14).

Davidson *et al.* found adenocarcinoma in 35% of subsequent biopsies from patients with a previous diagnosis of PIN, compared with 13% in a control group without PIN (Davidson *et al.*, 1995). High-grade PIN, patient age and serum PSA concentration are all highly significant predictors of cancer, but PIN alone increases the risk 15-fold above those without PIN and provides the highest risk ratio. Others have reported a high predictive value of PIN for cancer, ranging from 38% to 100% (Markham, 1989; Brawer *et al.*, 1991; Berner *et al.*, 1993; Weinstein and Epstein, 1993). These data underscore the strong association of PIN and adenocarcinoma, and indicate that diagnostic follow-up is needed.

Biopsy remains the only definitive method for detecting PIN and early invasive cancer. If all procedures fail to identify coexistent carcinoma, close surveillance and follow-up are indicated. Follow-up is suggested at 3- or 6-month intervals for 2 years, and thereafter at 12-month intervals for life. Identification of PIN in the prostate should not influence or dictate therapeutic decisions.

6.4 SERUM PSA AND PIN

PIN has little or no influence on serum PSA concentration and does not cause clinically suspicious elevations (Ronnett *et al.*, 1993; Alexander *et al.*, 1996). Some studies found a positive correlation of PSA and PIN, but this is the result of the confounding influence of cancer volume on serum PSA (Brawer and Lange, 1989).

6.5 HISTOCHEMISTRY AND IMMUNOHISTOCHEMISTRY OF PIN

Virtually all histochemical and immunohistochemical studies of high-grade PIN have indicated that it is more closely related to carcinoma than to benign epithelium (McNeal *et al.*, 1988a; Perlman and Epstein, 1990; Humphrey, 1991; Nagle *et al.*, 1991; Maygarden, Strom and Ware, 1992; Colombel *et al.*, 1993; Montironi *et al.*, 1993b; Bostwick, Vonk and Picado, 1994; Myers *et al.*, 1994; Bostwick, Pacelli and Lopez-Beltran, 1996). There is increased cytoplasmic expression of p160^{ERBB3} and p185^{ERBB2} in PIN and cancer when compared to normal or hyperplastic epithelium (Myers *et al.*, 1994) similar to other biomarkers in the prostate, including epidermal growth factor, epidermal growth factor receptor (Maygarden, Strom and Ware, 1992), type IV collagenase (Boag and Young, 1993), Lewis Y antigen (Perlman and Epstein, 1990) and TGF-alpha. Increased cell proliferation is the most likely explanation for this phenotypic similarity of PIN and cancer (Gainnulis *et al.*, 1993; Montironi *et al.*, 1993b), suggesting that the basal cells are the regenerative or stem cells of the prostate.

Other biomarkers show progressive loss of expression with increasing grades of PIN and cancer, including markers of secretory differentiation such as prostate-specific antigen, secretory proteins, cytoskeletal proteins, glycoproteins and neuroendocrine cells. McNeal *et al.* found that reduction of cytoplasmic differentiation markers during the preinvasive phase may be followed by abrupt re-expression at the site of microinvasion (McNeal *et al.*, 1988b). Bostwick *et al.* demonstrated a progressive decrease in the number of neuroendocrine cells from normal epithelium to high-grade PIN and carcinoma (Bostwick, Vonk and Picado, 1994). These results indicate that there is progressive impairment of cell differentiation and regulatory control with advancing stages of prostatic carcinogenesis. Changes in cytoskeletal proteins in PIN may affect transport of cell products, accounting for

Table 6.2 Prostatic intraepithelial neoplasia: differential diagnosis

Normal anatomic structures and embryonic rests
- Seminal vesicles and ejaculatory ducts
- Cowper glands
- Paraganglionic tissue
- Mesonephric remnants
- Ectopic prostatic tissue of the urethra

Hyperplasia
- Benign epithelial hyperplasia
- Cribriform hyperplasia (including clear cell hyperplasia)
- Atypical basal cell hyperplasia
- Postatrophic hyperplasia
- Simple lobular atrophy
- Sclerosing adenosis

Metaplasia and reactive changes
- Urothelial metaplasia
- Infarction-induced atypia
- Inflammation-induced atypia
- Radiation-induced atypia
- Nephrogenic metaplasia of the prostatic urethra

Carcinoma
- Acinar adenocarcinoma
- Urothelial dysplasia and carcinoma
- Cribriform pattern of prostatic adenocarcinoma
- Ductal (endometrioid) prostatic adenocarcinoma

the differences in secretory protein distribution.

6.6 NEOVASCULARIZATION IN PIN

Growth and metastasis of prostate cancer require angiogenesis (Bigler, Deering and Brawer, 1993). The number of microvessels in high-grade PIN is greater than that in benign or hyperplastic prostatic epithelium, but less than that in adenocarcinoma (Montironi *et al.*, 1993c). The microvessels in PIN are shorter than those in benign epithelium, with irregular contours and open lumens, increased number of endothelial cells and greater distance from the basement membrane.

6.7 DIFFERENTIAL DIAGNOSIS OF PIN

The microscopic differential diagnosis of PIN includes lobular atrophy, postatrophic hyperplasia, atypical basal cell hyperplasia, cribriform hyperplasia and metaplastic changes associated with radiation, infarction, prostatitis, ductal carcinoma and urothelial carcinoma (Table 6.2).

Inflammatory reactive atypia of the benign epithelium is the most frequent mimic of PIN, and caution is warranted in diagnosing PIN in the presence of prominent acute or chronic inflammation. Many of these mimics display architectural and cytological abnormalities, including nucleolomegaly, and caution is warranted in the diagnosis of PIN. Cribriform adenocarcinoma, ductal carcinoma and urothelial carcinoma involving prostatic ducts and acini are malignant lesions which may be confused with PIN.

REFERENCES

Alexander, E., Qian, J., Wollan, P. *et al.* (1996) Prostatic intraepithelial neoplasia does not raise serum prostate-specific antigen. *Urology*, **47**, 693–698.

Arakawa, A., Song, S., Scardino, P. T. and Wheeler, T. M. (1995) High grade prostatic intraepithelial neoplasia in prostates removed following irradiation failure in the treatment of prostatic adenocarcinoma. *Pathol. Res. Pract.*, **191**, 868–872.

Berner, A., Danielson, H. E., Pettersen, E. O. *et al.* (1993) DNA distribution in the prostate. Normal gland, benign and premalignant lesions, and subsequent adenocarcinomas. *Anal. Quant. Cytol. Histol.*, **15**, 247–252.

Bigler, S. A., Deering, R. E. and Brawer, M. K. (1993) Comparison of microscopic vascularity in benign and malignant prostate tissue. *Hum. Pathol.*, **24**, 220–226.

Boag, A. H. and Young, I. D. (1993) Immunohistochemical analysis of type IV collagenase expression in prostatic hyperplasia and adenocarcinoma. *Mod. Pathol.*, **6**, 65–68.

Bostwick, D. G. (1995) High grade prostatic intraepithelial neoplasia. The most likely precursor of prostate cancer. *Cancer*, **75**, 1823–1836.

Bostwick, D. G. and Brawer, M. K. (1987) Prostatic intra-epithelial neoplasia and early invasion in prostate cancer. *Cancer*, **59**, 788–794.

Bostwick, D. G., Pacelli, A. and Lopez-Beltran, A. (1996) Molecular biology of prostatic intraepithelial neoplasia. *Prostate*, **29**, 117–134.

Bostwick, D. G., Qian, J. and Frankel, K. (1995) The incidence of high grade prostatic intraepithelial neoplasia in needle biopsies. *J. Urol.*, **154**, 1791–1794.

Bostwick, D. G., Amin, M. B., Dundore, P. *et al.* (1993) Architectural patterns of high grade prostatic intraepithelial neoplasia. *Hum. Pathol.*, **24**, 298–310.

Bostwick, D. G., Dousa, M. K., Crawford, B. G. and Wollan, P. C. (1994) Neuroendocrine differentiation in prostatic intraepithelial neoplasia and adenocarcinoma. *Am. J. Surg. Pathol.*, **18**, 1240–1246.

Brawer, M. K. and Lange, P. H. (1989) Prostate-specific antigen and premalignant change. Implications for early detection. *CA-A. Cancer J.*, **39**, 361–375.

Brawer, M. K., Bigler, S. A., Sohlberg, O. E. *et al.* (1991) Significance of prostatic intraepithelial neoplasia on prostate needle biopsy. *Urology*, **38**, 103–107.

Colombel, M., Symmans, F., Gil, S. *et al.* (1993) Detection of the apoptosis-suppressing oncoprotein bcl-2 in hormone-refractory human prostate cancers. *Am. J. Pathol.*, **143**, 390–400.

Davidson, D., Bostwick, D. G., Qian, J. *et al.* (1995) Prostatic intraepithelial neoplasia is predictive of adenocarcinoma. *J. Urol.*, **154**, 1295–1299.

De La Torre, M., Haggman, M., Brandstedt, S. *et al.* (1993) Prostatic intraepithelial neoplasia and invasive carcinoma in total prostatectomy specimens: distribution, volume and DNA ploidy. *Br. J. Urol.*, **72**, 207–213.

Ferguson, J., Zincke, H., Ellison, E. *et al.* (1994) Decrease of prostatic intraepithelial neoplasia (PIN) following androgen deprivation therapy in patients with stage T3 carcinoma treated by radical prostatectomy. *Urology*, **44**, 91–95.

Gainnulis, I., Montironi, R., Galluzzi, C. M. *et al.* (1993) Frequency and location of mitoses in prostatic intraepithelial neoplasia (PIN). *Anticancer Res.*, **13**, 2447–2452.

Helpap, B. (1988) Observations on the number, size and location of nucleoli in hyperplastic and neoplastic prostatic disease. *Histopathology*, **13**, 203–211.

Humphrey, P. A. (1991) Mucin in severe dysplasia in the prostate. *Surg. Pathol.*, **4**, 137–143.

McNeal, J. E. and Bostwick, D. G. (1986) Intraductal dysplasia: a premalignant lesion of the prostate. *Hum. Pathol.*, **17**, 64–71.

McNeal, J. E., Leav, I., Alroy, J. and Skutelsky, E. (1988a) Differential lectin staining of central and peripheral zones of the prostate and alterations in dysplasia. *Am. J. Clin. Pathol.*, **89**, 41–48.

McNeal, J. E., Alroy, J., Leav, I. *et al.* (1988b) Immunohistochemical evidence for impaired cell differentiation in the premalignant phase of prostate carcinogenesis. *Am. J. Clin. Pathol.*, **90**, 23–32.

McNeal, J. E., Villers, A., Redwine, E. A. *et al.* (1991) Microcarcinoma in the prostate: its association with duct–acinar dysplasia. *Hum. Pathol.*, **22**, 644–652.

Markham, C. W. (1989) Prostatic intraepithelial neoplasia. Detection and correlation with invasive cancer in fine-needle biopsy. *Urology (Suppl)*, **24**, 57–61.

Maygarden, S. J., Strom, S. and Ware, J. L. (1992) Localization of epidermal growth factor receptor by immunohistochemical methods in human prostatic carcinoma, prostatic intraepithelial neoplasia, and benign hyperplasia. *Arch. Pathol. Lab. Med.*, **116**, 269–273.

Mettlin, C., Lee, F., Drago, J. *et al.* (1991) The American Cancer Society National Prostate Cancer Detection Project. Findings on the detection of early prostate cancer in 2425 men. *Cancer*, **67**, 2949–2958.

Montironi, R., Braccischi, A., Matera, G. *et al.* (1990) Quantitation of prostatic intra-epithelial neoplasia. Analysis of the nuclear size, number and location. *Pathol. Res. Pract.*, **187**, 307–314.

Montironi, R., Magi Galluzzi, C., Scarpelli, M. *et al.* (1993a) Occurrence of cell death (apoptosis) in prostatic intra-epithelial neoplasia. *Virchows Arch. Pathol. Anat.*, **423**, 351–357.

Montironi, R., Magi Galluzzi, C., Diamanti, L. *et al.* (1993b) Prostatic intra-epithelial neoplasia. Expression and location of proliferating cell nuclear antigen (PCNA) in epithelial, endothelial and stromal nuclei. *Virchows Arch. Pathol. Anat.*, **422**, 185–192.

Montironi, R., Magi Galluzzi, C., Diamanti, L. *et al.* (1993c) Prostatic intra-epithelial neoplasia. Qualitative and quantitative analyses of the blood capillary architecture on thin tissue sections. *Pathol. Res. Pract.*, **189**, 542–548.

Myers, R. B., Srivastava, S., Oelschlager, D. K. *et al.* (1994) Expression of p160erbB-3 and p185erbB-2 in prostatic intraepithelial neoplasia and prostatic adenocarcinoma. *J. Nat. Cancer Inst.*, **86**, 1140–1144.

Nagle, R. B., Brawer, M. K., Kittelson, J. *et al.* (1991) Phenotypic relationships of prostatic intraepithelial neoplasia to invasive prostatic carcinoma. *Am. J. Pathol.*, **138**, 119–128.

Perlman, E. J. and Epstein, J. I. (1990) Blood group antigen expression in dysplasia and adenocarcinoma of the prostate. *Am. J. Surg. Pathol.*, **14**, 810–818.

Qian, J., Wollan, P. and Bostwick, D. G. (1996) The extent and multicentricity of high grade prostatic intraepithelial neoplasia in clinically localized prostatic adenocarcinoma. *Hum. Pathol.*, (in press).

Ronnett, B. M., Carmichael, M. J., Carter, H. B. *et al.* (1993) Does high grade prostatic intraepithelial neoplasia result in elevated serum prostate specific antigen levels? *J. Urol.*, **150**, 386–389.

Sakr, W. A., Haas, G. P., Cassin, B. J. *et al.* (1993) The frequency of carcinoma and intraepithelial neoplasia of the prostate in young male patients. *J. Urol.*, **150**, 379–385.

Weinstein, M. H. and Epstein, J. I. (1993) Significance of high grade prostatic intraepithelial neoplasia on needle biopsy. *Hum. Pathol.*, **24**, 624–629.

7

ADENOCARCINOMA

Prostate cancer is the most common cancer of men in the United States, and is second only to lung cancer as a cause of cancer death. In 1996, 41 400 Americans died of prostate cancer and 317 000 new cases were diagnosed (Parker *et al.*, 1996). For all men, the overall lifetime probability of developing clinical evidence of prostate cancer is one in six (Parker *et al.*, 1996). Despite an 80% prevalence at autopsy by age 80 years, the clinical incidence is much lower, indicating that most men die with prostate carcinoma rather than of prostate carcinoma (Seidman *et al.*, 1985; Scardino, 1989; Nomura and Kolonel, 1991; Bostwick *et al.*, 1992; Morra and Das, 1992). Little is known about the causes of prostate cancer despite its high incidence and prevalence.

The incidence of prostatic adenocarcinoma has risen dramatically in the past decade, probably owing to early detection programs which employ digital rectal examination, serum PSA and transrectal ultrasonography. As competing causes of mortality such as lung cancer and heart disease decline, men are living longer and increasing their risk of developing clinically apparent prostate cancer.

Prostate cancer has no specific presenting symptoms, and is usually clinically silent, although it may cause lower urinary tract symptoms mimicking nodular hyperplasia. Cancer is often initially manifest in metastatic sites such as cervical lymph nodes and bone. The diagnosis is made in the following clinical instances:

- routine surveillance for prostatic adenocarcinoma in men over 40 years of age – digital rectal examination shows a nodular or diffusely enlarged prostate (clinical stage T 2 or 3); serum PSA concentration is greater than 4 ng/ml (clinical stage T1c); or transrectal ultrasound (TRUS) and biopsies are positive for malignancy (lesion-directed, random or systematic sextant needle biopsies);
- incidental carcinoma in transurethral resection specimens (clinical stage T1 carcinoma);
- metastatic adenocarcinoma of unknown primary;
- carcinoma of the prostate presenting as a perirectal or perivesicular mass – prostate carcinoma very rarely produces an eccentric or circumferential rectal perirectal mass with or without mucosal involvement of the rectum.

7.1 DIAGNOSIS OF CARCINOMA

7.1.1 Gross pathology

Gross identification of prostatic adenocarcinoma is often difficult in radical prostatectomy specimens, and definitive diagnosis requires microscopic examination. In transurethral resection specimens, adenocarcinoma is rarely grossly identified unless extensive, because of the confounding macroscopic features of nodular hyperplasia.

Adenocarcinoma tends to be multifocal, with a predilection for the peripheral zone (McNeal *et al.*, 1988). Grossly apparent tumor foci are at least 5 mm in greatest dimension, and appear yellow-white with a firm consistency due to stromal desmoplasia. Some tumors appear as yellow granular masses, which stand in contrast with the normal spongy prostatic parenchyma. Similar gross findings may be seen in tuberculosis, granulomatous prostatitis and extensive acute and chronic prostatitis.

7.1.2 Microscopic features

Most prostatic adenocarcinomas are composed of acini arranged in one or more patterns. The diagnosis relies on a combination of architectural and cytological findings. The light-microscopic features are usually sufficient for diagnosis, but rare cases may benefit from immunohistochemical studies.

(a) Architectural features of adenocarcinoma

Architectural features are assessed at low- to medium-power magnification. The arrangement of the acini is diagnostically useful and is the basis of Gleason grading (Chapter 8). Malignant acini usually have an irregular haphazard arrangement, randomly scattered in the stroma in clusters or single acini (Figures 7.1 and 7.2). The spacing between malignant acini often varies widely (Figure 7.3).

Variation in acinar size is a useful criterion, particularly when there are small irregular abortive acini with primitive lumens at the periphery of a focus of well-differentiated carcinoma. The acini in suspicious foci are usually small or medium-sized, with irregular

contours that stand in contrast with the smooth, round to elongate contours of benign and hyperplastic acini. Comparison with the adjacent benign prostatic acini is always of value (Figure 7.4). Well-differentiated carcinoma and the large gland variant of Gleason grade 2 are particularly difficult to separate from benign acini in needle biopsies because of the relatively uniform size and spacing of acini (Figure 7.5) (Chapter 8).

The stroma in cancer frequently contains young collagen, which appears lightly eosinophilic, although desmoplasia may be prominent. There is sometimes splitting or distortion of muscle fibers in the stroma, but this is a difficult feature to appreciate and cannot be relied upon, due to the resemblance to benign acini. An understanding of the Gleason grading system is of value in interpretation of small foci because of its reliance on architectural patterns (Chapter 8).

(b) Cytological features of adenocarcinoma

The cytological features of adenocarcinoma include nuclear and nucleolar enlargement, and these are present in the majority of malignant cells (Figures 7.6–7.9).

Every cell has a nucleolus, so one searches for 'prominent' nucleoli that are at least 1.25–1.50 µm in diameter or larger; however, we do not routinely measure nucleoli for diagnosis, so this determination is based on comparison with benign epithelial cells elsewhere in the specimen (Bostwick *et al.*, 1993). The identification of two or more nucleoli is virtually diagnostic of malignancy, according to Helpap (1988), particularly when the nucleoli are eccentrically located in the nucleus; we find this criterion useful, but employ it sparingly. Artifacts often obscure the nuclei and nucleoli, and overstaining of nuclei by hematoxylin creates one of the most common and difficult problems encountered in interpretation of suspicious foci. Differences in fixation and handling of biopsy specimens influence nuclear size

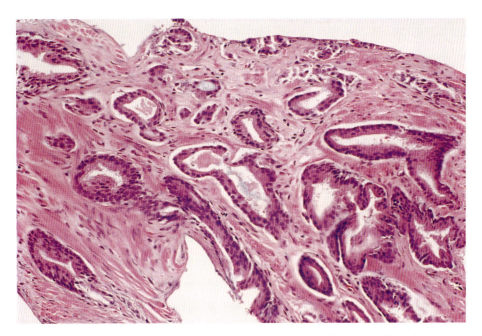

Figure 7.1 Gleason pattern 3 adenocarcinoma, large acinar type, consisting of an irregular aggregate of rigid angulated acini with variability of size, shape and spacing. The epithelium may separate from the adjacent stroma, creating an artifactual space in some acini.

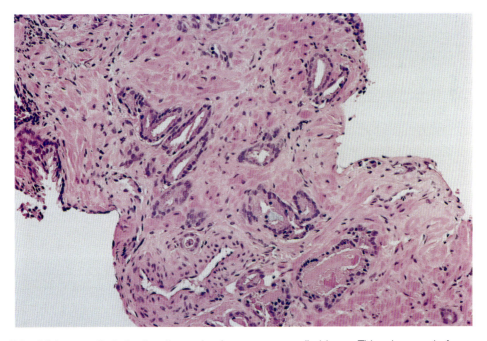

Figure 7.2 Minimum criteria for the diagnosis of cancer on needle biopsy. This microscopic focus contains acini with variation in size, shape and spacing.

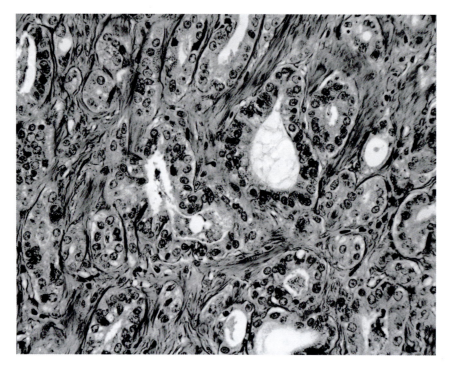

Figure 7.3 Adenocarcinoma (Gleason pattern 3) showing variation in acinar size, shape, and spacing.

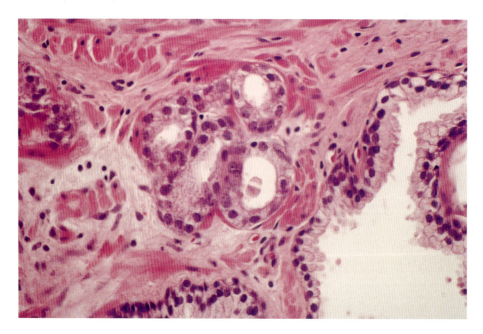

Figure 7.4 Minimum criteria for the diagnosis of cancer on needle biopsy. This tight cluster of small acini stands in contrast with the adjacent benign acini.

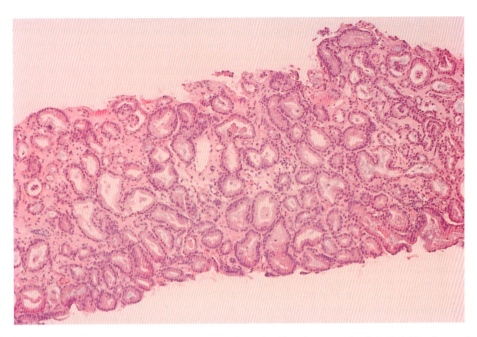

Figure 7.5 Well-differentiated adenocarcinoma consists of uniformly spaced acini mimicking hyperplastic epithelium.

and chromasia, so comparison with cells from the same specimen is optimal (internal control). Many pathologists prefer pale staining with eosin, but this approach fails to accentuate nucleoli, which are often enlarged. In such cases, with nuclear hyperchromasia and pale eosinophil staining, we often increase the light source and magnification of suspicious foci in an effort to identify hidden enlarged nucleoli.

The basal cell layer is absent in adenocarcinoma, an important feature which is difficult to evaluate in routine sections. Compressed stromal fibroblasts can mimic basal cells, but are usually only seen focally at the periphery of acini. An intact basal cell layer is present with benign acini, whereas carcinoma entirely lacks a basal cell layer. Sometimes, small foci of adenocarcinoma cluster around large benign acini that have an intact basal cell layer, compounding the difficulty. In problem cases, it may be useful to employ monoclonal antibodies directed against high-molecular-weight cytokeratin (e.g. clone 34βE12) to evaluate the

basal cell layer, but we use this infrequently (in less than 5% of cases) and only as an adjunct to the light-microscopic findings; this should not be the basis for a diagnosis of malignancy, particularly in small suspicious foci. This stain is of greatest utility in confirming the benignancy of a suspicious focus by demonstrating an immunoreactive basal cell layer.

Nucleoli are found in virtually all cells, and the prognostic significance of nucleolar enlargement in prostatic carcinoma has been demonstrated by various methods, including scanning electron microscopy and computerized image analysis. Nucleolar diameter is a powerful discriminant of cancer when compared with benign prostatic epithelium (Tannenbaum *et al.*, 1982), and nucleolar prominence separates AAH from carcinoma (Keleman, Buschmann and Weisz-Carrington, 1990); however, Keleman and coworkers considered a nucleolus prominent when the diameter was 3 μm or greater, considerably larger than that observed by Böcking and colleagues (1.88 μm) (Böcking, Kiehn and Heinzel-Wach,

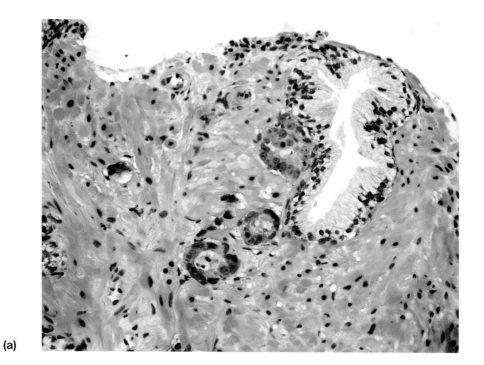

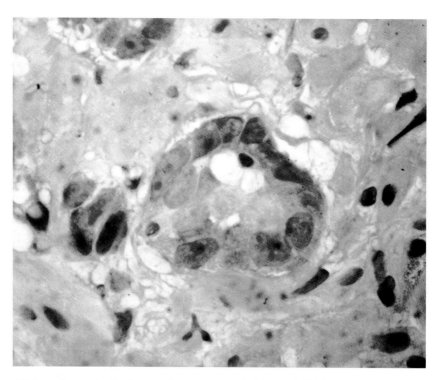

Figure 7.6 Minimal diagnosis of adenocarcinoma on needle biopsy. **(a)** This is the only diagnostic focus in the biopsy, with four acinar structures that stand in contrast with the adjacent benign acinar epithelium. **(b)** There is marked nuclear and nucleolar enlargement which was considered sufficient for the diagnosis of adenocarcinoma. The patient underwent radical prostatectomy, and the specimen revealed extensive bilateral Gleason 3 + 4 = 7 adenocarcinoma. (Source: case courtesy of Dr Deborah Davidson, Lincoln, NE.)

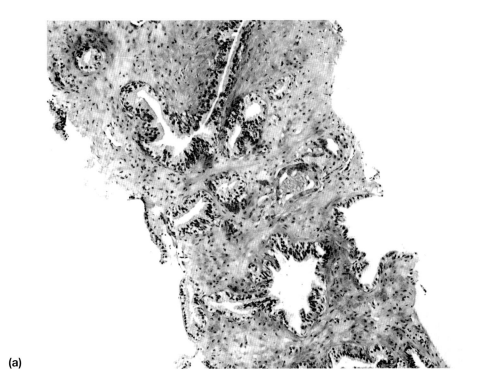

(a)

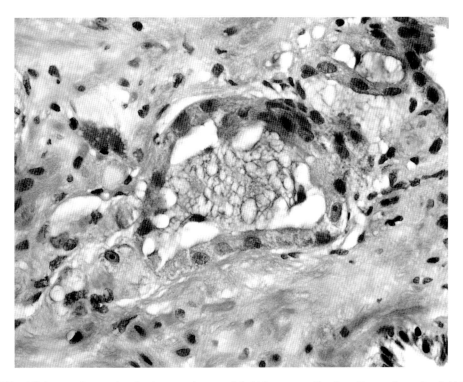

(b)

Figure 7.7 Minimum diagnosis of adenocarcinoma. **(a)** At low magnification, the malignant acini blend with the stroma and may be easily overlooked. **(b)** At high magnification, the malignant acini are lined by cells with enlarged nuclei and prominent nucleoli, and the lumens contain abundant mucin; these features were in contrast with the adjacent benign acini.

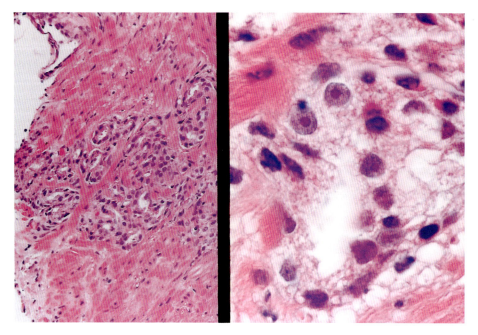

Figure 7.8 Minimum criteria for the diagnosis of adenocarcinoma. This minute focus of closely packed small acini contains cells with enlarged prominent eosinophilic nucleoli.

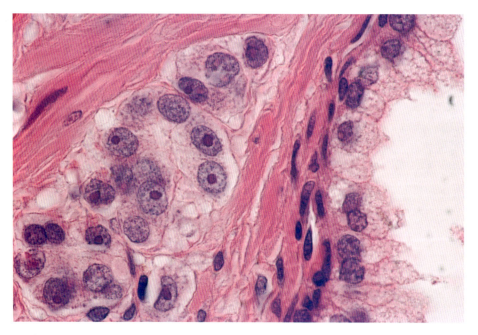

Figure 7.9 This focus of adenocarcinoma (left) displays marked nuclear and nucleolar enlargement when compared with adjacent benign epithelium (right).

1982), Gleason(1 µm; Gleason, 1985), Tannenbaum *et al.* (2.4 µm² surface area; Tannenbaum *et al.*, 1982), Deschenes and Weidner (AAH, 0.79 µm; Gleason grades 2 and 3 cancer, 1.60 µm; Deschenes and Weidner, 1990), Montironi *et al.* (1991), and Bostwick, Cupp and Oesterling (1993). Conversely, Layfield and Goldstein (1991) failed to find any nucleoli > 1.8 µm in diameter in benign or low-grade malignant fine needle aspirates. Interestingly, one study found no significant difference in nucleolar diameter between AAH and normal and hyperplastic epithelium (Keleman, Buschmann and Weisz-Carrington, 1990).

(c) Luminal mucin

Acidic sulfated and non-sulfated mucin is often seen in acini of adenocarcinoma, appearing as amorphous or delicate thread-like faintly basophilic secretions in routine sections (Figure 7.10).

This mucin stains with alcian blue, and is best demonstrated at pH 2.5, whereas the normal prostatic epithelium contains periodic-acid–Schiff-reactive neutral mucin. Acidic mucin is not specific for carcinoma, and may be found in PIN, AAH, sclerosing adenosis, and rarely in nodular hyperplasia (Ro *et al.*, 1988a, b; Humphrey, 1991; Epstein and Fynheer, 1992; Goldstein, Qian and Bostwick, 1995).

(d) Crystalloids

Crystalloids are sharp, needle-like eosinophilic structures which are often present in the lumens of well-differentiated and moderately differentiated carcinoma (Figure 7.11) (Holmes, 1977; Del Rosario *et al.*, 1993). They are not specific for carcinoma, and can be found in AAH, PIN, nodular hyperplasia and benign prostatic epithelium.

Special stains highlight the presence of crystalloids, which are otherwise inapparent by light microscopy (Ro *et al.*, 1988b; Molberg,

Mikhail and Vuitch, 1994; Tressera *et al.*, 1994). Crystalloids stain red with trichrome stain, blue with toluidine blue and violet with phosphotungstic hematoxylin; no staining is observed with PAS, alcian blue, Prussian blue and Congo red. Immunohistochemical stains for PSA and PAP are negative.

The pathogenesis of crystalloids is uncertain, but they probably result from abnormal protein and mineral metabolism within benign and malignant acini. Ultrastructurally, they are composed of electron-dense material that lacks the periodicity of crystals, and X-ray microanalysis reveals abundant sulfur, calcium and phosphorus, and a small amount of sodium (Del Rosario *et al.*, 1993). Hard, proteinaceous secretions are almost always present in adjacent acini and are probably the source of the crystalloids.

The presence of crystalloids in metastatic adenocarcinoma of unknown site of origin is strong presumptive evidence of prostatic origin, although it is an uncommon finding and is not conclusive (Molberg, Mikhail and Vuitch, 1994; Tressera *et al.*, 1994).

(e) Collagenous micronodules

Collagenous micronodules, consisting of microscopic nodular masses of paucicellular eosinophilic fibrillar stroma which impinge on acinar lumens (Figure 7.12) (McNeal *et al.*, 1991; Bostwick, Wollan and Adlakha, 1995), are a specific but infrequent and incidental finding in prostatic adenocarcinoma.

They are usually present in mucin-producing adenocarcinoma and result from extravasation of acidic mucin into the stroma. Collagenous micronodules are present in about 13% of cases of adenocarcinoma and are not observed in benign epithelium, nodular hyperplasia or PIN. They are an infrequent finding, present in 0.6% of needle biopsies and 12.7% of prostatectomies. Collagenous micronodules are a useful but infrequent diagnostic clue in prostatic adenocarcinoma and may be particularly valuable in challenging needle

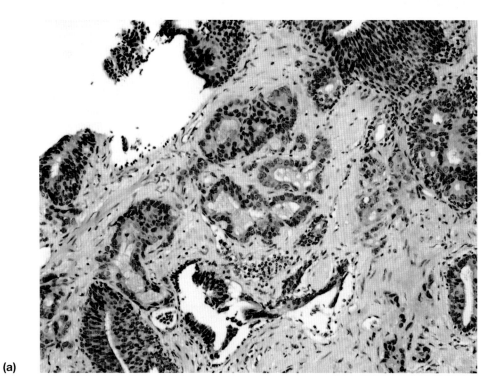

(a)

(b)

Figure 7.10 Luminal mucin in a small focus of adenocarcinoma. **(a)** There is a small focus of distorted angulated acini with variable spacing. Compare with **(b)**, showing nuclear enlargement and distortion and luminal mucin; the patient underwent radical prostatectomy, and the specimen revealed bilateral Gleason 3 + 4 = 7 adenocarcinoma.

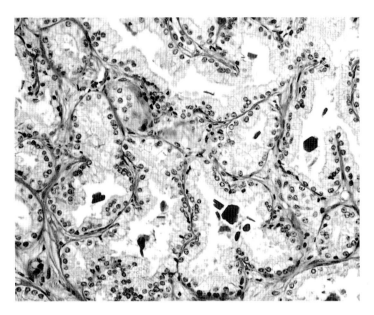

Figure 7.11 Crystalloids in Gleason pattern 1 adenocarcinoma. We consider the presence of crystalloids to be a 'soft' criterion for malignancy because they can be seen in AAH and other benign conditions.

biopsy specimens (Bostwick, Wollan and Adlakha, 1995).

(f) Perineural invasion

Perineural invasion is common in adenocarcinoma, and may be the only evidence of malignancy in biopsy specimens (Figure 7.13). This finding is strong presumptive evidence of malignancy, but is not pathognomonic because it occurs present rarely with benign acini (Figure 7.14) (Hasson and Maksem, 1980; McIntire and Franzina, 1986; Bastacky, Walsh and Epstein, 1993). Complete circumferential growth, intraneural invasion and ganglionic invasion are found only with cancer.

Perineural invasion indicates tumor spread along the path of least resistance, and does not represent lymphatic invasion. When present in needle biopsy specimens , perineural invasion is not an independent predietor of extraprostatic extension (Egan *et al.*, 1997). This finding should be included in the pathology report, according to the Cancer Committee of the College of American Pathologists (Henson *et al.*, 1994). However, we have recently discontinued this practice because it is of no apparent value (Egan *et al.*, 1997).

(g) Vascular/lymphatic invasion

Microvascular invasion is a strong indicator of malignancy and its presence correlates with histological grade, although it is sometimes difficult to distinguish from fixation-associated retraction artifact of acini (Figure 7.15) (Bahnson *et al.*, 1989; Salamao, Graham and Bostwick, 1995).

Microvascular invasion may also be an important predictor of outcome, and carries a fourfold greater risk of tumor progression and death (Bahnson *et al.*, 1989). The Cancer Committee of the College of American Pathologists (Henson *et al.*, 1994) recommends reporting microvascular invasion in all prostatic specimens, presumably using routine light-microscopic examination; despite this recommendation, this finding is not measured in

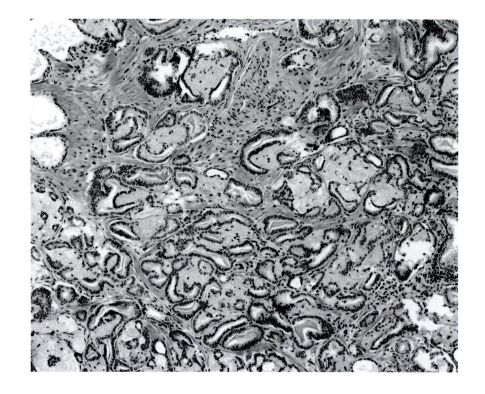

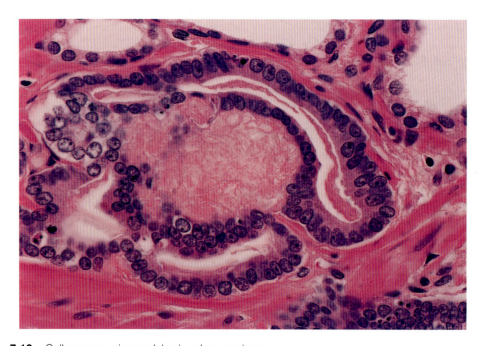

Figure 7.12 Collagenous micronodules in adenocarcinoma.

prostatic biopsies by most laboratories, including ours. Immunohistochemical stains directed against endothelial cells such as Factor-VIII-related antigen or *Ulex europaeus* may increase the detection rate (Salamao, Graham and Bostwick, 1995).

Microvascular invasion is defined as the unequivocal presence of tumor cells within endothelial-lined spaces. We do not require the presence of a cellular reaction in the adjacent stroma with hemosiderin and fibrin deposition to diagnose microvascular invasion. Also, we do not differentiate vascular and lymphatic channels because of the difficulty and lack of reproducibility among different observers by routine light-microscopic examination (Salamao, Graham and Bostwick, 1995).

Microvascular invasion is most often confused with perineural invasion and with cell clusters within empty spaces without a lining as a result of retraction artifact. Equivocal foci and spaces without an identifiable endothelial lining are not considered evidence of perineural invasion. Microvascular invasion is present in 38% of radical prostatectomy specimens, and is commonly associated with extraprostatic extension and lymph node metastases (62% and 67% of cases respectively) (Bahnson *et al.*, 1989; Salamao, Graham and Bostwick, 1995). However, it is not an independent predictor of progression when stage and grade are included in the multivariate analysis (Bahnson *et al.*, 1989).

(h) Microvessel density (angiogenesis)

There is a significant increase in microvessel density in prostatic intraepithelial neoplasia (Montironi *et al.*, 1993) and adenocarcinoma when compared with normal prostatic tissue (Weidner *et al.*, 1993; Brawer *et al.*, 1994; Siegal, Yu and Brawer, 1995; Bostwick *et al.*, 1996). Mean blood vessel count is higher in tumors with metastases than in those without metastases (Hall *et al.*, 1994; Vesalainen *et al.*, 1994). Increased microvessel density in prostatic carcinoma is probably related to the production of angiogenesis-associated growth factors (Brown *et al.*, 1995; Sinha *et al.*, 1995; Vartanian and Weidner, 1995), as in other organs (Folkman, 1992). The cumulative data suggest that microvascular invasion and increased microvessel density contribute to extraprostatic spread of adenocarcinoma. This factor is an important independent predictor of pathological stage (Bostwick *et al.*, 1996).

7.1.3 Differential diagnosis

In recent years, there has been a growing recognition of the diversity of acinar changes in the prostate that mimic adenocarcinoma. The diagnostic difficulty has been compounded by the success of early detection methods which often yield biopsies with small foci. In a retrospective study of transurethral resections and needle biopsies obtained at the Mayo Clinic between 1960 and 1968, we found that about 2% of cases were overdiagnosed as adenocarcinoma (Bostwick, D. G., unpublished observations). The most common mimics of cancer in this series were postatrophic hyperplasia, atypical adenomatous hyperplasia, basal cell hyperplasia, prostatic intraepithelial neoplasia and, rarely, sclerosing adenosis. Each of these lesions and other mimics of cancer are described in detail in other chapters (Table 7.1).

7.2 EIGHT COMMON PROBLEMS IN NEEDLE BIOPSY INTERPRETATION

7.2.1 Atypical small acinar proliferation versus adenocarcinoma

In up to 2.5% of needle biopsies, there is a localized proliferation of small acini which is suspicious for carcinoma but falls below the diagnostic threshold. This problem is often due to the small size of the focus; although we do not use quantitative criteria for malignancy in the prostate, very small foci with less than a dozen malignant acini are evaluated

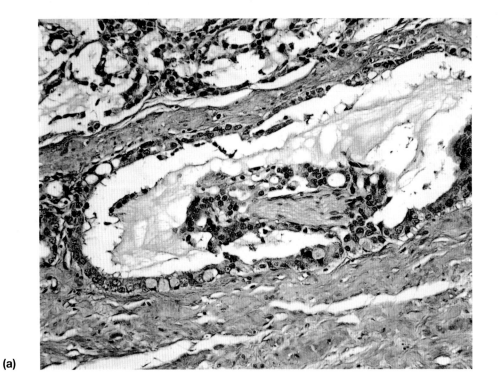

(a)

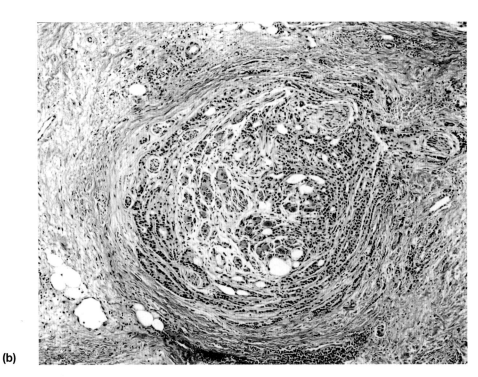

(b)

Figure 7.13 Perineural invasion by adenocarcinoma. **(a)** The nerve twig is hidden in the center of this large acinus of mucinous carcinoma. **(b)** Periprostatic ganglion (center) is surrounded and infiltrated by high-grade adenocarcinoma.

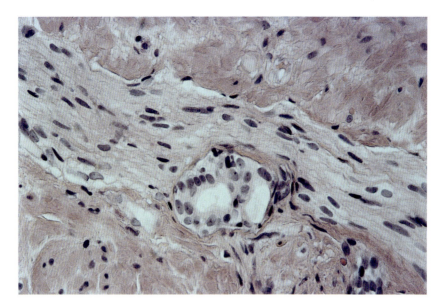

Figure 7.14 Benign prostatic acini abut a large nerve twig.

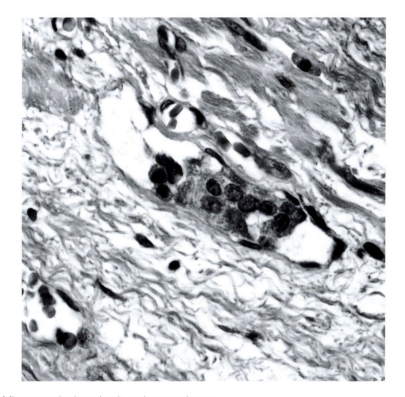

Figure 7.15 Microvascular invasion by adenocarcinoma.

Table 7.1 Prostatic adenocarcinoma: differential diagnosis

- Adenoid basal cell carcinoma
- Atrophy
  - *Simple lobular atrophy*
  - *Cystic atrophy*
  - *Sclerotic atrophy*
  - *Postatrophic hyperplasia*
- Atypical adenomatous hyperplasia
- Basal cell hyperplasia (typical and atypical)
- Cowper glands
- Direct extension from rectal carcinoma
- Florid hyperplasia of mesonephric remnants
- Metastatic carcinoma
- Nephrogenic adenoma of the prostatic urethra
- Paraganglia
- Seminal vesicles
- Sclerosing adenosis
- Verumontanum mucosal gland hyperplasia
- Xanthoma

cautiously and usually with intradepartmental consultation. We have rarely diagnosed adenocarcinoma with as few as three malignant acini and only when there was frank cytological anaplasia that was in stark contrast with the adjacent benign epithelium, there was no inflammation near the focus of concern, serial sections were obtained and the possibility of seminal vesicle or ejaculatory duct epithelium was excluded.

Other causes of difficulty with small suspicious foci include the presence of distorted acini that lack convincing cytological features, prominent inflammation in which the adjacent benign acini show distortion and inflammatory reactive atypia with nuclear and nucleolar enlargement (Figure 7.16).

In such cases, it is appropriate to sign the case out as 'atypical small acinar proliferation suspicious for but not diagnostic of malignancy.'

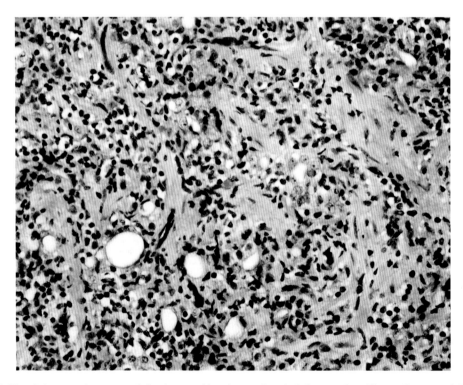

Figure 7.16 Adenocarcinoma partially obscured by dense chronic inflammation. The malignant acini seem to blend with the lymphocytes, creating diagnostic difficulty. We urge caution in such cases unless the evidence for maligancy is substantial and unequivocal.

We consider this a valid diagnostic category based on our 'absolute uncertainty' regarding the diagnosis: the diagnosis of carcinoma cannot be made but the possibility cannot be definitively excluded. In view of the serious consequences of the diagnosis of carcinoma, it is prudent to render this diagnosis only when there is absolute confidence in the histological findings. Other supportive evidence is useful, including patient age, serum PSA concentration and keratin 34βE12 expression, but none is a substitute for the light-microscopic findings; we usually evaluate these other findings only after microscopic examination in order to avoid bias. A wide variety of small acinar proliferations may mimic adenocarcinoma, particularly in small specimens.

We classify suspicious small acinar proliferations as 'suspicious, favor benign', 'suspicious', and 'highly suspicious'. The expected clinical response to each of these diagnoses is identical: patient follow-up with consideration of repeat biopsy. This classification may appear cumbersome, but we find it useful to stratify our level of suspicion as a teaching tool.

7.2.2 Atypical small acinar proliferation versus atypical adenomatous hyperplasia versus adenocarcinoma

Needle biopsies are much more likely to contain a suspicious atypical small acinar proliferation than AAH. We rarely use the diagnosis of AAH in needle biopsies and only when most or all of the focus of concern is present for evaluation and nodular hyperplasia is present; this conservative approach to the diagnosis of AAH avoids overdiagnosis of AAH and underdiagnosis of cancer. There is a temptation to diagnose all small acinar proliferations as AAH, an approach that would eliminate the value of this diagnostic category. For this reason, the participants in the consensus statement on AAH (Bostwick *et al.*, 1993) felt that this diagnosis should be reserved for small acinar proliferations that are in intimate association with nodular hyperplasia.

AAH is distinguished from well differentiated carcinoma by the presence of inconspicuous nucleoli, lack of basophilic mucin and fragmented basal cell layer. Both may arise in association with nodular hyperplasia, but the small acini of AAH almost always appear on the nodule edge and merge with the larger acini, unlike cancer, which is random in its spatial relation with nodules.

7.2.3 Prostatic intraepithelial neoplasia versus large gland variant of Gleason grade 3 carcinoma

The large gland variant of Gleason grade 3 carcinoma, including the cribriform variant, does not have a circumferential basal cell layer and is usually associated with areas of small acinar adenocarcinoma. In equivocal cases, the diagnosis may be aided by staining with basal-cell-specific antibodies to high-molecular-weight-cytokeratin 34βE12. Small acini with abnormal cells almost always represent invasive carcinoma rather than PIN.

7.2.4 Clear cell pattern of carcinoma versus benign clear cell foci

Numerous forms of adenocarcinoma contain clear cytoplasm. Adenocarcinoma arising in the transition zone characteristically contains clear cells and is well or moderately differentiated. Gleason grade 4 carcinoma may contain cells with clear cytoplasm, referred to as the 'hypernephroid' pattern. Androgen deprivation therapy induces abundant clear cell change in benign and malignant acini, and the diagnosis of adenocarcinoma in such cases may be difficult. The clear cell pattern of carcinoma may be confused with histiocytes, vacuolated stromal smooth muscle cells and metaplastic cells. Cribriform carcinoma with clear cell pattern may be difficult to separate from clear cell cribriform hyperplasia, but cancer always has significant cytological abnormalities.

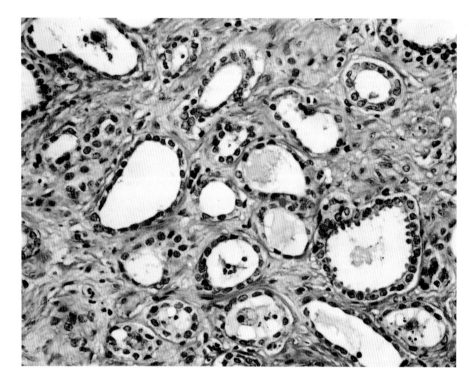

(a)

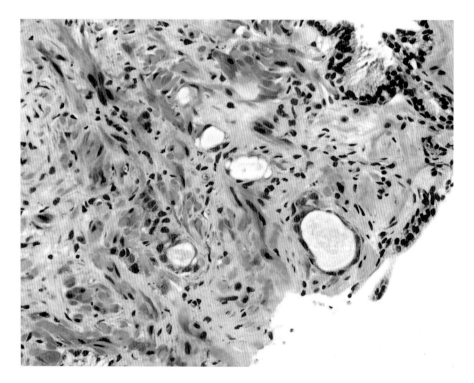

(b)

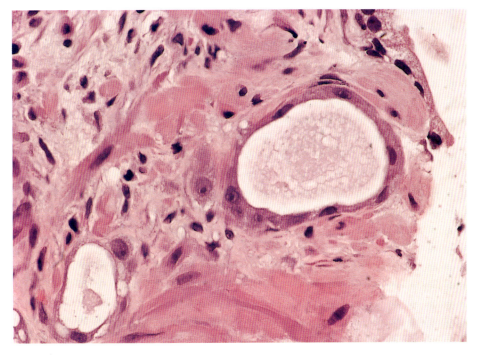

(c)

Figure 7.17 'Atrophic' pattern of adenocarcinoma. **(a)** These malignant acini are dilated, with some flattening of the lining epithelium, mimicking atrophy. Some of the cells contained slightly enlarged nuclei and prominent nucleoli. **(b)** In this case, the biopsy revealed less than ten shrunken acini with scant luminal mucin and attenuated epithelial lining, which, at high magnification **(c)** revealed enlarged nucleoli. This was considered highly suspicious of adenocarcinoma and the patient underwent repeat biopsy and subsequent radical prostatectomy, with large areas containing a similar pattern of adenocarcinoma merging with Gleason pattern 3 carcinoma.

7.2.5 Large acinar variant of grade 3 carcinoma versus benign glands

One of the more difficult problems in prostatic needle biopsy interpretation is the diagnosis of large acini as malignant, particularly if they are abundant and replace a sizable portion of the specimen (Chapter 8). Small, irregular malignant acini often stand in contrast with the adjacent benign acini architecturally and can be readily identified at low-power magnification, whereas large malignant acini may merge with adjacent benign acini and can be overlooked. The cytological features of malignancy are invariably present in large malignant acini, but are not often appreciated at scanning magnification. Appreciation of this pattern of carcinoma can avoid this problem.

7.2.6 Atrophic pattern of carcinoma versus postatrophic hyperplasia

Atrophic acini occasionally mimic adenocarcinoma and, conversely, adenocarcinoma occasionally mimics atrophy. The atrophic pattern of carcinoma is uncommon and invariably present only locally within moderately differentiated carcinoma but the limited sampling by needle biopsy may yield a pure specimen of atrophic, shrunken malignant acini (Figure 7.17) (Egan *et al.*, 1997).

The acini contain dilated lumens with a flattened attenuated epithelial lining, but at least some of the neoplastic cells retain diagnostic cytological features of nuclear and nucleolar enlargement. Pale wispy blue luminal mucin may be present in carcinoma, but is a rare

125

finding in atrophic acini. If the focus is small and has marginal cytological findings, the best diagnosis is suspicious but not diagnostic of malignancy. The variation in acinar size and spacing without fusion in the atrophic pattern of cancer is best considered to be Gleason pattern 3.

7.2.7 Urothelial carcinoma with microglandular pattern versus ductal carcinoma

Small, round lumens may occasionally punctuate solid aggregates of urothelial carcinoma, imparting a microglandular pattern that may be mistaken for prostatic adenocarcinoma. Most cases of urothelial carcinoma in or near the prostate involve the prostatic urethra, and the cribriform pattern of ductal (endometrioid) carcinoma is the main differential diagnostic consideration. These cancers are treated differently, so this distinction is clinically important. The degree of cytological atypia of these two types of cancer may overlap, so this is not a useful distinguishing feature, although ductal carcinoma is more likely to have prominent nucleoli. The presence of glandular differentiation, including cytoplasmic blebs and mucin production, is more likely in ductal carcinoma. Immunohistochemical stains for PSA and PAP will stain ductal carcinoma but not urothelial carcinoma.

7.2.8 Androgen deprivation-treated cancer versus benign clear cell change

It is always useful to have the clinical history, but all too often the pathologist must interpret specimens without this information. The changes induced by androgen deprivation therapy are distinctive, uniform and diffuse, and affect benign and malignant acini; knowledge of these changes is critical in avoiding this diagnostic pitfall. These changes include prominent clear cell change, nuclear shrinkage and nuclear hyperchromasia (see Chapter 10). If abundant tumor is available for evaluation, there are usually some neoplastic cells that retain diagnostic cytological features of nucleomegaly and nucleolomegaly. Benign clear cell change is usually focal and lacks cytological atypia.

7.3 NEEDLE BIOPSY FINDINGS

7.3.1 The biopsy report

In a landmark report in 1994, Henson and colleagues from the Cancer Committee of the College of American Pathologists (CAP) described the essential features that should be included in prostate specimens, including needle biopsies, TURP specimens and prostatectomies (Table 7.2) (Henson, Hutter and Farrow, 1994). This important statement was based on consensus, editing by legal counsel and extensive field-testing by a large random sample of practicing pathologists in the CAP.

We have incorporated almost all of the CAP recommendations into our abbreviation system for prostate specimen interpretation (Table 7.3).

These abbreviations are used to shorten pathologists' transcription time, accelerate secretarial transcription time, reduce typographic errors through computerization, create uniform nomenclature and style for the benefit of clinicians and pathology quality assurance and standardize the approach to common prostate biopsy problems. The disadvantages of this abbreviation system are the potential for misinterpretation and erroneous reporting of the abbreviations, as well as simplification of histopathological findings by 'forcing' all cases into the abbreviation template. Some critics claim that such systems are more work than they are worth, but we find it useful. It should be noted that the abbreviations are meant only as a guide, recognizing that some cases will not fit any category; there is a temptation to use the system for cases in which it may not apply, because of its ease of use, but this should be avoided.

Table 7.2 Protocol for examination of biopsy specimens*

Patient identification
- Name
- Age
- Race
- Identification number

Clinical history (appropriate clinical information should be provided to the pathologist for optimal pathological evaluation)
- Previous diagnosis
- Treatment
- Clinical stage (digital rectal examination findings)
- Serum PSA concentration
- Imaging study findings (TRUS)

Type of operation
Gross examination
- Specimen fresh or in fixative
- Size, number of pieces and orientation*
- Recognizable gross features
- Amount submitted for histological processing (total or partial)

Microscopic features/diagnosis
- Tumor (versus no tumor)
  - Histological type (not determinable or as appropriate; include mixtures)
  - Gleason grade (score)
  - Extent of tumor (amount of specimen involved)
  - Perineural invasion (we exclude this because of recent data – Egan *et al.*, 1997)
  - Extraprostatic extension
- Other lesions
  - High-grade PIN
  - Therapy-associated changes
- Special studies
  - Immunohistochemistry
  - DNA ploidy analysis (flow cytometry; digital image analysis)
  - Other (histochemistry, morphometry)

Based on the Practice Protocol of the Cancer Committee of the College of American Pathologists (Henson, Hutter and Farrow, 1994), with modifications suggested at the International Consultation on Prostatic Intraepithelial Neoplasia and Pathological Staging of Prostate Cancer (*Cancer*, 1996, **78**, 366–368).

  * Amount in TURP specimens is at least 12 g (about six cassettes for the first 30 g and one cassette for every 10 g thereafter.

7.3.2 Volume of adenocarcinoma in needle biopsy

Can the amount of cancer in the needle biopsy predict the volume of tumor in the prostate? Stamey *et al.* developed algorithms to maximize accuracy of preoperative volume estimates by combining serum PSA concentration with ultrasonographic assessment of prostatic volume as measured by 2 mm axial step sections, biopsy Gleason grade and amount of adenocarcinoma in sextant biopsies; they found an excellent correlation ($r = 0.76$) for organ-confined adenocarcinoma and noted that digital rectal examination added no additional information to the multiple regression analysis (Stamey *et al.*, 1993). Conversely, we studied 162 patients with prostatic adenocarcinoma treated at Mayo Clinic and compared the tumor burden on needle biopsy

127

Table 7.3   Mayo Clinic prostate biopsy abbreviations

Tissue sites/normal

P	Prostate
SV	Seminal vesicle
EJ	Ejaculatory ducts
SK	Skeletal muscle
BPT	Benign prostatic tissue
FO	Fragments of
NEON	No evidence of neoplasm

Inflammation

CINF1 CINF2, CINF3
   (Mild, moderate, severe) chronic inflammation
AINF1, AINF2, AINF3
   (Mild, moderate, severe) acute inflammation
GRAN1, GRAN2, GRAN3
   (Mild, moderate, severe) granulomatous inflammation

Atrophy and hyperplasia

A1, A2, A3	(Mild, moderate, severe) atrophy
AAH	Atypical adenomatous hyperplasia
BCH	Basal cell hyperplasia
ABCH	Atypical basal cell hyperplasia
BPH	Nodular hyperplasia
PAH	Postatrophic hyperplasia

Prostatic intraepithelial neoplasia

HGPIN   High-grade prostatic intraepithelial neolasia is present

Atypical small acinar proliferations

ASAPB	Atypical small acinar proliferation, favor benign; malignancy cannot be definitively excluded
ASAPS	Atypical small acinar proliferation suspicious for but not diagnostic of malignancy
ASAPH	Atypical small acinar proliferation highly suspicious for but not diagnostic of malignancy
R	Repeat biopsy may be of value if clinically indicated (This code is rarely used)

Carcinoma

CA	Adenocarcinoma
CAG	Adenocarcinoma (Gleason #) involving #% of the specimen

Needle biopsy examples

BPT. A1. AINF1. Benign prostatic tissue. Mild atrophy. Mild acute inflammation
CA G 3 + 4, 20% Adenocarcinoma (Gleason 3 + 4 = 7) involving about 20% of the specimen.
ASAPS. HGPIN. CINF1. Atypical small acinar proliferation suspicious for but not diagnostic of malignancy. High-grade prostatic intraepithelial neoplasia. Mild chronic inflammation.

TURP examples

BPH. AAH. Nodular hyperplasia with atypical adenomatous hyperplasia
CA G 2 + 2, < 5% BPH. Adenocarcinoma (Gleason 2 + 2 = 4) involving less than 5% of the specimen. Nodular hyperplasia

with that of matched, step-sectioned, whole-mount radical prostatectomies (Figure 7.18).

Linear regression analysis revealed a weak correlation of the amount of tumor in the needle biopsy and radical prostatectomy specimens ($r = 0.39$) (Cupp *et al.*, 1995). Low tumor burden on needle biopsy did not appear predictive of low volume prostatic adenocarcinoma, whether measured as percentage of biopsy cores involved, percentage of adenocarcinoma area in biopsy cores, millimetres of adenocarcinoma in the entire biopsy, or millimetres of adenocarcinoma per core. Patients with less than 30% of cores involved had a mean volume of 6.06 ml (range 0.19–16.8 ml), indicating that the amount of tumor on transrectal needle biopsy was not a good predictor of tumor volume for the individual

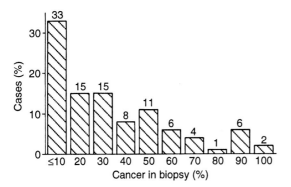

Figure 7.18 Distribution of cancer in 316 biopsies. Note that 33% of cases had a small amount of tumor (10% or less of specimen). (Source: redrawn from Bostwick, 1994.)

patient and should not influence therapeutic decisions. This study was limited by the variability in needle biopsy sampling, with the number of cores ranging from four to 10 (mean 5.7 cores) (Cupp *et al.*, 1995). The combined results from these studies indicate that biopsy extent of tumor provides some predictive value for extent in radical prostatectomy specimens and should be reported.

Some investigators claim that there is a strong correlation between tumor burden in sextant core biopsies and lymph node metastases (Hammerer, Huland and Sparenberg, 1992; Terris, McNeal and Stamey, 1992; Stamey *et al.*, 1993). Hammerer *et al.* found lymph node metastases in 52 of 57 patients (91% specificity) and 10 of 14 patients (71% sensitivity) when adenocarcinoma replaced two core biopsies and 80% of a third from the sextant sample (Hammerer *et al.*, 1992). They noted that the addition of grade to tumor volume improved the sensitivity and specificity.

7.4 PROSTATE-SPECIFIC ANTIGEN (PSA) AND EARLY DETECTION OF CANCER

PSA is the most important, accurate and clinically useful biochemical marker in the prostate. It is manufactured by the secretory epithelial cells and empties into the ductal system, where it catalyzes the liquefaction of the seminal coagulum after ejaculation. Serum levels are normally below about 4.0 ng/ml (monoclonal), but vary according to patient age and race; any process that disrupts the normal architecture of the prostate allows diffusion of PSA into the stroma and microvasculature. Elevated serum PSA concentration is seen with prostatitis, infarcts, hyperplasia and transiently following biopsy, but the most clinically important elevations are seen with prostatic adenocarcinoma. Cancer produces less PSA per cell than benign epithelium, but the greater number and density of malignant cells and the stromal disruption associated with cancer account for the elevated serum PSA concentration. Serum PSA concentration correlates positively with clinical stage, tumor volume, histological grade and the presence of extraprostatic extension and seminal vesicle invasion; despite these strong correlations, its value is limited in predicting stage for an individual patient. It may also predict the presence of lymph node metastases, bone metastases and survival after androgen deprivation therapy. PSA has contributed to an increase in the early detection rate of cancer and is now advocated for annual routine use in men over age 40 years who are at increased risk and all men over 50 years. It is a test with high sensitivity and specificity that is rapid, inexpensive, minimally invasive and acceptable to patients.

In addition to serum PSA concentration, other derivatives of serum PSA have recently been described that may increase the predictive value by accounting for confounding variables such as patient age, prostate volume and cancer volume: age-specific reference ranges, PSA density, PSA velocity, PSA cancer density and PSA doubling times. Serum PSA detects a heterogeneous group of cancers (clinical stage T1c) that are clinically important and potentially curable. The immunohistochemical expression of PSA in tissue sections allows determination of prostatic origin of some metastatic adenocarcinomas, although extraprostatic expression of PSA has been reported in a number of tissues and tumors, including periurethral gland adenocarcinoma in women, rectal carcinoid and extramammary Paget's disease. In the future, serum PSA assays will be standardized, with development of primary PSA reference material and quality control preparations that will focus on the ratio of alpha$_1$-antichymotrypsin-bound PSA to free PSA.

The major form of measurable PSA in the serum is a complex between the PSA molecule and alpha$_1$-antichymotrypsin (Lilja, 1993). PSA may also be complexed with alpha$_2$-macroglobulin and other acute phase proteins, or may exist in a free uncomplexed form that is enzymatically inactive. There is a higher proportion of complexed PSA in the serum of patients with cancer than in other patients, and this serum fractionation may be diagnostically useful (Lilja, 1993). New microassays for serum PSA allow detectability as low as 0.1 ng/ml (Vessella and Lange, 1993). The half-life of PSA in serum is 2–3 days (Stamey et al., 1987).

PSA is an important tool in the detection and management of prostate cancer. Elevation of PSA correlates with tumor recurrence and progression after surgery, radiation therapy and androgen ablation therapy (Ercole et al., 1987; Lange et al., 1989; Stamey et al., 1989; Dundas, Porter and Venner, 1990; Babaian and Camps, 1991). Persistent elevation of PSA is associated with persistent carcinoma (Dundas, Porter and Venner, 1990). Because PSA is a sensitive marker for tumor recurrence after treatment, it is useful for the early detection of metastases (Stamey et al., 1990).

Serum PSA concentration is of proven value in detecting many cases of early prostate cancer. Catalona et al. identified cancer in 2.2% of a large series of men with PSA level greater than 4.0 ng/ml (Catalona et al., 1991). The positive predictive value for PSA between 4.1 and 10.0 ng/ml was 22.4–26.5% and for PSA above 10.0 ng/ml was 50–67% (Catalona et al., 1991, 1994; Brawer et al., 1994). A large multi-institutional study of 6630 men over 50 years of age revealed PSA greater than 4.0 ng/ml in 15%;

PSA was superior to digital rectal examination in detecting cancer (4.6% vs. 3.2% respectively) and the combination of these two tests was even better (5.8%) (Catalona et al., 1994).

7.4.1 PSA expression in carcinoma

Immunohistochemical staining for PSA is useful in identifying poorly differentiated prostate cancer in close proximity to the bladder and the rectum; it can also verify prostatic origin of metastatic carcinoma. The intensity of PSA immunoreactivity often varies from field to field within a tumor, and the correlation of staining intensity with tumor differentiation is inconsistent. PSA expression is generally greater in low-grade tumors than in high-grade tumors, but there is significant heterogeneity from cell to cell. Up to 1.6% of poorly differentiated cancers will be negative for both PSA and PAP (Ellis et al., 1984; Svanholm, 1986; Keillor and Aterman, 1987). The presence of PSA-immunoreactive tumor cells in poorly differentiated carcinoma suggests that these tumors retain subpopulations of cells with properties of normal secretory prostatic epithelial cells.

7.4.2 PSA expression: primary versus metastases

The histological appearance and biochemical assessment of metastatic prostatic adenocarcinoma do not always mirror the primary tumor. Metastases are frequently composed of only one of the patterns seen in the primary tumor, and are usually moderately or poorly differentiated (Kramer et al., 1981; Brawn et al., 1990). In a recent study, Bovenberg et al. evaluated the immunoreactivity of three monoclonal antibodies against different epitopes of the PSA molecule in metastatic prostate cancer, and found that the expression of PSA was similar but not identical to the primary tumor (Bovenberg et al., 1993). Similar results were obtained in another study of a variety of cytoplasmic markers in breast and gastric carcinoma, including cytokeratin, carcino-embryonic antigen, epithelial membrane antigen and human milk fat globule (Estaban and Battifora, 1990). Fidler suggested that prostatic adenocarcinoma, like other hetero-geneous tumors, is composed of populations of cells with differing immunological proper-ties and metastatic potential (Fidler, 1978). These findings show that, when cancer metas-tasizes, it often retains expression of antigenic-ity and cellular differentiation. The cascade theory of metastases predicts that generalized metastases do not usually occur directly from the primary tumor but from prior metastases, allowing for additional heterogeneity. The conservation of PSA expression in metastases has important implications for the use of radio-pharmaceuticals for *in vivo* imaging and treat-ment of cancer utilizing PSA.

7.5 CLINICAL AND PATHOLOGICAL STAGING OF CANCER

Current clinical and pathological staging of early prostatic adenocarcinoma separates patients into two groups: those with palpable tumors and those with non-palpable tumors (Figure 7.19) (Schröder *et al.*, 1992; Bostwick, Myers and Oesterling, 1994). This reliance on palpability of the tumor as determined by digital rectal examination is unique among organ staging systems, and is hampered by the low sensitivity, low specificity and low posi-tive predictive value of digital rectal examination (Friedman *et al.*, 1991).

Recent refinements in staging have led to the introduction of a new stage of non-palpable adenocarcinoma detected by elevated serum PSA concentration, referred to as stage T1c or B0; however, this new stage was introduced without supportive clinical evidence and recent studies show that it does not identify a distinct group of patients (Oesterling *et al.*, 1993; Epstein *et al.*, 1994; Scaletscky *et al.*, 1994).

Two principal clinical staging systems are currently in widespread use: the TNM system and the American system (modified Whit-more–Jewett) (Figure 7.19; Table 7.4) (Schröder

et al., 1992; Bostwick, Myers and Oesterling, 1994).

These two systems are similar, although the TNM system contains a greater number of sub-divisions for most stages. The 1992 revision of the TNM system is the international standard for prostatic adenocarcinoma staging (Schröder *et al.*, 1992; Bostwick, Myers and Oesterling, 1994). Efforts directed toward standardization of staging, including guidelines for pathologi-cal evaluation of specimens, will allow com-parison of results from different centers.

7.5.1 Extraprostatic extension

Cancer within adipose tissue is indicative of extraprostatic extension (EPE; capsular invasion; capsular penetration; capsular per-foration); this is a rare finding in biopsy speci-mens. Similarly, tumor within the muscular wall or in intimate contact with the epi-thelium of the seminal vesicles indicates extraprostatic extension, which should be documented in the biopsy report. Some biopsies target the seminal vesicles in an effort to document unequivocal extraprosta-tic extension, recognizing that this may alter treatment decisions.

7.5.2 Clinical understaging of transition zone adenocarcinoma with transurethral resection

Clinical understaging with transurethral resec-tion of the prostate is a recognized problem in prostatic adenocarcinoma. The sensitivity of transurethral resection in detecting stage T1 (A) carcinoma is only 28%, and up to 60% of patients with stage T1a (A1) tumors who undergo repeat transurethral resection have residual adenocarcinoma, with 26% of these being upstaged (Blute, Zincke and Farrow, 1986; Epstein *et al.*, 1986; Greene *et al.*, 1991a, b; Bostwick, Myers and Oesterling, 1994). Despite the limitation of examining trans-urethral resection specimens to stage some prostatic adenocarcinomas, this remains the

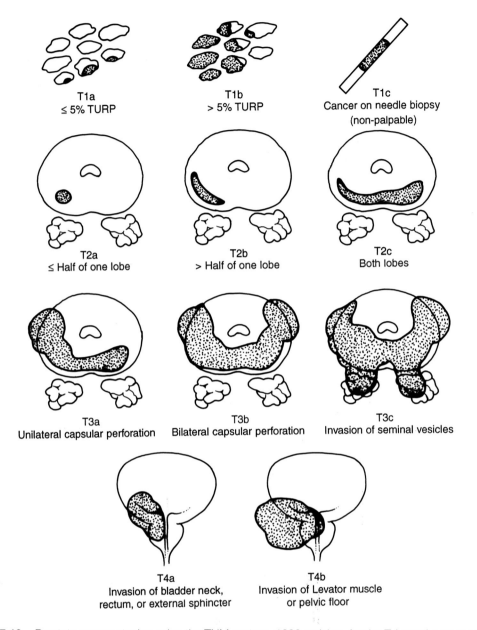

Figure 7.19 Prostate cancer staging using the TNM system, 1992 revision, for the T (tumor) category. Black indicates extent of cancer. (Source: redrawn from Bostwick and Eble, 1996.)

standard of care. Prostate cancer staging is unique among organ-staging systems in relying on the presence or absence of palpability and by substaging T2 (B) adenocarcinomas based upon the proportion of organ induration identified.

Clinical understaging was identified in 59% of cases and overstaging in 5% in a series of 311 serially sectioned radical retropubic prostatectomies removed for clinically localized prostatic adenocarcinoma (Bostwick, Myers and Oesterling, 1994). This substantial error rate

Table 7.4 Staging of prostatic adenocarcinoma

	American	*TNM†*
Non-palpable cancer		
≤ 5% of TURP tissue*	A1	T1a
> 5% of TURP tissue*	A2	T1b
Cancer detected by biopsy (e.g. elevated PSA)	B0	T1c
Palpable or visible cancer clinically confined within the capsule		
≤ Half of one lobe	B1	T2a
> Half of one lobe, but not both lobes	B1	T2b
Both lobes	B2	T2c
Cancer with local extracapsular extension		
Unilateral	C1	T3a
Bilateral	C1	T3b
Seminal vesicle invasion	C2	T3c
Invasion of bladder neck, rectum, or external sphincter	C2	T4a
Invasion of levator muscle or pelvic wall	C2	T4b
Metastatic cancer		
Single regional lymph, ≤ 2 cm in greatest dimension	D1	N1‡
Single regional lymph node, 2–5 cm, or multiple regional lymph nodes ≤ 5 cm	D1	N2
Single regional lymph node, > 5 cm	D1	N3
Distant metastasis	D2	M1
Non-regional lymph node(s)	D2	M1a
Bone(s)	D2	M1b
Other sites	D2	M1c

* Different definitions exist for substaging A1 and A2 cancers

† N_o or $N_x M_o$ for T1–T4

‡ N_x–regional lymph nodes are not assessable; M_x–distant metastasis is not assessable.

STAGE GROUPINGS FOR TNM STAGING SYSTEMS (G = grade on 1–4 scale)

Stage 0	T1a	N0	M0	G1
Stage I	T1a	N0	M0	G2,3,4
	T1b	N0	M0	Any G
	T1c	N0	M0	Any G
	T1	N0	M0	Any G
Stage II	T2	N0	M0	Any G
Stage III	T3	N0	M0	Any G
Stage IV	T4	N0	M0	Any G
	Any T	N1,2,3	M0	Any G
	Any T	Any M	M1	Any G

must be accounted for when evaluating recurrence and survival rates, especially when comparing studies of clinically staged patients followed with active surveillance (watchful waiting) and surgically (pathologically) staged patients.

Imaging studies to assess tumor volume and extent would be valuable in clinical staging. However, the current accuracy of such methods limits the utility of these methods. The accuracy of correctly identifying extra-prostatic extension is 63% with TRUS (Rifkin *et*

133

al., 1990), 71% with body coil magnetic resonance imaging (MRI) (Rifkin *et al.*, 1990), and 83% with endorectal and surface coil MRI (Ramchandani and Schnall, 1993).

7.5.3 Pathological staging of stage T1 (A) adenocarcinoma

Staging of adenocarcinoma in transurethral resection specimens is not standardized and numerous methods have been developed to objectively measure tumor volume and define substages T1a (A1) and T1b (A2) (Bostwick and Choi, 1992). The pathologist's 'eyeball' estimate of tumor volume correlates well with morphometrically determined measures and the predictive ability is similar to that of other methods of tumor quantitation (Cantrell *et al.*, 1981; Foucar *et al.*, 1990). Also, percentage tumor was slightly more predictive of tumor progression than absolute tumor volume for both stage A and stage B tumors (Partin *et al.*, 1989; Christenson *et al.*, 1990). Some methods employ additional factors such as tumor grade in an effort to stratify patients more precisely, but this 'blending of stage and grade seems somewhat incongruous', according to one report (Weems and Morris, 1992). Nevertheless, the distinction between the two substages of stage T1 (A) is critically important in clinical practice, particularly in patients who are considering watchful waiting as an option.

7.5.4 PSA-detected prostate cancer: stage T1c

Prior to widespread clinical use of PSA, most organ-confined cancers were identified by digital rectal examination (clinical stage T2 or higher) or at the time of transurethral resection (clinical stage T1). We observed more than a sevenfold increase in PSA-detected cancers at our institution in the 3-year period from 1988–1991 (14 versus 118 cases) (Oesterling *et al.*, 1993). These cancers are designated clinical stage T1c in the 1992 revision of the TNM classification (Schröder *et al.*, 1992).

There is no equivalent pathological stage for clinical stage T1c, and such tumors are invariably upstaged at surgery, usually to pathological stage T2 or T3. Oesterling *et al.* undertook a retrospective case–control study of 208 patients undergoing radical prostatectomy for clinical stage T1c cancer and 208 matched cases of clinical stage T2a + b cancer in order to define the characteristics of PSA-detected cancers (Oesterling *et al.*, 1993). These two groups of tumors had similar maximum tumor diameter, frequency of multifocality, tumor grade, DNA content, pathological stage and tumor location; however, T1c cancer had higher serum PSA, greater tumor volume, higher frequency of positive surgical margins and greater prostate size. These findings indicate that PSA detects a heterogeneous group of cancers that are clinically important and potentially curable. Other studies have confirmed these results (Epstein *et al.*, 1994).

7.6 TUMOR TRACK SEEDING

Traditional transperineal 14-gauge needle biopsy is more likely to cause cancer tracking through the capsule than contemporary transrectal 18-gauge biopsy. The external diameter of the 14-gauge needle is 2.08 mm, compared with 1.27 mm for the 18-gauge needle; since the volume of a cylinder is πr^2 times length, the 14-gauge needle makes a wound 2.7 times as large as that made by the 18-gauge needle. Previous reports have described tracking, seeding and implantation, with palpable perineal tumor nodules resulting from transperineal 14-gauge biopsy in 0.29% (Ryan and Peeling, 1990) to 1.0% (Moul *et al.*, 1989; Haddad, 1990) of malignant biopsies and 0.09% of all transperineal biopsies (Ryan and Peeling, 1990). Risk factors for tumor tracking and perineal implantation include large volume of tumor within the prostate and high tumor grade; however, exceptions are noted, including tracking in two cases of well-differentiated adenocarcinoma and one case of leiomyosarcoma (Blackard, Soucheray and Gleason, 1971; Greenstein *et al.*, 1989; Moul *et al.*, 1989; Zablow, 1989; Baech, Gote and Raahave, 1990; Haddad, 1990; Ryan and Peeling, 1990; Bastacky, Walsh and Epstein, 1991; Blight, 1992). Perineal implantation occurs from 1 month to 7 years after biopsy, but usually within 1 year. Perineal seeding and implantation carries a poor prognosis despite the use of adjuvant radiation therapy or androgen deprivation therapy (Ryan and Peeling, 1990). Interestingly, rare implantation tumor nodules have been identified after transrectal biopsy of benign tissue, presumably due to tumor seeding that was not identified in the biopsy specimen (Blight, 1992).

The biopsy technique appears to be a critical factor for tracking and seeding, with increased risk following complete removal of the needle sheath and obturator with each pass rather than removal of only the obturator (Ryan and Peeling, 1990). In one study, there was microscopic cancer tracking in seven needle biopsies (2% of cases) based on examination of 350 prostatectomies with palpable organ-confined carcinoma, but none was associated with local tumor recurrence at the site of tracking; four of seven cases were from patients undergoing transrectal needle biopsy (Bastacky, Walsh and Epstein, 1991). These authors noted that tumor tracking consisted of malignant acini embedded in dense fibrous tissue with hemosiderin deposition and extension away from the biopsy site. Conversely, no cases of tumor tracking were found in a contemporary series of 311 totally embedded radical prostatectomies with cancer following transrectal 18-gauge biopsy, suggesting that transrectal biopsy is associated with no risk of local cancer seeding and implantation (Bostwick, Vonk and Picado, 1994). Thus, the risk for cancer seeding with the thin needle is much lower than that reported historically with transperineal large needle biopsy. Based on these findings, we believe that sextant biopsies for detection of small volume cancers amenable to watchful waiting pose little or no risk of tumor seeding.

REFERENCES

Babaian, R. J. and Camps, J. L. (1991) The role of prostate-specific antigen as part of the diagnostic triad and as a guide when to perform a biopsy. *Cancer*, **68**, 2060–2063.

Baech, J., Gote, H. and Raahave, D. (1990) Perineal seeding of prostatic carcinoma after Trucut biopsy. *Urol. Int.*, **45**, 370–371.

Bahnson, R. R., Dresner, S. M., Gooding, W. and Becich, M. J. (1989) Incidence and prognostic significance of lymphatic and vascular invasion in radical prostatectomy specimens. *Prostate*, **15**, 149–155.

Bastacky, S. S., Walsh, P. C. and Epstein, J. I. (1991) Needle biopsy associated tumor tracking of adenocarcinoma of the prostate. *J. Urol.*, **145**, 1003–1007.

Bastacky, S. I., Walsh, P. C. and Epstein, J. I. (1993) Relationship between perineural tumor invasion on needle biopsy and radical prostatectomy capsular penetration in clinical stage B adenocarcinoma of the prostate. *Am. J. Surg. Pathol.*, **17**, 336–341.

Blackard, C. E., Soucheray, J. A. and Gleason, D. F. (1971) Prostatic needle biopsy with perineal extension of adenocarcinoma. *J. Urol.*, **106**, 401–403.

Blight, E. M. Jr (1992) Seeding of prostate adenocarcinoma following transrectal needle biopsy. *Urology*, **39**, 297–298.

Blute, M. L., Zincke, H. and Farrow, G. M. (1986) Long-term followup of young patients with Stage A adenocarcinoma of the prostate. *J. Urol.*, **136**, 840–843.

Böcking, A., Kiehn, J. and Heinzel-Wach, M. (1982) Combined histologic grading of prostatic carcinoma. *Cancer*, **50**, 288–294.

Bostwick, D. G. and Choi, C. (1992) Prognostic factors in early prostate cancer. *Urol. Annu.*, **6**, 63–101.

Bostwick, D. G., Cupp, M. R. and Oesterling, J. E. (1993) Tumor volume in prostate cancer: Correlation of needle biopsy and radical prostatectomy findings. *Mod. Pathol.*, **6**, 57A.

Bostwick, D. G. and Eble, J. N. (1996) *Urologic Surgical Pathology*, Mosby-Yearbook, St Louis, MO.

Bostwick, D. G., Myers, R. P. and Oesterling, J. E. (1994) Staging of prostate cancer. *Sem. Surg. Oncol.*, **10**, 60–73.

Bostwick, D. G., Vonk, K. and Picado, A. (1994) Pathologic changes in the prostate following contemporary 18 gauge needle biopsy: no apparent risk of local cancer seeding. *J. Urol. Pathol.*, **2**, 203–211.

Bostwick, D. G., Cooner, W. H., Denis, L. *et al.* (1992) The association of benign prostatic hyperplasia and cancer of the prostate. *Cancer*, **70**, 291–301.

Bostwick, D. G., Wollan, P. and Adlakha, K. (1995) Collagenous micronodules in prostate cancer: a specific but infrequent diagnostic finding. *Arch. Pathol. Lab. Med.*, **119**, 444–447.

Bostwick, D. G., Srigley, J., Grignon, D. *et al.* (1993) Atypical adenomatous hyperplasia of the prostate: morphologic criteria for its distinction from well-differentiated carcinoma. *Hum. Pathol.*, **24**, 819–832.

Bostwick, D. G., Wheeler, T. M, Blute, M. *et al.* (1996) Optimized microvessel density analysis improves expression in prostate cancer and its metastases. *Urology*, **48**, 47–57.

Bovenberg, S. A., van der Zwet, C. J. J., van der Kwast, T. H. *et al.* (1993) Prostate-specific antigen expression in prostate cancer and its metastases. *J. Urol. Pathol.*, **1**, 55–62.

Brawer, M. K., Deering, R. E., Brown, M. *et al.* (1994) Predictors of pathologic stage in prostatic carcinoma. The role of neovascularity. *Cancer*, **73**, 678–687.

Brawn, P., Kuhl, D., Johnson, C. *et al.* (1990) Stage D1 prostate carcinoma: The histologic appearance of nodal metastases and its relationship to survival. *Cancer*, **65**, 538–543.

Brown, L. F., Yeo, K. T., Berse, B., *et al.* (1995) Vascular permeability factor (vascular endothelial growth factor) is strongly expressed in the normal male genital tract and is present in substantial quantities in semen. *J. Urol.*, **154**, 576–579.

Cantrell, B. B., DeKlerk, D. P., Eggleston, J. C. *et al.* (1981) Pathological factors that influence prognosis in stage A prostatic cancer: the influence of extent versus grade. *J. Urol.*, **125**, 516–519.

Catalona, W. J., Smith, D. S., Ratliff, T. L. *et al.* (1991) Measurement of prostate-specific antigen in serum as a screening test for prostate cancer. *N. Engl. J. Med.*, **324**, 1156–1161.

Catalona, W. J., Richie, J. P., Ahmann, F. R. *et al.* (1994) Comparison of digital rectal examination and serum prostate specific antigen in the early detection of prostate cancer: results of a multicenter clinical trial of 6630 men. *J. Urol.*, **151**, 1283–1290.

Christenson, W. N., Parfitt, A. W., Walsh, P. C. and Epstein, J. I. (1990) Pathologic findings in clinical stage A2 prostate cancer. Relation of tumor volume, grade, and relation to pathologic stage. *Cancer*, **65**, 1021–1027.

Cupp, M. R., Bostwick, D. G., Myers, R. P. *et al.* (1995) The volume of prostate cancer in the biopsy specimen cannot reliably predict the quantity of cancer in the radical prostatectomy specimen on an individual basis. *J. Urol.*, **153**, 1543–1548.

Del Rosario, A. D., Bui, H. X., Abdulla, M. and Ross, J. S. (1993) Sulfur-rich prostatic intraluminal crystalloids: a surgical pathologic and electron probe x-ray microanalytic study. *Hum. Pathol.*, **24**, 1159–1167.

Deschenes, J. and Weidner, N. (1990) Nucleolar organizer regions (NOR) in hyperplastic and neoplastic prostate disease. *Am. J. Surg. Pathol.*, **14**, 1148–1155.

Dundas, G. S., Porter, A. T. and Venner, P. M. (1990) Prostate-specific antigen. Monitoring the response of carcinoma of the prostate to radiotherapy with a new tumor marker. *Cancer*, **66**, 45–48.

Egan, M., Pacelli, A. and Bostwick, D. G. (1997) Atrophic pattern of prostatic carcinoma. Submitted.

Egan, M., Wollan, P., Bostwick, D. G. (1997) Perineural invasion by prostate cancer is not an independent predictive factor of stage. In preparation.

Ellis, D. W., Leffers, S., Davies, J. S. *et al.* (1984) Multiple immunoperoxidase markers in benign hyperplasia and adenocarcinoma of the prostate. *Am. J. Clin. Pathol.*, **81**, 279–283.

Epstein, J. I. and Fynheer, J. (1992) Acid mucin in the prostate: can it differentiate adenosis from adenocarcinoma? *Hum. Pathol.*, **23**, 1321–1325.

Epstein, J. I., Paull, G., Eggleston, J. C. and Walsh, P. C. (1986) Prognosis of untreated stage A1 prostatic carcinoma: a study of 94 cases with extended followup. *J. Urol.*, **136**, 837–839.

Epstein, J. I., Walsh, P. C., Carmichael, M. and Brendler, C. B. (1994) Pathologic and clinical findings to predict tumor extent of nonpalpable (stage T1c) prostate cancer. *J. A. M. A.*, **271**, 368–374.

Ercole, C. J., Lange, P. H., Mathisen, M. *et al.* (1987) Prostatic specific antigen and prostatic acid phosphatase in the monitoring and staging of patients with prostatic cancer. *J. Urol.*, **138**, 1181–1184.

Estaban, J. M. and Battifora, H. (1990) Tumor immunophenotype: comparison between primary neoplasm and its metastases. *Mod. Pathol.*, **3**, 192–196.

Fidler, I. J. (1978) Tumor heterogeneity and the biology of cancer invasion and metastasis. *Cancer Res*, **38**, 2651–2657.

Folkman, J. (1992) The role of angiogenesis in tumor growth. *Semin. Cancer Biol.*, **3**, 65–71.

Foucar, E., Haake, G., Dalton, L. *et al.* (1990) The area of cancer in transurethral resection specimens as a prognostic indicator in carcinoma of the prostate: a computer-assisted morphometric study. *Hum. Pathol.*, **21**, 586–592.

Friedman, G. D., Hiatt, R. A., Quesenberry, C. P. and Selby, J. V. (1991) Case–control study of screening for prostate cancer by digital rectal examinations. *Lancet* **337**, 1526–1529.

Gleason, D. F. (1985) Atypical hyperplasia, benign hyperplasia, and well-differentiated adenocarcinoma of the prostate. *Am. J. Surg. Pathol.*, **9**, 53–67.

Goldstein, N., Qian, J. and Bostwick, D. G. (1995a) Mucin expression in atypical adenomatous hyperplasia of the prostate. *Hum. Pathol.*, **26**, 887–891.

Greene, D. R., Wheeler, T. M., Egawa, S. *et al.* (1991a) Relationship between clinical stage and histological zone of origin in early prostate cancer: morphometric analysis. *Br. J. Urol.*, **68**, 499–509.

Greene, D. R., Egawa, S., Neerhut, G. *et al.* (1991b) The distribution of residual cancer in radical prostatectomy specimens in stage A prostate cancer. *J. Urol.*, **145**, 324–329.

Greenstein, A., Merimsky, E., Baratz, M. and Braf, Z. (1989) Late appearance of perineal implantation of prostatic carcinoma after perineal needle biopsy. *Urology*, **33**, 59–60.

Haddad, F. S. R. E. (1990) Risk factors for perineal seeding of prostate cancer after needle biopsy. *J. Urol.*, **143**, 587–588.

Hall, M. C., Troncoso, P., Pollack, A. *et al.* (1994) Significance of tumor angiogenesis in clinically localized prostate carcinoma treated with external beam radiotherapy. *Urology*, **44**, 869–875.

Hammerer, P., Huland, H. and Sparenberg, S. (1992) Digital rectal examination, imaging, and systematic-sextant biopsy in identifying operable lymph node-negative prostatic carcinoma. *Eur. Urol.*, **22**, 281–287.

Hasson, M. O. and Maksem, J. (1980) The prostatic perineural space and its relation to tumor spread. An ultrastructural study. *Am. J. Surg. Pathol.*, **4**, 143–148.

Helpap, B. (1988) Observations on the number, size and location of nucleoli in hyperplastic and neoplastic prostatic disease. *Histopathology*, **13**, 203–211.

Henson, D. E., Hutter, R. V. P. and Farrow, G. M. (1994) Practice protocol for the examination of specimens removed from patients with carcinoma of the prostate gland. A publication of the Cancer Committee, College of American Pathologists. *Arch. Pathol. Lab. Med.*, **118**, 779–783.

Holmes, E. J. (1977) Crystalloids of prostatic carcinoma: relationship to Bence–Jones crystals. *Cancer*, **39**, 2073–2080.

Humphrey, P. A. (1991) Mucin in severe dysplasia in the prostate. *Surg. Pathol.*, **4**, 137–143.

Keillor, J. S. and Aterman, K. (1987) The response of poorly differentiated prostatic tumors to staining for prostate specific antigen and prostatic acid phosphatase: a comparative study. *J. Urol.*, **137**, 894–898.

Keleman, P. R., Buschmann, R. J. and Weisz-Carrington, P. (1990) Nucleolar prominence as a diagnostic variable in prostatic carcinoma. *Cancer*, **65**, 1017–1020.

Kramer, S. A., Farnham, R. J., Glenn, J. F. *et al.* (1981) Comparative morphology of primary and secondary deposits of prostatic adenocarcinoma. *Cancer*, **48**, 271–273.

Lange, P. H., Ercole, C. J., Lightner, D. J. *et al.* (1989) The value of serum PSA determinations before and after radical prostatectomy. *J. Urol.*, **141**, 873–879.

Layfield, L. J. and Goldstein, N. S. (1991) Morphometric analysis of borderline atypia in prostatic aspiration biopsy specimen. *Anal. Quant. Cytol. Histol.*, **13**, 288–292.

Lilja, H. (1993) Significance of different molecular forms of serum PSA: the free, noncomplexed form of PSA versus that complexed to alpha-1-antichymotrypsin. *Urol. Clin. North Am.*, **20**, 681–686.

McIntire, T. L. and Franzina, D. A. (1986) The presence of benign prostate glands in perineural spaces. *J. Urol.*, **135**, 507–509.

McNeal, J. E., Redwine, E. A., Freiha, F. S. and Stamey, T. A. (1988) Zonal distribution of prostatic adenocarcinoma. Correlation with histologic pattern and direction of spread. *Am. J. Surg. Pathol.*, **12**, 897–906.

McNeal, J. E., Alroy, J., Villers, A. *et al.* (1991) Mucinous differentiation in prostatic adenocarcinoma. *Hum. Pathol.*, **22**, 979–988.

Molberg, K. H., Mikhail, A. and Vuitch, F. (1994) Crystalloids in metastatic prostatic adenocarcinoma. *Am. J. Clin. Pathol.*, **101**, 266–268.

Montironi, R., Braccischi, A., Matera, G. *et al.* (1991) Quantitation of the prostatic intra-epithelial neoplasia. Analysis of the nucleolar size, number and location. *Pathol. Res. Pract.*, **187**, 307–314.

Montironi, R., Magi Galluzzi, C. M., Damanti, L. *et al.* (1993) Qualitative and quantitative analyses of the blood capillary architecture on thin tissue sections. *Path. Res. Pract.*, **189**, 542–548.

Morra, M. N. and Das, S. (1993) Prostate cancer. Epidemiology and etiology, in *Cancer of the Prostate*, (eds S. Das and E. D. Crawford), Marcel Dekker, New York, pp. 1–12.

Moul, J. W., Miles, B. J., Skoog, S. J. and McLeod, D. G. (1989) Risk factors for perineal seeding of prostate cancer after needle biopsy. *J. Urol.*, **142**, 86–88.

Myers, R. P., Neves, R. J., Farrow, G. M. and Utz, D. C. (1982) Nucleolar grading of prostatic adenocarcinoma: light microscopic correlation with disease progression. *Prostate*, **3**, 423–432.

Nomura, A. M. Y. and Kolonel, L. N. (1991) Prostate cancer: a current perspective. *Am. J. Epidemiol.*, **13**, 200–227.

Oesterling, J. E., Suman, V. J., Zincke, H. and Bostwick, D. G. (1993) PSA-detected (clinical stage T1c or B0) prostate cancer: pathologically significant tumors. *Urol. Clin. N. Am.*, **20**, 687–693.

Parker, S. L., Tong, T., Bolden, S. and Wingo, P. A. (1996) Cancer statistics, 1996. *CA Cancer J. Clin.*, **65**, 5–27.

Partin, A. W., Epstein, J. I. and Cho, R. (1989) Morphometric measurement of tumor volume and per cent of gland involvement as predictors of pathological stage in clinical stage B prostate cancer. *J. Urol.*, **141**, 341–346.

Ramchandani, P. and Schnall, M. D. (1993) Magnetic resonance imaging of the prostate. *Sem. Roentgenol.*, **28**, 74–82.

Rifkin, M. D., Zerhouni, E. A., Garsonis, C. A. *et al.* (1990) Comparison of magnetic resonance imaging and ultrasonography in staging early prostate cancer: results of a multi-institutional cooperative trial. *N. Engl. J. Med.*, **323**, 621–627.

Ro, J. Y., El-Naggar, A., Ayala, A. G. *et al.* (1988a) Signet-ring-cell carcinoma of the prostate: electron microscopic and immunohistochemical studies of eight cases. *Am. J. Surg. Pathol.*, **12**, 453–460.

Ro, J. Y., Grignon, D. J., Troncoso, P. and Ayala, A. G. (1988b) Mucin in prostatic adenocarcinoma. *Sem. Diag. Pathol.*, **5**, 273–283.

Ryan, P. G. and Peeling, W. B. (1990) Perineal prostatic tumour seedling after 'Tru-Cut' needle biopsy: case report and review of the literature. *Eur. Urol.*, **17**, 189–192.

Salamao, D., Graham, S. D. and Bostwick, D. G. (1995) Microvascular invasion in prostate cancer correlates with pathologic stage. *Arch. Pathol. Lab. Med.*, **119**, 1050–1054.

Scaletscky, R., Koch, M. O., Eckstein, C. W. *et al.* (1994) Tumor volume and stage in carcinoma of the prostate detected by elevations in prostate specific antigen. *J. Urol.*, **152**, 129–131.

Scardino, P. T. (1989) Early detection of prostate cancer. *Urol. Clin. North Am.*, **16**: 635–655.

Schröder, F. H., Hermanek, P., Denis, L. *et al.* (1992) The TNM classification of prostate carcinoma. *Prostate*, **4**, 129–138.

Seidman, H., Mushinski, M. H., Gelb, S. K. and Silverberg, E. (1985) Probabilities of eventually developing or dying of cancer – United States. *CA*, **35**, 36–56.

Siegal, J. A., Yu, E. and Brawer, M. K. (1995) Topography of neovascularity in human prostate carcinoma. *Cancer*, **75**, 2545–2551.

Sinha, A. A., Gleason, D. F., Staley, N. A. *et al.* (1995) Cathepsin B in angiogenesis of human prostate: An immunohistochemical and immunoelectron microscopic analysis. *Anat. Record*, **241**, 353–362.

Stamey, T. A., Yang, N., Hay, A. R. *et al.* (1987) Prostate-specific antigen as a serum marker for adenocarcinoma of the prostate. *N. Engl. J. Med.*, **317**, 909–916.

Stamey, T. A., Kabalin, J. N. K., McNeal, J. E. *et al.* (1989) Prostate-specific antigen in the diagnosis and treatment of adenocarcinoma of the prostate. II. Radical prostatectomy treated patients. *J. Urol.*, **141**, 1076–1083.

Stamey, T. A., Freiha, F. S., McNeal, J. E. *et al.* (1993) Localized prostate cancer. Relationship of tumor volume to clinical significance for treatment of prostate cancer. *Cancer*, **71**, 933–938.

Svanholm, H. (1986) Evaluation of commercial immunoperoxidase kits for prostate specific antigen and prostatic specific acid phosphatase. *Acta Pathol. Microbiol. Immunol. Scand. [A]*, **94**, 7–15.

Tannenbaum, M., Tannenbaum, S., DeSnactis, P. N. and Olsson, C. A. (1982) Prognostic significance of nucleolar surface area in prostate cancer. *Urology*, **19**, 546–551.

Terris, M. K., McNeal, J. E. and Stamey, T. A. (1992) Detection of clinically significant prostate cancer by transrectal ultrasound-guided systematic biopsies. *J. Urol.*, **148**, 829–832.

Tressera, F., Barastegui, C., Salas, A. and Ristol, J. (1994) Cristaloides intraluminales en el carcinoma de prostata: estudio morfologico e histoquimico. *Actas Urol. Esp.*, **18**, 749–754.

Vartanian, R. K. and Weidner, N. (1995) Endothelial cell proliferation in prostatic carcinoma and prostatic hyperplasia. Correlation with Gleason's score, microvessel density, and epithelial cell proliferation. *Lab. Invest.*, **73**, 844–850.

Vesalainen, S., Lipponen, P., Talja, M. *et al.* (1994) Tumor vascularity and basement membrane structure as prognostic factors in T1-2MO prostatic adenocarcinoma. *Anticancer Res.*, **14**, 709–714.

Vessella, R. L. and Lange, P. H. (1993) Issues in the assessment of PSA immunoassays. *Urol. Clin. North Am.*, **20**, 607–620.

Weems, W. L. and Morris, J. S. (1992) The limits of resectability of prostate cancer. *Urol. Annu.*, **6**, 129–146.

Weidner, N., Carroll, P. *et al.* (1993) Tumor angiogenesis correlates with metastasis in invasive prostate carcinoma. *Am. J. Pathol.*, **143**, 401–407.

Zablow, A. I. (1989) Implantation of prostatic cancer after perineal needle biopsy. *Urology*, **33**, 449.

8

GRADING

Histological grade is a powerful predictive factor in prostatic adenocarcinoma, and is valuable even in contemporary 18-gauge needle biopsies. More than 40 grading systems have been proposed since the pioneering work of Broders more than 70 years ago (Broders, 1926). All systems successfully identify well-differentiated adenocarcinoma that progresses slowly and poorly differentiated adenocarcinoma that progresses rapidly (Bostwick, 1994b). However, grading systems are less successful in subdividing the majority of moderately differentiated adenocarcinomas that have intermediate clinical behavior. Some of the popular grading systems are compared in Table 8.1 (Gleason, 1966; Mostofi, 1975; Böcking et al., 1982; Gleason, 1990, 1992).

Problems with grading include interobserver and intraobserver variability, imprecise predictive value and lack of a single universal system. In biopsies, these problems are compounded by small sample size, tumor heterogeneity and undergrading of biopsy samples. Also, significant histological changes in adenocarcinoma occur as a result of radiation and androgen deprivation therapy, which make grading difficult and of questionable value (Chapter 10). This chapter describes the current role of grading in prostatic adenocarcinoma, correlation of biopsy grade with prostatectomy grade and clinical significance of grade. Emphasis is placed on the Gleason grading system, the most commonly used system (Gardner et al., 1988) .

8.1 GLEASON GRADING SYSTEM

The Gleason grading system (Veterans Administration Cooperative Urological Research Group grading system; VACURG system) is based on prospective study of more than 4000 patients between 1960 and 1975, and is the *de facto* grading standard in the United States and other parts of the world (Gleason, 1966, 1990, 1992). Other systems in use internationally are the World Health Organization (Mostofi, 1975) and Böcking (Böcking, Kiehn and Heinzel-Wach, 1982) systems. These systems are clinically useful, showing a positive correlation with tumor volume, preoperative serum PSA concentration, the likelihood of pelvic lymph node metastases, and tumor recurrence after surgery and radiation therapy.

The Gleason system is based on the degree of architectural differentiation (Table 8.2).

Tumor heterogeneity is accounted for by assigning a primary pattern for the dominant grade and a secondary pattern for the non-dominant grade; the histological score is

Table 8.1 Grading systems for prostate adenocarcinoma: brief summaries

Gleason	Mostofi (WHO)	Broders, 1926	Böcking	Gaeta	Helpap
Pattern 1: Lobular cluster of closely packed single, separate, round, uniform glands	*Grade 1*: Well differentiated, with slight nuclear anaplasia	*Grade 1*: 75–100% of tumor composed of glands	*Grade 1*: Uniform glands with or without nuclear and nucleolar variation	*Grade 1*: Single, separate glands; small nuclei with inconspicuous nucleoli	*Grade 1a*: Well-differentiated glands
Pattern 2: Same as pattern 1, except for less uniformity of gland spacing and shape, and tumor margin not well defined	Grade 2: Moderately to poorly differentiated, with moderate nuclear anaplasia	*Grade 2*: 50–75% of tumor composed of glands	*Grade 2*: Cribriform, without nuclear anaplasia, or pleomorphic glands and small glands with variable nuclear and nucleolar size	*Grade 2*: Small or medium glands; pleomorphic nuclei with nucleolomegaly	*Grade 1b*: Moderately differentiated glands
Pattern 3: Single, separate, irregular glands, including cribriform and papillary patterns	*Grade 3*: Poorly differentiated, with marked nuclear anaplasia, or undifferentiated carcinoma	*Grade 3*: 25–50% of tumor composed of glands	*Grade 3*: Cribriform, with enlarged nuclei and nucleoli, or sheets of cells without glands and variable nuclear and nucleolar size	*Grade 3*: Small glands, including cribriform and scirrhous patterns; pleomorphic nuclei with nucleomegaly	*Grade 2a*: Poorly differentiated, with moderate nuclear and nucleolar atypia, or mixed pattern with minor component
Pattern 4: Coalescing and fused glands form cords, including solid and cribriform patterns; may have hypernephroid appearance (clear cells)		*Grade 4*: 0–25% of tumor composed of glands		*Grade 4*: Sheets of cells without glands; nuclei and nucleoli of any size; mitotic figures >3 per high power field	*Grade 2b*: Poorly differentiated, with marked nuclear atypia, or mixed pattern, with chiefly cribriform pattern
Pattern 5: Few or no glands; tumor in sheets or comedo pattern					Grade 3: Solid trabecular pattern with marked atypia, with or without cribriform pattern

Table 8.2 Gleason grading system for prostatic adenocarcinoma: histological patterns (*Source*: from Bostwick, 1994b, with permission).

Pattern	Peripheral borders	Infiltrative appearance	Appearance of glands	Size of glands	Architecture of glands	Cytoplasm
1	Circumscribed, pushing, expansile	Minimal	Simple, round, monotonously replicated	Medium, regular	Closely-packed rounded masses	Similar to benign epithelium
2	Less circumscribed; early infiltration	Mild, with definite separation of glands	Simple, round, some variability in shape	Medium, less regular	Loosely-packed rounded masses	Similar to benign epithelium
3A	Infiltration	Marked	Angular, with variation in shape	Medium to large	Variable packed irregular masses	More basophilic than patterns 1 and 2
3B	Infilteration	Marked	Angular, with variation in shape	Small	Variable packed irregular masses	More basophilic than patterns 1 and 2
3C	Smooth, rounded	Marked	Papillary and cribriform	Irregular	Round to elongate masses	More basophiic than patterns 1 and 2
4A	Ragged infiltration	Marked	Microacinary, papillary, and cribriform	Irregular	Fused, with chains and cords	Dark
4B	Ragged infiltration	Marked	Microacinar, papillary, and cribriform	Irregular	Fused, with chains and cords	Clear ("hypernephroid")
5A	Smooth, rounded	Marked	Comedocarcinoma	Irregular	Round to elongate masses	Variable
5B	Ragged infiltration	Marked	Difficult to identify gland lumens	Fused sheets and masses		Variable

derived by adding these two values together. Early studies described the addition of the clinical stage (1–4 scale) to create the Gleason 'sum', but this did not achieve widespread use (Gleason *et al.*, 1974). Some contemporary reports use the term sum for Gleason score (Greene *et al.*, 1994).

The success of Gleason grading is due to four factors. First, histological patterns are identified by the degree of acinar differentiation without relying on morphogenetic or histogenetic models. Second, a simplified and standardized drawing is available which has been popular among pathologists throughout the world (Figure 8.1).

Third, Gleason and coworkers provided abundant prospective information that allowed objective development of this self-defining grading system, which combined nine separate patterns into five grades. Finally, unlike any other grading system in the body, the Gleason system provided for tumor heterogeneity by identifying primary and secondary patterns.

Gleason noted that more than 50% of adenocarcinomas in his series contained two or more patterns (Gleason, 1992). Similarly, Aihara *et al.* recently found an average of 2.7 different Gleason grades per case (range 1–5) in a series of 101 totally embedded prostatectomies and more than 50% of adenocarcinomas contained at least three different grades (Aihara *et al.*, 1994). The number of grades increases with increasing cancer volume and the most common finding is high-grade adenocarcinoma within a larger well or moderately differentiated adenocarcinoma (53% of cases).

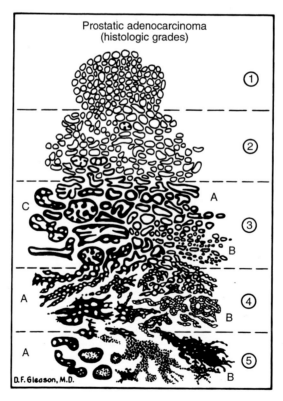

Figure 8.1 Standardized drawing for grading prostate cancer (Gleason grading system). See Table 8.2 for a description of the patterns.

8.2 GRADING NEEDLE BIOPSIES

The diagnostic features of the histological patterns of the Gleason grading system are presented in Table 8.2. Each pattern represents a blend of the growth pattern of the tumor and the amount of acinar differentiation. Recognition of these features in biopsies is frequently difficult due to small size and incomplete sampling. Grading of variants of adenocarcinoma such as mucinous carcinoma, signet-ring-cell carcinoma and small cell carcinoma are discussed in Chapter 9.

The primary grade is the most common or predominant grade. The secondary grade is the next most common, but should comprise at least 5% of the tumor. It is often hard to apply this rule when the amount of cancer in the specimen is small; in such cases, there may be no secondary pattern, and the primary grade is simply doubled. Most cancers are moderately differentiated, so biopsies usually contain Gleason pattern 3. We report cancer as 'Adenocarcinoma (Gleason $n + n = n$)' to avoid possible confusion of what constitutes grade and score. Some useful clues that we use for needle biopsies are shown in Table 8.3.

8.2.1 Gleason pattern 1 (grade 1)

Gleason pattern 1 adenocarcinoma is uncommon and difficult to diagnose, particularly in biopsies. It consists of a circumscribed mass of simple round acini that are uniform in size, shape, and spacing (Figure 8.2).

Circumscription is the single most important criterion to separate pattern 1 and pattern 2, but is usually difficult to identify in biopsies because most foci of cancer extend beyond the edge of the needle core. In such cases, it is best to consider the focus as pattern 2, recognizing that focal loss of the rounded circumscribed border disqualifies pattern 1.

The acini in pattern 1 are monotonously replicated, with round contours, evenly spaced acini, uniform round lumens and distinct cell membranes. Even spacing of the acini is an important but little-appreciated criterion for pattern 1 and pattern 2 cancer. The acini are usually separated from each other by a distance of less than one acinar diameter and may appear closely packed in some areas. Irregular spacing and separation of more than a few glands at the periphery suggests a higher grade.

The cells in Gleason pattern 1 tend to be rectangular, with pale or clear cytoplasm. Nuclear and nucleolar enlargement are moderate, but allow and often define separation from one of its closest mimics, atypical adenomatous hyperplasia (AAH). In small foci on needle biopsies, this distinction may be difficult, particularly when confounding factors such as crush artifact or drying artifact are present; however, AAH is rare in needle biopsies.

Acidic luminal mucin is usually scant and wispy in patterns 1 and 2 carcinoma. Crystalloids are observed in more than half of cases, more than in other patterns.

8.2.2 Gleason pattern 2 (grade 2)

Gleason pattern 2 is very similar to pattern 1 except for the lack of circumscription of the focus, indicating the ability of the cancer to spread through the stroma (Figure 8.3).

Slightly greater variation in acinar size and shape is observed, but the acinar contours are chiefly round and smoothly sculpted. Acinar packing is somewhat more variable than pattern 1, and separation is usually less than one acinar diameter. The cytological features of pattern 2 are indistinguishable from pattern 1.

8.2.3 Gleason pattern 3 (grade 3)

Pattern 3 is the most common pattern of prostatic adenocarcinoma, and encompasses a wide and diverse group of lesions (Figures 8.4 and 8.5).

This diversity is reflected in the three main variants: A, B and C. Pattern 3A, also referred to descriptively as the large gland variant of pattern 3, is easily distinguished from pattern

Table 8.3 Thirteen clues for Gleason grading in prostate needle biopsies – Gleason score (or sum) equals the sum of the primary and secondary Gleason grades (or patterns) (e.g. Gleason 3 + 4 = 7)

Clue no. 1: Small foci of cancer do not necessarily mean low-grade cancer
With the advent of serum PSA and sextant biopsy, small foci of carcinoma are frequently found in needle biopsies. However, these small foci are not low-grade simply because they are small. High-grade adenocarcinoma (Gleason pattern 4 and 5) often infiltrates as irregular ribbons or ragged masses immediately beneath the edge of the prostate, and a small portion may be sampled by biopsy, resulting in very few malignant acini in the specimen. In rare instances, the only evidence of carcinoma may be a few acini surrounding one or more small nerve twigs; this small focus is usually Gleason pattern 3 or 4 in our experience.

Clue no. 2: It probably isn't Gleason pattern 1
Gleason patterns 1 and 5 are the least common patterns in any prostate specimen, including radical prostatectomies and biopsies. Pattern 1 is usually present in the transition zone, an area infrequently sampled by needle biopsy. Further, these tumors are usually small. In a Mayo Clinic study of over 300 needle biopsies, only one had Gleason pattern 1 (secondary pattern 1; primary pattern 2).

Clue no. 3: To identify Gleason pattern 1, the cancer must be circumscribed
The most important difference between Gleason pattern 1 and 2 is the presence or absence of circumscription respectively. Contemporary needle biopsy rarely provides the entire focus of cancer for evaluation, precluding evaluation of the periphery for completeness of circumscription. Consequently, the default grade for partially sampled low-grade cancers with uniform spacing is pattern 2.

Clue no. 4: Gleason pattern 2 should satisfy the three 'R's': Round, Regularly spaced and Relatively uniform in size
Gleason pattern 2 cancer consists of predominately round acini without sharp angulation or distorted shape. Nearly as important as acinar roundness is spacing – pattern 2 acini have relatively uniform spacing throughout the focus, unlike pattern 3, with variable spacing.

Clue no. 5: Gleason pattern 2 acini may be close to one another but must have intervening stroma and no significant distortion of shape
If significant acinar crowding is present with some loss of intervening stroma between acini, it may be more accurately considered as pattern 3. Any significant distortion of adjacent malignant acini constitutes Gleason pattern 3.

Clue no. 6: It's probably Gleason pattern 3
The 'default' grade for prostatic adenocarcinoma is pattern 3, recognizing that the great majority of cancers fall in this pattern, which encompasses the center of the normal distribution curve. More than 80% of Gleason's original series was pattern 3. Don't be hesitant about assigning pattern 3 + 3 = 6 to a needle biopsy simply because the previous five cases with small foci of cancer were the same grade.

Clue no. 7: If there is a twofold or greater variation in acinar size, it's probably Gleason pattern 3 rather than pattern 2
When malignant acini are uniformly separated from one another, a twofold variation in acinar size distinguishes Gleason pattern 3 from pattern 2. Any variation in acinar size less than this may represent Gleason pattern 2 (exceptions to this exist; see Clue no. 8).

Clue no. 8: Despite relative uniformity of acinar size, significant acinar angulation or distortion indicates Gleason pattern 3 rather than pattern 2
Significant acinar angulation violates Clue no. 4 above, precluding pattern 2. Some areas of Gleason pattern 3 may have relatively uniform acinar size with or without crowding. This pattern often has acini that are smaller than pattern 2. The lack of acinar roundness in such cases separates pattern 3 from pattern 2.

Table 8.3 Continued

Clue no. 9: Fusion is fusion is fusion (Gleason pattern 4)
Acinar fusion separates most cases of Gleason pattern 4 and 3. This is a critical cut-point in grading prostate cancer, as pattern 4 indicates poorly differentiated cancer. Fortunately, this is one of the most reproducible cut-points, because of the requirement for acinar fusion in pattern 4. If a line can be drawn around individual acini, no mattern how tightly packed, then the acini are not fused and it is pattern 3 (see Clue no. 10).

Clue no. 10: If a line can be drawn between acini that have no intervening stroma (fusion) for a length of at least four times the width of the acinus, this constitutes Gleason pattern 4
Tangentially cut tubular and tortuous acini of Gleason 3 may mimic pattern 4, and such 'grade inflation' should be avoided. In difficult cases, if the length of 'fusion' of the acinus of concern is less than four times its width, we consider it pattern 3.

Clue no. 11: If it's cribriform and nearly solid, it's probably Gleason pattern 4
Cribriform acini are usually pattern 3 (with comedo necrosis, pattern 5). However, when the sieve-like openings lose their round, rigid, punched-out appearance and become collapsed and nearly solid, it is best considered pattern 4. Similarly, when the sieve-like masses lose their round contours, it often indicates transition to pattern 4.

Clue no. 12: The loss of most acinar lumens within fused acini indicates Gleason pattern 5
Most acinar lumens must be absent in order to separate Gleason pattern 5 from pattern 4. Tangential cutting and crush artifact may obscure or hide lumens. However, if most acini lack lumens, it constitutes pattern 5.

Clue no. 13: If in doubt, double the pattern to create the score.
With small foci of cancer, it is often best to simply double the Gleason pattern. We invariably do this when there is less than 5% of the needle biopsy involved with cancer unless there is an obvious secondary pattern (this almost never occurs).

3B, the small gland variant, and 3C, the cribriform variant. Mixtures of these patterns are frequently observed.

The hallmark of pattern 3 adenocarcinoma is prominent variation in size, shape and spacing of acini. We often use an arbitrary cut point of greater than twofold variation in acinar size to separate Gleason pattern 3 from pattern 2. Despite this variation, the acini remain discrete and separate, unlike the fused acini of pattern 4 (see below). Some acini of pattern 3 display apparent rigidity, with irregular, sharply angular contours and twisted, elongated forms that stand in contrast with the rounded contours of lower grades. Acinar spacing is often variable, usually more than one diameter apart; however, close packing may also be prominent without acinar fusion. Acini are haphazardly arranged in the stroma, some-times with prominent stromal fibrosis. The irregular size and spacing at the edges imparts a ragged appearance.

The large acinar pattern, 3A, differs from the small acinar pattern, 3B, by the average size of the acini (Figure 8.5). The cribriform pattern, 3C, is distinctive, consisting of aggregates of cells punctuated by fenestrations imparting a sieve-like appearance (Figure 8.5). Papillae may also be present. Ductal adenocarcinoma (endometrioid carcinoma) is included in this pattern (see Chapter 9).

Patterns 3B and 3C are progressively slightly more aggressive than 3A, but they often coexist and have similar cancer-specific death rates. Thus, separation of these subgrades is not necessary and could create additional problems with consistency of grading (Gleason, 1990).

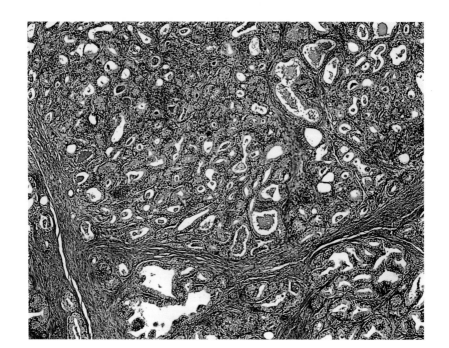

(a)

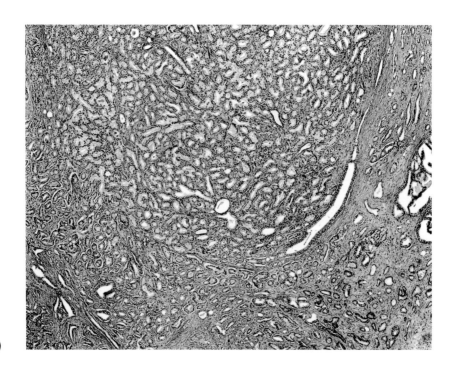

(b)

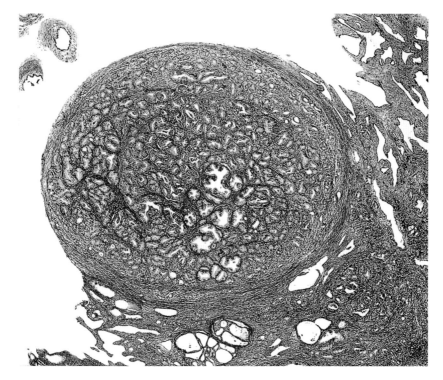

(c)

Figure 8.2 Gleason pattern 1 adenocarcinoma. **(a)** The proliferation is circumscribed without stromal infiltration; **(b)** Another case, consisting of a rounded nodule of adenocarcinoma (center) and surrounding pattern 2; **(c)** Transurethral resection contains a circumscribed round nodule of Gleason pattern 1 adenocarcinoma (center) and adjacent Gleason pattern 2 (bottom right).

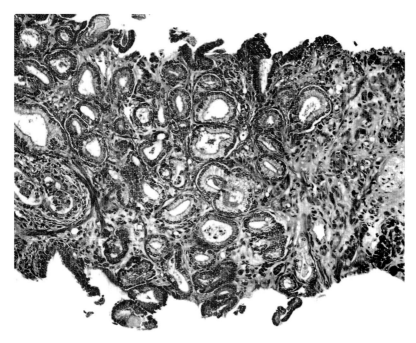

Figure 8.3 Gleason pattern 2 adenocarcinoma. Needle biopsy consists of a minute proliferation of relatively uniformly spaced medium size and large acini with nuclear and nucleolar features of malignancy.

149

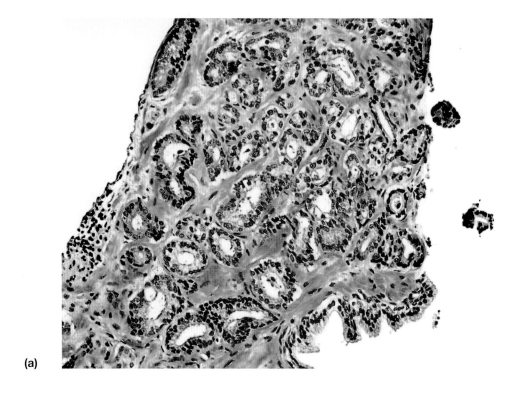

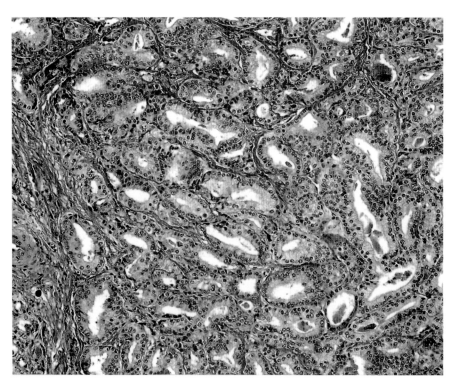

Figure 8.4 Gleason pattern 3 adenocarcinoma. **(a)** There is greater variation in size, shape, and spacing of acini than in pattern 2 carcinoma. **(b)** In this case, the acini are closely packed, but there is no significant fusion and each is distinct.

Table 8.4 Correlation of biopsy grade and prostatectomy grade

Author/year	No. of patients	Biopsy specimens	Grading system	Correlation of biopsy and prostatectomy grade (Gleason score) (%)				
				Exact	±1 unit	Needle higher	Needle lower	Other
14 Gauge Biopsies								
Kastendieck, 1980	120	Needle biopsies: 120	Glandular differentiation	63	–	–	–	
Catalona, Stein and Fair, 1982	66	Needle biopsies: 66	Well, moderately, poorly	59	–	8	33	*No correlation of grading error and clinical understaging
Lange and Narayan, 1983	72	Needle biopsies: 66 TURP: 6	Gleason score	74	–	14	39	*Grading error greatest with low-grade tumors
Garnett, Oyasu and Grayhack, 1984	115	Needle biopsies: 111 TURP: 4	Gleason score	30	72	32	38	*Grading error greatest with low-grade tumors
Mills and Fowler, 1986	53	Needle biopsies: 38 TURP: 15	Gleason score	51	74	4	45	*Grading error greatest with low-grade tumors and small amounts of tumor *No correlation of grading error and clinical understaging
18 Gauge Biopsies								
Spires et al., 1993	67	Needle biopsies: 67	Gleason score	58	94	–	–	*No correlation of grading error and clinical understaging
Bostwick, 1994c	316	Needle biopsies: 316	Gleason score	35	74	25	40	*Grading error greatest with low-grade tumors and small amounts of tumor *No correlation of grading error and clinical understaging
Humphrey et al., 1995	50	Needle biopsies: 50	Gleason score	26	86	26	48	

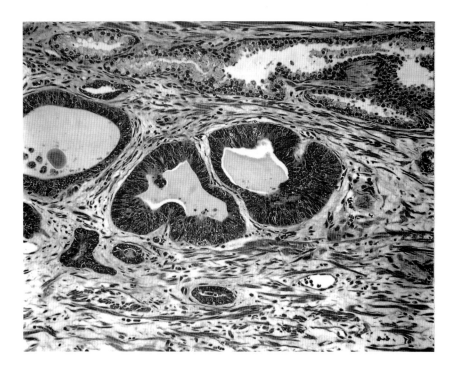

(a)

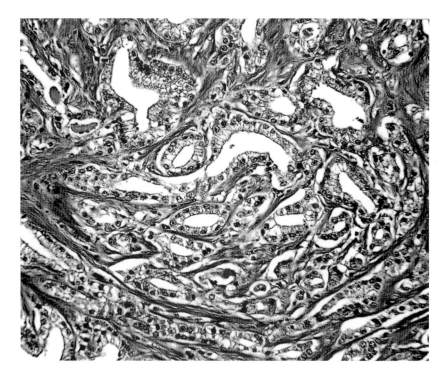

(b)

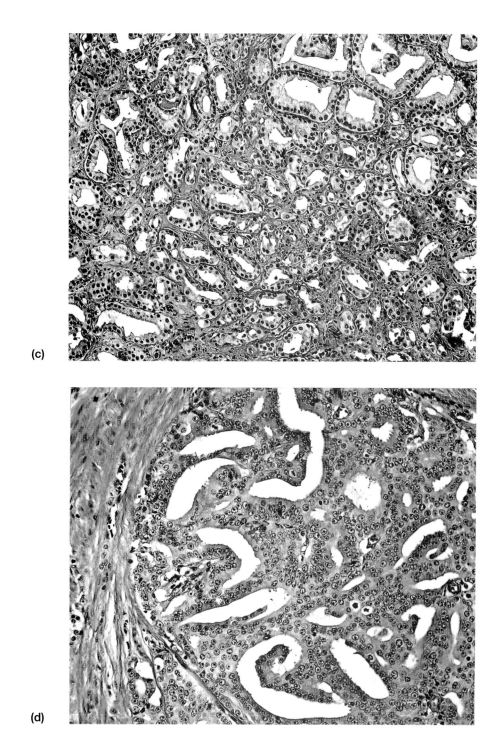

(c)

(d)

Figure 8.5 *Gleason pattern 3 adenocarcinoma.* **(a)** Large acinar pattern (Gleason 3A): these acini with dark cytoplasm mimick high-grade PIN, but lacked a basal cell layer and were part of a large carcinoma. **(b)** Another example of large acinar pattern, with closely packed malignant acini and pale cytoplasm. **(c)** Small acinar pattern (Gleason 3B); the acini show marked variation in size, shape and spacing but are not fused. **(d)** Cribriform pattern of Gleason pattern 3 (Gleason 3C); this focus was part of numerous cribriform structures in this needle core specimen. No basal cell layer was present at the periphery, effectively excluding cribriform PIN.

153

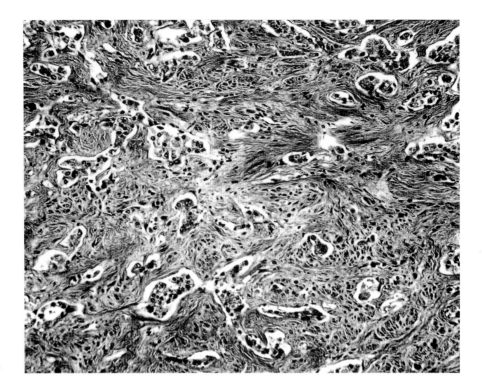

(a)

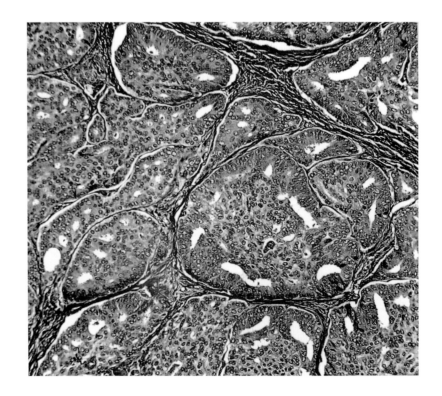

(b)

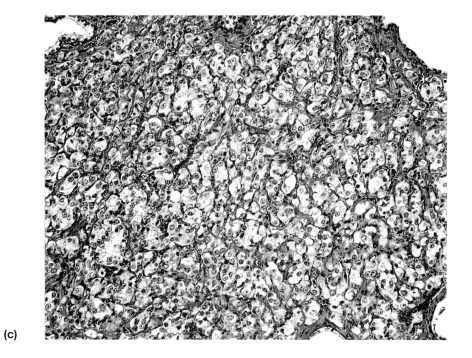

(c)

Figure 8.6 Gleason pattern 4 adenocarcinoma. **(a)** Ribbons and irregular nests and aggregates of malignant cells are embedded in dense fibrous (scirrhous) stroma; the nuclei are often shrunken and hyperchromatic, belying the high-grade architectural features (Gleason 4A). Compare with **(b)**, showing solid cribriform pattern (Gleason 4B). **(c)** Hypernephroid pattern of Gleason 4 contains abundant clear or pale cytoplasm.

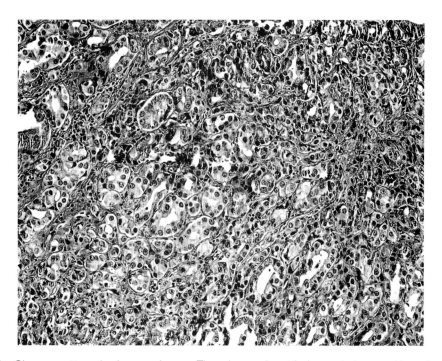

Figure 8.7 Gleason pattern 4 adenocarcinoma. There is prominent fusion and close packing of acini.

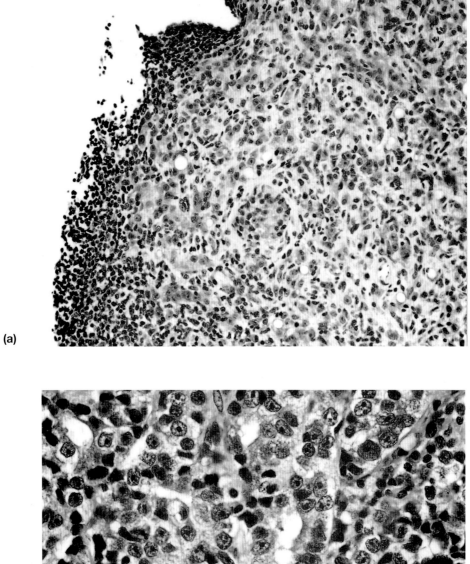

Figure 8.8 Gleason pattern 5 adenocarcinoma. **(a)** The tumor is growing in solid aggregates with only scattered gland lumina or vacuoles; the nuclei in this case were relatively uniform in size and shape at low magnification despite the high-grade architectural pattern. **(b)** At high magnification, cytological features of malignancy are identified, including nuclear and nucleolar enlargement.

8.2.4 Gleason pattern 4 (grade 4)

The characteristic finding of pattern 4 is fusion of acini, with ragged infiltrating cords and nests at the edges (Figures 8.6 and 8.7). Unlike the simple entwined acinar tubules of pattern 3, this pattern consists of an anastomosing network or spongework of epithelium.

The most common subtype, 4A, consists of cells with basophilic cytoplasm, unlike the clear or pale cytoplasm of 4B, the 'hypernephroid' pattern. Pattern 4 adenocarcinoma is considered poorly differentiated and is much more malignant than pattern 3.

8.2.5 Gleason pattern 5 (grade 5)

Pattern 5 adenocarcinoma is characterized by fused sheets and masses of haphazardly arranged acini in the stroma, often displacing or overrunning adjacent tissues (Figures 8.8 and 8.9).

In biopsy specimens, these cases raise the serious concern for anaplastic carcinoma or sarcoma. Cases with scattered acinar lumens indicative of glandular differentiation are included within this pattern. Comedocarcinoma is an important subtype of this pattern, consisting of luminal necrosis within an otherwise cribriform pattern; only a single acinus has to contain necrosis to apply this designation. Pattern 5 also includes rare histological variants such as signet-ring-cell carcinoma and small-cell undifferentiated carcinoma (Chapter 9).

8.2.6 Grading errors

Needle core biopsy underestimates tumor grade in 33–45% of cases and overestimates grade in 4–32% (Table 8.4) (Kastendieck, 1980; Catalona et al., 1982; Lange et al., 1983; Garnett et al., 1984; Mills and Fowler, 1986; Epstein and Steinberg, 1990; Bostwick, 1994c; Spires et al., 1994; Humphrey et al., 1995).

Grading errors are common in biopsies with small amounts of tumor and low-grade tumor, and are probably due to tissue sampling error, tumor heterogeneity and undergrading of needle biopsies. The accuracy of biopsy is highest for the primary Gleason pattern, but the secondary pattern also provides useful predictive information, particularly when combined with primary pattern to create the Gleason score (Figure 8.10). Gleason grading should be used for all needle biopsies (Bostwick, 1994b), even those with small amounts of tumor, according to the recommendations of Gleason (1992).

Kramer et al. compared Gleason score in 14-gauge needle biopsies with matched lymph node metastases, and found exact correlation in 17 of 42 cases (40%), ± 1 in 32 of 42 cases (76%), and ± 2 in 40 of 42 cases (95%) (Kramer et al., 1980, 1981). The lack of a more anaplastic pattern in the metastatic deposits implies that factors other than loss of differentiation are responsible for the ability of cancer cells to metastasize (Brawn et al., 1990; Cumming et al., 1990).

8.3 REPRODUCIBILITY OF GLEASON GRADING AND COMPARISON WITH OTHER GRADING SYSTEMS

Interobserver and intraobserver variability limit the reproducibility of grading in the prostate as in other organs with their grading systems (Bain, Koch and Hanson, 1982; Schröder et al., 1985a, b, c; Ten Kate et al., 1986; De Las Morenas et al., 1988; Gallee et al., 1990; Cintra and Billis, 1991; Di Loreto et al., 1991; Gleason, 1992). The subjective nature of grading precludes absolute precision, no matter how carefully the system is defined, yet the significant correlation of prostatic adenocarcinoma grade with virtually every outcome measure attests to the predictive strength and utility of grading in the hands of most investigators. Gleason noted exact reproducibility of score in 50% of needle biopsies and ± 1 score in 85%, similarly to others (Gleason, 1992; Bain, Koch and Hanson, 1982).

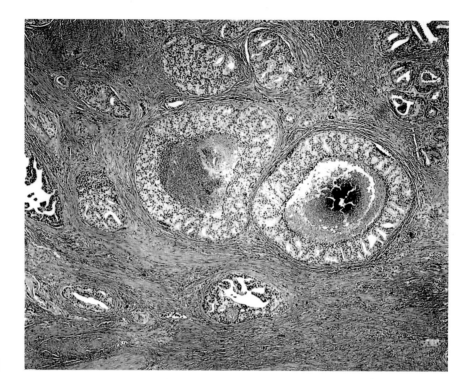

(a)

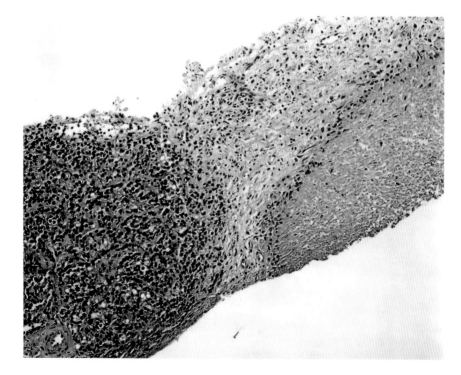

(b)

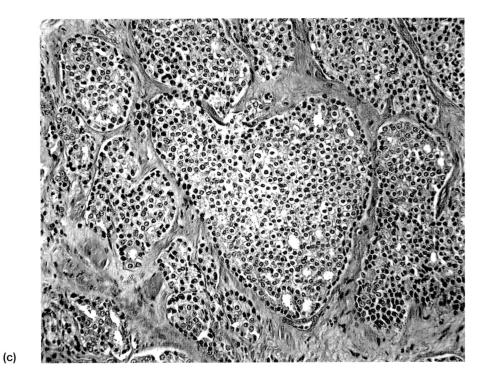

(c)

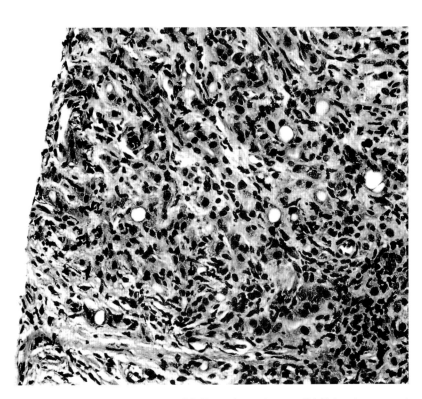

(d)

Figure 8.9 Gleason pattern 5 adenocarcinoma. **(a)** Comedocarcinoma. **(b)** Extensive necrosis adjacent to cancer. **(c)** Solid sheets of malignant cells occasionally punctuated by small fenestrations. **(d)** This focus of cancer was mistaken for granulation tissue with plump endothelial cells.

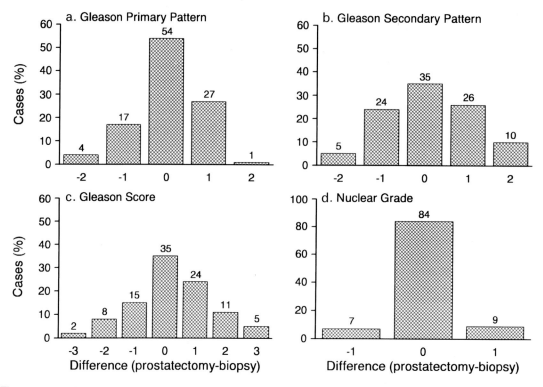

Figure 8.10 Distribution of grading differences between prostatectomy and biopsy in 316 matched cases. **(a)** Gleason primary pattern. **(b)** Gleason secondary pattern. (c) Gleason score (sum of primary and secondary patterns). **(d)** Nuclear grade. (Source: reprinted with permission from Bostwick, 1994c.)

Some investigators question the utility of grading because of the significant incidence of interobserver variability (Bain, Koch and Hanson, 1982; De Las Morenas *et al.*, 1988; Di Loreto *et al.*, 1991). One study found a high level of disagreement in grading among three pathologists evaluating 41 cases of well- to moderately differentiated adenocarcinoma (Di Loreto *et al.*, 1991). Another study compared the level of interobserver agreement with four grading systems in a consecutive series of 100 prostatic adenocarcinomas and found the Gleason grading system to be the least reproducible, with complete agreement of score in only 66% of cases (De Las Morenas *et al.*, 1988). To perform the analysis, the authors compressed the Gleason scores into three grade groups: 2–5, 6–7, and 8–10. Gallee *et al.* compared the prognostic accuracy of five grading systems (Broders, Gleason, M. D. Anderson,

Mostofi and Mostofi–Schröder), and found that the Gleason system had the lowest predictive ability for recurrence and death, whereas the Broders and Mostofi–Schröder systems had reasonable accuracy (Gallee *et al.*, 1990). Conversely, another report compared the level of intraobserver agreement with the Gleason, Mostofi and Böcking systems and found no significant differences; further, the level of variability was unaffected by type of specimen or amount of tissue examined (Cintra and Billis, 1991). Despite questions of reproducibility, the collective experience supports the clinical utility of grading prostatic adenocarcinoma.

Using a variety of architectural and nuclear features, Bibbo *et al.* developed a Bayesian belief network for grading prostatic adenocarcinoma, and attained agreement with Gleason grade in 241 of 256 microscopic fields (Bibbo *et al.*, 1990, 1993). Features used by the belief network included acinus formation, lumen area, acinar fusion, type of acinar fusion, acinar packing, acinar size, acinar uniformity, thickness of acinar epithelial layer, nuclear size, nuclear variability, nuclear shape, chromatin pattern and nucleolar size. These authors noted that four diagnostic clues allowed unique mapping of Gleason primary patterns and additional clues offered redundancy and robustness to the network.

8.4 PROPOSED MODIFICATIONS TO GLEASON GRADING

Numerous modifications have been proposed for Gleason grading to improve its discriminative capabilities, including nuclear grading and morphometric grading, grade compression, and measuring the amount of high-grade adenocarcinoma.

8.4.1 Nuclear and nucleolar grading

Nuclear and nucleolar enlargement are important diagnostic clues for the diagnosis of malignancy. Morphometric methods allow objective evaluation of nuclear size, roundness, shape, chromatin texture and other features. In an effort to create an objective method of grading prostatic adenocarcinoma, one study found that morphometric estimates of variation in nuclear size separated patients undergoing prostatectomy into two groups with differing survival rates (Blom et al., 1990). Other investigators have utilized morphometry to improve the predictive value of Gleason grading, but these methods are not used routinely (Diamond et al., 1982; Aragona et al., 1989; Robutti, Pilato and Betta,1989; Schultz et al., 1990; Irinopoulou, Rigaut and Benson, 1993).

Nuclear roundness has been the subject of considerable interest since the first report by Diamond et al. in 1982 (Epstein, Berry and Eggleston, 1984; Mohler, Partin and Coffey,

1987; Mohler et al., 1988a, b; Partin et al., 1989, 1992; Armas et al., 1991; Schaeffer et al., 1992). Average nuclear roundness accurately predicted prognosis in patients with untreated stage T1b (A2) prostatic adenocarcinoma and other clinical stage adenocarcinomas. However, many of these reports were limited by small sample size (less than 30 patients), use of the same patient cohort in multiple publications, failure to describe the morphological variations and nuclear roundness extremes, and patient selection bias. Nuclear roundness failed to identify patients with tumor recurrence following radiation therapy except in those with well-differentiated adenocarcinoma (Schaeffer et al., 1992).

Nucleolar grading of prostatic adenocarcinoma has also been proposed, but has not been adopted (grade 1: large and prominent nucleoli in virtually every cell; grade 2: intermediate; grade 3: very small nucleoli which are difficult to find) (Myers et al., 1982).

8.4.2 Grade compression

Many authors have simplified the Gleason grading system by compressing the scores into groups, usually creating three groups: 2–3–4, 5–6–7, and 8–9–10 (De Las Morenas et al., 1988). Unfortunately, grade compression diminishes the statistical strength of grading (Gleason, 1992). Further, the choice of grouping is often problematic; the most important 'cut-point' is between Gleason score 6 and 7 due to the emergence of poorly differentiated adenocarcinoma (pattern 4) in score 7, yet many studies combine these scores. Gleason argued against grade compression except in studies with a small number of patients in which grouping is unavoidable; in such cases, a cut-point between scores 6 and 7 is preferred (Gleason, 1992; Oesterling et al., 1987). The probability of lymph node metastases is significantly greater in patients with score 7 adenocarcinoma than in those with score 6 (Thomas et al., 1982; McNeal et al., 1990).

8.4.3 Volume of high-grade adenocarcinoma

The volume of high-grade adenocarcinoma appears to be an important prognostic factor; as tumor volume increases, the frequency and volume of high-grade tumor increase (McNeal *et al.*, 1986, 1990; Bostwick *et al.*, 1993; Bostwick, 1994a). Gleason grade stratifies adenocarcinoma into three subgroups with different levels of aggressiveness; Gleason pattern 1 and 2 adenocarcinoma is almost always small, usually less than 1 ml, indolent, localized and frequently located in the transition zone, whereas pattern 3 adenocarcinoma is variable in size and very common. Pattern 4 and 5 adenocarcinomas are usually larger and more aggressive than lower-grade tumors, and likely to extend beyond the prostate or metastasize (McNeal *et al.*, 1990). One study of 209 radical prostatectomies from patients with clinical stage T1 and T2 adenocarcinomas reported that the volume of high-grade adenocarcinoma (Gleason grades 4 and 5) had the highest predictive value for lymph node metastases, greater even than tumor volume (McNeal *et al.*, 1990). Of 38 patients with more than 3.2 ml of high-grade adenocarcinoma, 22 (58%) had pelvic lymph node metastases compared with only one of 171 patients (0.6%) with smaller volumes of high-grade adenocarcinoma. The extent of solid undifferentiated carcinoma shows a strong correlation with tumor progression according to one report of 24 cases (Gaffney, Sullivan and O'Brien, 1992). Gleason score and percentage of pattern 4 and 5 adenocarcinoma show a positive correlation with tumor volume (Bostwick, 1994a). In addition, poorly differentiated adenocarcinoma was the strongest predictor of tumor progression and cancer-specific survival in a series of 107 patients with clinically localized prostatic adenocarcinoma (Egawa *et al.*, 1993). The cumulative data suggest that the volume of high-grade adenocarcinoma is of prognostic significance, refuting Gleason's contention that prostatic carcinoma behaves according to the average of histological grades. However,

many of these studies grouped the Gleason scores, raising questions of grade compression.

Histological dedifferentiation of prostatic adenocarcinoma has been reported by numerous investigators, but these studies included only cases with more than one resection, probably selecting for adenocarcinomas that are more aggressive and thus more likely to require repeat operation (Brawn, 1983; Cumming *et al.*, 1990; McNeal *et al.*, 1990). Dedifferentiation occurs in 65% of repeat transurethral resections (Brawn, 1983; Cumming *et al.*, 1990). Dedifferentiation to high-grade adenocarcinoma appears to be unusual in low-grade (Gleason patterns 1–3) and small-volume (1 ml) adenocarcinoma, occurring in only 2.4% of patients in 7 years according to one study (Whittemore, Keller and Betensky, 1991).

8.5 CLINICAL SIGNIFICANCE OF GRADING

8.5.1 Correlation of grade and PSA

Adenocarcinoma associated with an elevated serum PSA is more likely to be of higher grade, larger volume and more advanced pathological stage than adenocarcinoma associated with a normal serum PSA concentration (Partin *et al.*, 1990; Tomita *et al.*, 1993; Blackwell *et al.*, 1994). There is a significant positive correlation between serum PSA and primary Gleason grade, percentage Gleason patterns 4 and 5, nuclear grade and DNA content (Blackwell *et al.*, 1994). Adenocarcinomas with Gleason scores of 7 or greater have a significantly higher median serum PSA and median cancer volume than cancers with lower (less than 7) Gleason scores. Also, patients with adenocarcinoma consisting of greater than 30% Gleason patterns 4 and 5 have a significantly higher median serum PSA and cancer volume than those with less than 30% Gleason patterns 4 and 5. Further, the median serum PSA concentration is greater in tumors with Gleason pattern greater than 3 than in those with

Gleason pattern less than 3 after controlling for tumor volume in 5 ml increments.

Serum PSA is of limited usefulness for staging localized prostatic adenocarcinoma because of the influence of tumor grade (Partin *et al.*, 1990). Although individual cells in poorly differentiated adenocarcinoma produce less PSA than cells in well-differentiated and moderately differentiated adenocarcinoma, they are usually present in such large numbers (greater tumor volume) and replace more of the prostate that serum PSA concentration is higher.

8.5.2 Correlation of grade and pathological stage

Grade is one of the strongest and most useful predictors of pathological stage and other clinical and pathological features, according to numerous univariate and multivariate studies (reviewed in Bostwick, 1994b). This predictive ability applies to extraprostatic extension, seminal vesicle invasion, lymph node metastases and bone metastases. Some investigators claim that Gleason score of 8 or higher on biopsy is strongly predictive of lymph node metastases and suggest dispensing with staging lymph node dissection in these cases. Despite the ability of grade to predict pathological stage, the predictive value is not sufficiently high to permit its application for individual patients, particularly in those with moderately differentiated adenocarcinoma.

8.5.3 Correlation of grade and tumor location

Grade may be related to the site of origin of adenocarcinoma within the prostate (McNeal *et al.*, 1988, 1992; Greene *et al.*, 1991, 1994). Adenocarcinoma arising in the transition zone of the prostate appears to be lower grade and less aggressive clinically than the more common adenocarcinoma arising in the peripheral zone. The majority of transition zone adenocarcinomas arise adjacent to nodular hyperplasia, with one-third actually originating within nodules. These adenocarcinomas are better differentiated than those in the peripheral zone, accounting for the majority of Gleason pattern 1 and 2 tumors.

8.5.4 Correlation of grade with recurrence and survival

Virtually every measure of recurrence and survival is strongly correlated with grade, including crude survival, tumor-free survival following treatment, metastasis-free survival and cause-specific survival (reviewed in Bostwick, 1994b). Gleason score is the strongest predictor of time to recurrence after radical prostatectomy (Humphrey *et al.*, 1993).

Schröder *et al.* calculated the impact on cancer-specific survival of 12 histopathological features used in grading prostatic adenocarcinoma (Schröder *et al.*, 1985a, b, c). In their analysis of 346 patients treated by radical perineal prostatectomy, they found that four features provided independent predictive value: acinar arrangement (architecture), nuclear size, nuclear shape and the presence of mitotic figures.

REFERENCES

Aihara, M., Wheeler, T. M., Ohori, M. and Scardino, P. T. (1994) Heterogeneity of prostate cancer in radical prostatectomy specimens. *Urology*, **43**, 60–66.

Aragona, F., Franco, V., Rodolico, V. *et al.* (1989) Interactive computerized morphometric analysis of the differential diagnosis between dysplasia and well differentiated adenocarcinoma of the prostate. *Urol. Res.*, **17**, 35–40.

Armas, O. A., Pizov, G., Pitcock, R. V. *et al.* (1991) Nuclear morphology of prostatic carcinoma: Comparison of computerized image analysis (CAS 200) versus video planimetry (DynaCELL). *Mod. Pathol.*, **4**, 763–767.

Bain, G., Koch, M. and Hanson, J. (1982) Feasibility of grading prostatic carcinomas. *Arch. Pathol. Lab. Med.*, **106**, 265–267.

Bibbo, M., Kim, D. H., Galera-Davidson, G. *et al.* (1990) Architectural, morphometric and photometric features and their relationship to the main subjective diagnostic clues in the grading of prostatic cancer. *Anal. Quant. Cytol. Histol.*, **12**, 85–90.

Bibbo, M., Bartels, P. H., Pfeifer, T. *et al.* (1993) Belief network for grading prostate lesions. *Anal. Quant. Cytol. Histol.*, **15**, 124–135.

Blackwell, K. L., Bostwick, D. G., Zincke, H. *et al.* (1994) Combining prostate specific antigen with cancer and gland volume to predict more reliably pathologic stage: the influence of prostate specific antigen cancer density. *J. Urol.*, **151**, 1565–1570.

Blom, J. H., Ten Kate, F. J., Schröder, F. H. and van der Heul, R. O. (1990) Morphometrically estimated variation in nuclear size. A useful tool in grading prostatic cancer. *Urol. Res.*, **18**, 93–99.

Böcking, A., Kiehn, J. and Heinzel-Wach, M. (1982) Combined histologic grading of prostatic carcinoma. *Cancer*, **50**, 288–294.

Bostwick, D. G. (1994a) The significance of tumor volume in prostate cancer. *Urol. Annu.*, **8**, 1–22.

Bostwick, D. G. (1994b) Grading prostate cancer. *Am. J. Clin. Pathol.*, **102** (Suppl 1), S38–S56.

Bostwick, D. G. (1994c) Gleason grading of prostatic needle biopsies: correlation with grade in 316 matched prostatectomies. *Am. J. Surg. Pathol.*, **18**, 796–803.

Bostwick, D. G., Graham, S. D. Jr, Napalkov, P. *et al.* (1993) Staging of early prostate cancer: a proposed tumor volume-based prognostic index. *Urology*, **41**, 403–411.

Brawn, P. N. (1983) The differentiation of prostatic carcinoma. *Cancer*, **52**, 246–251.

Broders, A. C. (1926) Carcinoma grading and practical application. *Arch. Pathol. Lab. Med.*, **2**, 376–381.

Catalona, W. J., Stein, A. J. and Fair, W. R. (1982) Grading errors in prostatic needle biopsies: relation to the accuracy of tumor grade in predicting pelvic lymph node metastases. *J. Urol.*, **127**, 919–922.

Cintra, M. L. and Billis, A. (1991) Histologic grading of prostatic adenocarcinoma: intraobserver reproducibility of the Mostofi, Gleason and Bocking grading systems. *Int. Urol. Nephrol.*, **23**, 449–454.

Cumming, J. A., Ritchie, A. W., Goodman, C. M. *et al.* (1990) Dedifferentiation with time in prostate cancer and the influence of treatment on the course of the disease. *Br. J. Urol.*, **65**, 271–274.

De Las Morenas, A., Siroky, M. B., Merriam, J. and Stilmant, M. M. (1988) Prostatic adenocarcinoma: reproducibility and correlation with clinical stages of four grading systems. *Hum. Pathol.*, **19**, 595–597.

Diamond, D. A., Berry, S. J., Jewett, H. J. *et al.* (1982) A new method to assess metastatic potential of human prostate cancer: relative nuclear roundness. *J. Urol.*, **128**, 729–734.

Di Loreto, C., Fitzpatrick, B., Underhill, S. *et al.* (1991) Correlation between visual clues, objective architectural features and interobserver agreement in prostate cancer. *Am. J. Clin. Pathol.*, **96**, 70–75.

Egawa, S., Go, M., Kuwao, S. *et al.* (1993) Long-term impact of conservative management on localized prostate cancer. A twenty-year experience in Japan. *Urology*, **42**, 520–526.

Epstein, J. I. and Steinberg, G. D. (1990) The significance of low-grade prostate cancer on needle biopsy. A radical prostatectomy study of tumor grade, volume, and stage of the biopsied and multifocal tumor. *Cancer*, **66**, 1927–1932.

Epstein, J. I., Berry, S. J. and Eggleston, J. C. (1984) Nuclear roundness factor. A predictor of progression in untreated stage A2 prostate cancer. *Cancer*, **54**, 1666–1671.

Gaffney, E. F., O'Sullivan, S. N. and O'Brien, A. (1992) A major solid undifferentiated carcinoma pattern correlates with tumor progression in locally advanced prostatic carcinoma. *Histopathology*, **21**, 249–255.

Gallee, M. P., Ten Kate, F. J., Mulder, P. G. *et al.* (1990) Histological grading of prostatic carcinoma in prostatectomy specimens. Comparison of prognostic accuracy of five grading systems. *Br. J. Urol.*, **65**, 368–375.

Gardner, W. A. Jr, Coffey, D., Karr, J. P. *et al.* (1988) A uniform histopathologic grading system for prostate cancer. *Hum. Pathol.*, **19**, 119–120.

Garnett, J. E., Oyasu, R. and Grayhack, J. T. (1984) The accuracy of diagnostic biopsy specimens in predicting tumor grades by Gleason's classification of radical prostatectomy specimens. *J. Urol.*, **131**, 690–693.

Gleason, D. F. (1966) Classification of prostatic carcinomas. *Cancer Chemother. Rep.*, **50**, 125–128.

Gleason, D. F. (1990) Histologic grading of prostatic carcinoma, in *Pathology of the Prostate*, (ed. D. G. Bostwick), Churchill Livingstone, New York, pp. 83–93.

Gleason, D. F. (1992) Histologic grading of prostate cancer: a perspective. *Hum. Pathol.*, **23**, 273–279.

Gleason, D., Mellinger, G. and the Veterans Administration Cooperative Urological Research Group (1974) Prediction of prognosis for prostatic adenocarcinoma by combined histological grading and clinical staging. *J. Urol.*, **111**, 58–64.

Greene, D. R., Wheeler, T. M., Egawa, S. *et al.* (1991) Relationship between clinical stage and histological zone of origin in early prostate cancer: morphometric analysis. *Br. J. Urol.*, **68**, 499–509.

Greene, D. R., Rogers, E., Wessels, E. C. *et al.* (1994) Some small prostate cancers are nondiploid by nuclear image analysis: correlation of deoxyribonucleic acid ploidy status and pathological features. *J. Urol.,* **151**, 1301–1307.

Humphrey, P. A., Frazier, H. A., Vollmer, R. T. and Paulson, D. F. (1993) Stratification of pathologic features in radical prostatectomy specimens that are predictive of elevated initial postoperative serum prostate-specific antigen levels. *Cancer,* **71**, 1821–1827.

Irinopoulou, T., Rigaut, J. P. and Benson, M. C. (1993) Toward objective prognostic grading of prostatic carcinoma using image analysis. *Anal. Quant. Cytol. Histol.,* **15**, 341–344.

Kastendieck, H. (1980) Morphologie des Prostatacarcinoms in Stanzbiopsien und totalen Prostatektomien. Untersuchungen zur Frage der Relevanz bioptischer Befundaussagen. *Pathologe,* **2**, 31–43.

Kramer, S. A., Spahr, J., Brendler, C. B. *et al.* (1980) Experience with Gleason's histopathologic grading in prostatic cancer. *J. Urol.,* **124**, 223–225.

Kramer, S. A., Farnham, R., Glenn, J. F. and Paulson, D. F. (1981) Comparative morphology of primary and secondary deposits of prostatic adenocarcinoma. *Cancer,* **48**, 271–273.

Lange, P. H. and Narayan, P. (1983) Understaging and undergrading of prostate cancer. *Urology,* **21**, 113–118.

McNeal, J. E. (1992) Cancer volume and site of origin of adenocarcinoma in the prostate: relationship to local and distant spread. *Hum. Pathol.,* **23**, 258–266.

McNeal, J. E., Bostwick, D. G., Kindrachuk, R. A. *et al.* (1986) Patterns of progression in prostate cancer. *Lancet,* **1**, 60–63.

McNeal, J. E., Redwine, E. A., Freiha, F. S. and Stamey, T. A. (1988) Zonal distribution of prostatic adenocarcinoma. Correlation with histologic pattern and direction of spread. *Am. J. Surg. Pathol.,* **12**, 897–906.

McNeal, J. E., Villers, A. A., Redwine, E. A. *et al.* (1990) Histologic differentiation, cancer volume, and pelvic lymph node metastasis in adenocarcinoma of the prostate. *Cancer,* **52**, 246–251.

Mills, S. E. and Fowler, J. E. (1986) Gleason histologic grading of prostatic carcinoma. Correlations between biopsy and prostatectomy specimens. *Cancer,* **57**, 346–349.

Mohler, J. L., Partin, A. W. and Coffey, D. S. (1987) Correlation of prognosis to nuclear roundness and to flow cytometric light scatter. *Anal. Quant. Cytol. Histol.,* **9**, 156–164.

Mohler, J. L., Partin, A. W., Lohr, W. D. and Coffey, D. S. (1988a) Nuclear roundness factor measurement for assessment of prognosis of patients with prostatic carcinoma. I. Testing of a digitization system. *J. Urol.,* **139**, 1080–1084.

Mohler, J. L., Partin, A. W., Epstein, J. I. *et al.* (1988b) Nuclear roundness factor measurement for assessment of prognosis of patients with prostatic carcinoma. II. Standardization of methodology for histologic sections. *J. Urol.,* **139**, 1085–1090.

Mostofi, F. K. (1975) Grading of prostatic carcinoma. *Cancer Chemother. Rep.,* **59**, 111–117.

Myers, R. P., Neves, R. J., Farrow, G. M. and Utz, D. C. (1982) Nucleolar grading of prostatic adenocarcinoma: light microscopic correlation with disease progression. *Prostate,* **3**, 423–432.

Oesterling, J. E., Brendler, C. B., Epstein, J. I. *et al.* (1987) Correlation of clinical stage, serum prostatic acid phosphatase and preoperative Gleason grade with final pathological stage in 275 patients with clinically localized adenocarcinoma of the prostate. *J. Urol.,* **138**, 92–98.

Partin, A. W., Walsh, A. C., Pitcock, R. V. *et al.* (1989) A comparison of nuclear morphometry and Gleason grade as a predictor of prognosis in stage A2 prostate cancer: a critical analysis. *J. Urol.,* **142**, 1254–1258.

Partin, A. W., Carter, H. B., Chan, D. W. *et al.* (1990) Prostate specific antigen in the staging of localized prostate cancer: influence of tumor differentiation, tumor volume, and benign hyperplasia. *J. Urol.,* **143**, 747–752.

Partin, A. W., Steinberg, G. D., Pitcock, R. V. *et al.* (1992) Use of nuclear morphometry, Gleason histologic scoring, clinical stage, and age to predict disease-free survival among patients with prostate cancer. *Cancer,* **70**, 161–168.

Robutti, F., Pilato, F. P. and Betta, P.-G. (1989) A new method of grading malignancy of prostate carcinoma using quantitative microscopic nuclear features. *Pathol. Res. Pract.,* **185**, 701–703.

Schaeffer, J., Tegeler, J. A., Kuban, D. A. *et al.* (1992) Nuclear roundness factor and local failure from definitive radiation therapy for prostatic carcinoma. *Int. J. Radiat. Biol. Phys.,* **24**, 431–434.

Schröder, F. H., Blom, J. H. M., Hop, W. C. J. *et al.* (1985a) Grading of prostatic cancer: I. An analysis of the prognostic significance of single characteristics. *Prostate,* **6**, 81–100.

Schröder, F. H., Blom, J. H. M., Hop, W. C. J. *et al.* (1985b) Grading of prostatic cancer: II. The prognostic significance of the presence of multiple architectural patterns. *Prostate,* **6**, 403–415.

Schröder, F. H., Hop, W. C. J., Blom, J. H. M. *et al.* (1985c) Grading of prostate cancer: III. Multivariate analysis of prognostic parameters. *Prostate,* **7**, 13–20.

Schultz, D. S., Harry, T., Wong, K. L. *et al.* (1990) Computer-assisted grading of adenocarcinoma in prostatic aspirates. *Anal. Quant. Cytol. Histol.*, **12**, 91–97.

Spires, S. E., Cibull, M. L., Wood, D. P. Jr *et al.* (1994) Gleason histologic grading in prostatic carcinoma: correlation of 18-gauge core biopsy with prostatectomy. *Arch. Pathol. Lab. Med.*, **118**, 705–708.

Ten Kate, F. J. W., Gallee, M. P. W., Schmitz, P. I. M. *et al.* (1986) Problems in grading of prostatic carcinoma. Interobserver reproducibility of five different grading systems. *World J. Urol.*, **4**, 147–152.

Thomas, R., Lewis, R., Sarma, D. *et al.* (1982) Aid to accurate clinical staging – histopathologic grading in prostatic cancer. *J. Urol.*, **128**, 726–728.

Tomita, T., Dalton, T., Kwok, S. *et al.* (1993) Profile of prostatic-specific antigen in prostatic carcinomas. *Mod. Pathol.*, **6**, 259–264.

Whittemore, A. S., Keller, J. B. and Betensky, R. (1991) Low-grade, latent prostate cancer volume: predictor of clinical cancer incidence? *J. Nat. Cancer Inst.*, **83**, 1231–1235.

9

VARIANTS OF PROSTATIC ADENOCARCINOMA

The biological behavior of histological variants of adenocarcinoma may differ from typical acinar adenocarcinoma, and proper clinical management depends on accurate diagnosis and separation from tumors arising in other sites. Unusual tumors arising in the prostate also raise questions of histogenesis (Table 9.1).

9.1 DUCTAL CARCINOMA

Ductal carcinoma (adenocarcinoma with endometrioid features; papillary carcinoma; endometrioid carcinoma) accounts for about 0.8% of prostatic adenocarcinomas (Tannenbaum, 1975a; Bostwick, Kindrachuk and Rouse, 1985; Lee, 1994). It typically arises as a polypoid or papillary mass within the prostatic urethra and large periurethral prostatic ducts, and histologically resembles endometrial adenocarcinoma of the female uterus (Figure 9.1) (Melicow and Pachter, 1967; Zaloudek, Williams and Kempson, 1976; Greene *et al.*, 1979; Cantrell *et al.*, 1981; Walter *et al.*, 1982; August and Oyasu, 1983; Kuhajda *et al.*, 1984; Bostwick, Kindrachuk and Rouse, 1985; Walther *et al.*, 1985; Epstein and Woodruff, 1986; Sufrin *et al.*, 1986; Witters *et al.*, 1986; Wernert *et al.*, 1987; Cueva *et al.*, 1988; Ro *et al.*, 1988a; Christenson *et al.*, 1991; Aydin, 1993; Lee, 1994). Most refer to this tumor as adenocarcinoma with endometrioid features

Table 9.1 Variants of prostatic carcinoma

Adenocarcinoma and associated tumors	*Gleason primary pattern*
Ductal carcinoma (endometrioid carcinoma)	3 (no necrosis); 5 (necrosis)
Mucinous carcinoma	4
Signet ring cell carcinoma	5
Sarcomatoid carcinoma	5
Adenocarcinoma with neuroendocrine cells	Variable
Neuroendocrine carcinoma	5 (small cell carcinoma)
Squamous and adenosquamous carcinoma	Variable; usually high-grade
Adenocarcinoma with oncocytic features	Variable
Lymphoepithelioma-like carcinoma	5
Adenoid cystic carcinoma/basal cell carcinoma	Variable; usually high-grade

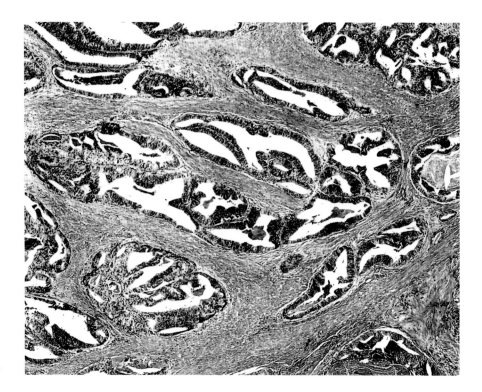

(a)

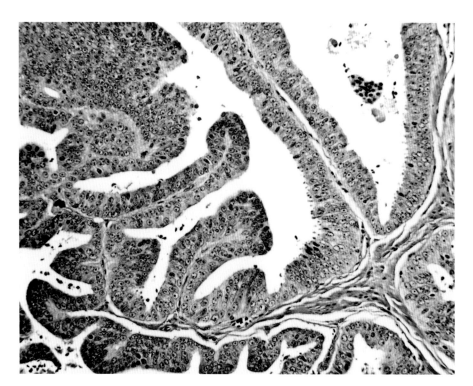

(b)

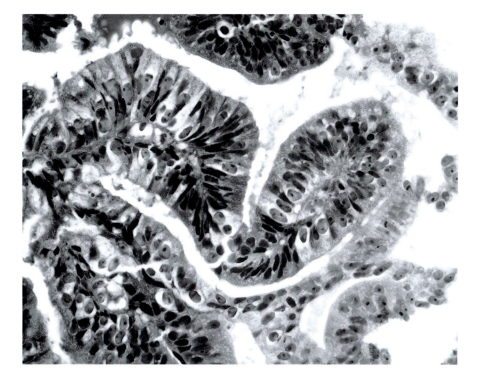

(c)

Figure 9.1 Ductal adenocarcinoma with papillary pattern (Gleason pattern 3). **(a)** The periurethral ducts are replaced by malignant glandular epithelium with some papillary projections. **(b)** The papillae are lined by uniform malignant cells with prominent nucleoli. **(c)** In another case, there was prominent cytoplasmic granularity within the tumor cells due to large neuroendocrine granules.

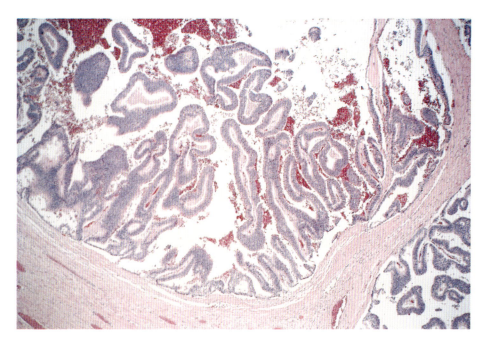

Figure 9.2 Ductal adenocarcinoma. This papillary proliferation filled the large periurethral prostatic ducts and protruded into the urethra.

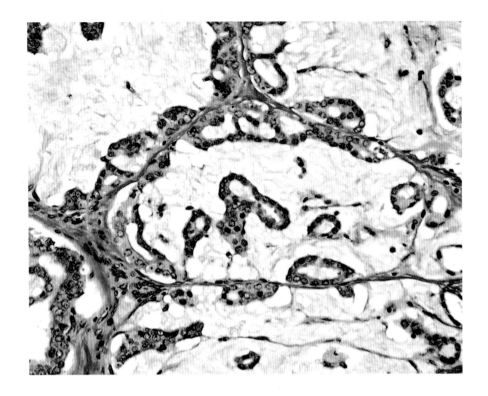

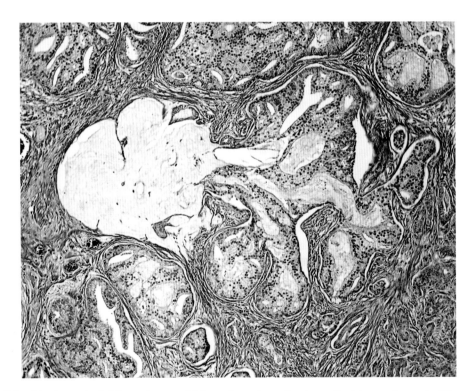

Figure 9.3 Mucinous (colloid) carcinoma. **(a)** Irregular acinar structures float in mucin pools. The nuclei are small, with indistinct nucleoli, and may be mistaken for benign cells. **(b)** Mucinous carcinoma is present focally within a typical cribriform adenocarcinoma.

170

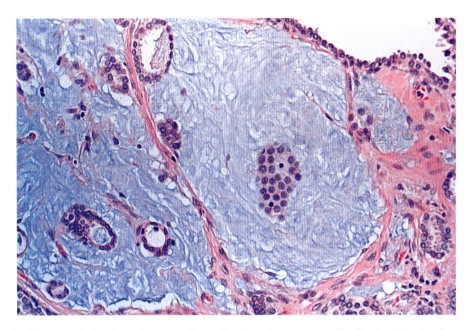

Figure 9.4 Mucinous (colloid) carcinoma, with pools of mucin punctuated by floating islands of cancer cells.

or simply ductal carcinoma. The term 'endometrial' should not be used in the prostate.

The clinical symptoms of pure ductal carcinoma and mixed ductal–acinar carcinoma are similar to typical acinar carcinoma. Cystoscopically, ductal carcinoma consists of multiple friable polypoid 'worm-like' white masses protruding from ducts at or near the mouth of the prostatic utricle at the apex of the verumontanum. The prostate is usually enlarged, with palpable induration or nodularity in the majority of cases. At the time of presentation, most patients have tumors confined to the prostate or urethra, with concurrent invasive acinar prostatic adenocarcinoma in at least 77% of cases. The prognosis of ductal carcinoma appears to be the same as typical acinar adenocarcinoma, although conflicting results have been found.

Serum concentrations of PSA and PAP may be normal at the time of diagnosis except in patients with bone metastases. Ductal carcinoma usually involves the large periurethral prostatic ducts and verumontanum, consisting of masses of complex papillae or acini lined by variably stratified columnar epithelium. Two

architectural patterns have been observed: papillary and cribriform (Figure 9.2) (Ro *et al.*, 1988a).

These patterns coexist in about half of cases, and both have nuclear abnormalities and frequent mitotic figures. Ductal carcinoma invariably displays intense cytoplasmic immunoreactivity for PAP and PSA. Focal CEA immunoreactivity is occasionally present.

The differential diagnosis of ductal carcinoma includes urothelial carcinoma of the prostate, large gland variant of Gleason pattern 3 adenocarcinoma, ectopic prostatic tissue, benign polyp, nephrogenic metaplasia, proliferative papillary urethritis, inverted papilloma and accentuated mucosal folds. There is usually evidence of acinar differentiation in ductal carcinoma, allowing separation from urothelial carcinoma; in difficult cases or those with small samples, immunohistochemical stains for PSA and PAP are useful (positive in ductal carcinoma and negative in urothelial carcinoma). The presence of urothelial abnormalities in the adjacent urethral mucosa is strong evidence of urothelial cancer, but is not definitive. Benign mimics

171

are distinguished from ductal carcinoma by the absence of dysplasia.

9.2 MUCINOUS CARCINOMA (COLLOID CARCINOMA)

Pure mucinous carcinoma of the prostate is rare (Figures 9.3 and 9.4) (Proia, McCarty and Woodard, 1981; Epstein and Lieberman. 1985; Odom, Donatucci and Dedshon, 1986; Krogh and Lund, 1988; Ro *et al.*, 1989; Ro *et al.*, 1990; Ishizu *et al.*, 1991; McNeal *et al.*, 1991; Teichman, Shabaik and Demby, 1994; Van de Voorde *et al.*, 1994), although typical acinar adenocarcinoma often produces mucin focally, particularly following high-dose estrogen therapy.

The clinical presentation of mucinous carcinoma is similar to typical acinar carcinoma, and there are no apparent differences in patient age, stage at presentation, cancer volume, serum PSA concentration or pattern of metastases (Epstein and Lieberman, 1985; Ro *et al.*, 1989; McNeal *et al.*; 1991). This tumor may not respond well to endocrine therapy (Efros *et al.*, 1992) or radiation therapy and is highly aggressive (Ishizu *et al.*, 1991; Teichman, Shabaik and Demby, 1994).

Focal mucinous differentiation is observed in at least one-third of cases of prostatic carcinoma, but the diagnosis of mucinous carcinoma requires that at least 25% of the tumor consists of pools of extracellular mucin (Elbadawi *et al.*, 1979). Mucinous carcinoma consists of tumor cell nests and clusters floating in mucin, similar to mucinous carcinoma of the breast. In biopsies, rarely there may be only pools of mucin without identifiable tumor cells, but serial sectioning usually reveals malignant cells on deeper levels. Three patterns of mucinous carcinoma have been described: acinar carcinoma with luminal distension, cribriform carcinoma with luminal distension and 'colloid carcinoma', with cell nests embedded in mucinous lakes (McNeal *et al.*, 1991). Other histological patterns of adenocarcinoma are usually present, including cribriform and comedocarcinoma patterns.

The cells of mucinous carcinoma have enlarged nuclei and display the entire spectrum of cytological abnormalities observed in typical adenocarcinoma. In some cases, the nuclei are low-grade, with uniform finely granular chromatin and inconspicuous nucleoli, but their presence within mucin pools is diagnostic of malignancy. Signet-ring cells are usually not seen in mucinous carcinoma (Uchijima *et al.*, 1990). McNeal and coworkers consider 'colloid' carcinoma a variant of Gleason grade 4 carcinoma (McNeal *et al.*, 1991).

Collagenous micronodules are an incidental finding in mucin-producing carcinoma, and probably result from extracellular acid mucin (Bostwick, Wollan and Adlakha, 1995). The number of collagenous micronodules is correlated with the amount of mucin produced by the tumor, including luminal mucin and extraacinar mucin. These micronodules are of no prognostic significance.

Mucinous carcinoma stains with PAS, alcian blue and mucicarmine, like other prostatic mucin, but we rarely use these in practice. Most studies have found neutral mucin in benign acini and acidic mucin in malignant acini, although benign acini rarely produce small quantities of acidic mucin (Franks, O'Shea and Thompson, 1964; Taylor, 1979; Ro *et al.*, 1988c; Pinder and McMahon, 1990; Grignon and O'Malley, 1993). Some have suggested that acidic mucin is a useful supportive feature in the diagnosis of adenocarcinoma, present in about 60% of cases, but this has been refuted (Ro *et al.*, 1988c; Hukill and Vidone, 1967; Taylor, 1979; Grignon and O'Malley, 1993). Acidic mucin has also been described in atypical adenomatous hyperplasia, mucinous metaplasia, prostatic intraepithelial neoplasia, sclerosing adenosis and basal cell hyperplasia (Humphrey, 1991; Epstein and Fynheer, 1992; Goldstein, Qian and Bostwick, 1995). The cells of mucinous carcinoma contain PSA and PAP, but usually do not produce CEA. The differential diagnosis includes mucinous carcinoma of the rectum, urinary bladder or Cowper glands. These distinctions are important because of significant differences in treatment and prognosis. Immunohistochemical stains for PSA and PAP are positive, at least focally, in mucinous carcinoma of the prostate and confirm prostatic origin.

9.3 SIGNET-RING-CELL CARCINOMA

Signet-ring-cell carcinoma of the prostate is rare (Figure 9.5) (Giltman, 1981; Kums and van Helsdingen, 1985; Ro *et al.*, 1988b; Hejka and England, 1989; Remmele, Weber and Harding, 1988; Uchijima *et al.*, 1990; Alline and Cohen, 1992; Catton, Hartwick and Srigley, 1992; Guerin, Hasan and Keen, 1993; Segawa and Kakehi, 1993; Smith *et al.*, 1994). The clinical presentation is similar to typical acinar adeno-carcinoma except that all are high stage. The prognosis is poor.

The diagnosis of signet-ring-cell carcinoma requires that 25% or more of the tumor is composed of signet-ring cells, although some authors require 50% (Figure 9.5). Most often it is a minor component of Gleason pattern 5 carcinoma. Tumor cells show distinctive nuclear displacement by clear cytoplasm. Signet-ring cells are present in 2.5% of cases of acinar adenocarcinoma, but rarely in sufficient numbers to be considered signet-ring-cell carcinoma (Guerin, Hasan and Keen, 1993). Almost all reported cases are associated with other forms of poorly-differentiated prostatic adenocarcinoma, including cribriform carcinoma, comedocarcinoma and solid (Gleason grade 5) carcinoma. Tumor cells diffusely infiltrate through the stroma, invading perineural and vascular spaces and often perforating the prostatic capsule.

Histochemical and immunohistochemical results with mucin, lipid, PSA, PAP and CEA stains are variable, and the signet-ring-cell appearance may result from cytoplasmic lumens, mucin granules and fat vacuoles.

The differential diagnosis of signet-ring-cell carcinoma of the prostate includes similar tumors arising in other sites, particularly the gastrointestinal tract and stomach. Prostatic origin should be considered in metastatic signet-ring-cell carcinoma of supraclavicular

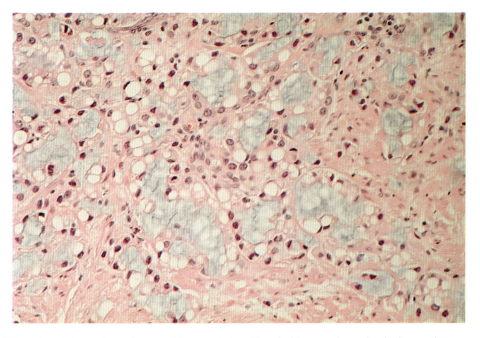

Figure 9.5 Signet-ring-cell carcinoma of the prostate with pale-blue mucinous luminal secretions.

lymph nodes, which exhibits negative mucin staining; PSA and PAP immunostaining may be useful. The characteristic cytoplasmic clearing of prostatic signet-ring-cell carcinoma is rarely mucicarminophilic, in contrast with mucicarmine-positive signet-ring-cell carcinoma of the bladder, urachus, stomach and other sites. Artifactual changes mimicking signet-ring-cell carcinoma can occur in lymphomas, benign lymphocytes and vacuolated smooth muscle cells, causing diagnostic difficulty (Alguacil-Garcia, 1986). In these cases, PSA and PAP staining of the suspicious cells is negative, and CD45 (leukocyte common antigen) and smooth muscle actin immunoreactivity is observed within the inflammatory cells and smooth muscle cells respectively.

9.4 CARCINOMA WITH NEUROENDOCRINE DIFFERENTIATION

Virtually all prostatic adenocarcinomas contain at least a small number of neuroendocrine cells, but special studies such as histochemistry and immunohistochemistry are usually necessary to identify them (Capella *et al.*, 1981; Abrahamsson *et al.*, 1986, 1987; Di Sant' Agnese, 1992; Turbat-Herrera *et al.*, 1988; Bonkhoff *et al.*, 1991; Aprikian *et al.*, 1993; Berner *et al.*, 1993; Bostwick *et al.*, 1994). About 10% of adenocarcinomas contain cells with large eosinophilic granules (formerly referred to as adenocarcinoma with Paneth-cell-like change), usually consisting of only rare foci of scattered cells and small clusters which may be overlooked (Haratake, Akio and Kenji, 1987; Frydman *et al.*, 1992; Weaver, Fadi and Abdul-Karim Srigley, 1992; Weaver *et al.*, 1992; Adlakha and Bostwick, 1994). Cells with large eosinophilic granules in the normal epithelium and adenocarcinoma resemble Paneth cells of the intestine and other sites by light microscopy, but they differ from Paneth cells by their neuroendocrine differentiation (producing chromogranin, neuron-specific enolase and serotonin expression) and their lack of

lysozyme (Figure 9.6) (Adlakha and Bostwick, 1994).

The clinical features of adenocarcinoma with neuroendocrine differentiation are similar to typical acinar adenocarcinoma. Neuroendocrine differentiation may indicate a poor prognosis in prostate cancer (Cohen *et al.*, 1990; Cohen, Glezerson and Haffejee, 1991), but this has been disputed (Wright *et al.*, 1992; Aprikian *et al.*, 1993; Bostwick *et al.*, 1994). The neuroendocrine component of prostatic carcinoma may be resistant to hormonal therapy. Di Sant' Agnese suggested an autocrine mechanism for stimulation of growth of tumor cells with epithelial and neuroendocrine differentiation (Di Sant' Agnese, 1992).

The number of neuroendocrine cells in benign prostatic epithelium and adenocarcinoma is greater than the number of cells with large eosinophilic granules, indicating that there are neuroendocrine cells with granules that are not apparent on hematoxylin-and-eosin-stained sections. Neuroendocrine differentiation typically consists of scattered cells which are inapparent by light microscopy but immunoreactive for neuroendocrine markers.

PSA and PAP immunoreactivity is present in cells with large eosinophilic granules (Azumi, Shibuya and Ishikura, 1984; Cohen, Glezerson and Haffejee, 1992; Aprikian *et al.*, 1993; Adlakha and Bostwick, 1994). Androgen receptor immunoreactivity is also present in cells with neuroendocrine differentiation (Abrahamsson *et al.*, 1993).

The differential diagnosis of adenocarcinoma with neuroendocrine differentiation is the same as typical acinar adenocarcinoma. Areas with neuroendocrine differentiation may be misinterpreted as poorly differentiated adenocarcinoma.

9.5 NEUROENDOCRINE CARCINOMA (SMALL CELL CARCINOMA AND CARCINOID)

Most cases of neuroendocrine carcinoma have typical local signs and symptoms of prostatic adenocarcinoma, although paraneoplastic

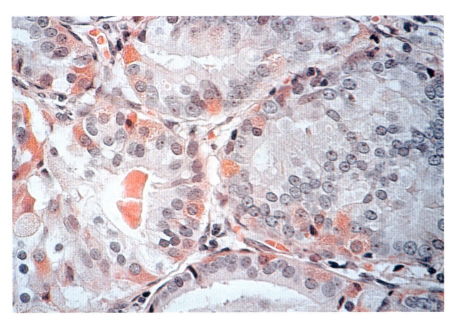

Figure 9.6 Prostatic adenocarcinoma with cells with large eosinophilic granules. (Source: case courtesy of Dr Michael Weaver, Cleveland, OH.)

syndromes are frequent in these patients. Cushing's syndrome is most common, invariably in association with ACTH immunoreactivity in tumor cells (Ghali and Gargia, 1984; Tetu *et al.*, 1987); other clinical conditions include malignant hypercalcemia (Mahadevia *et al.*, 1983; Barkin *et al.*, 1984), syndrome of inappropriate antidiuretic hormone (SIADH) secretion (Wenk *et al.*, 1977; Ghandur-Mnaynmah, Satterfield and Block, 1986) and myasthenic (Eaton–Lambert) syndrome (Tetu *et al.*, 1989). Small-cell carcinoma is aggressive and rapidly fatal (Ro *et al.*, 1987a; Moore, Reinberg and Zhang, 1992; Oesterling, Hauzear and Farrow, 1992; Abbas *et al.*, 1995). In one study, androgen receptor expression in small-cell carcinoma was predictive of a poorer outcome (median survival, 10 months) than in cases without expression (median, more than 30 months), regardless of treatment (Ferguson *et al.*, 1995).

Neuroendocrine carcinoma of the prostate varies histopathologically from carcinoid-like pattern (low-grade neuroendocrine carcinoma) to small-cell undifferentiated (oat cell) carcinoma (high-grade neuroendocrine carcinoma) (Figure 9.7) (Wasserstein and Goldman, 1979; Ansari *et al.*, 1981; Azumi, Shibuya and Ishikura, 1984; Schron, Gipson and Mendelsohn, 1984; Almagro *et al.*, 1986; Stratton, Evans and Lambert, 1986; Ro *et al.*, 1987a, b).

These tumors are morphologically identical to their counterparts in the lung and other sites. Typical acinar adenocarcinoma is present, at least focally, in many cases, and transition patterns may be seen (Figure 9.8). In cases with solid Gleason 5 pattern suggestive of neuroendocrine carcinoma, immunohistochemical stains are recommended.

Mixed patterns may be observed, including one case with small-cell carcinoma, adenocarcinoma, typical carcinoid and spindle-cell carcinoma (Egan, Youngkin and Bostwick, 1996).

A wide variety of secretory products may be detected within the malignant cells, including serotonin, calcitonin, ACTH, human chorionic gonadotrophin, thyroid stimulating hormone, bombesin, calcitonin-gene-related peptide and inhibin (Azumi, Shibuya and Ishikura, 1984; Ro *et al.*, 1987b; Oesterling, Hauzear and

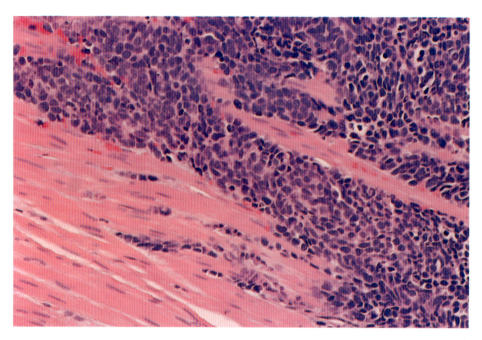

Figure 9.7   Small-cell undifferentiated (oat cell) carcinoma of the prostate. The architectural and cytological features are identical to its counterpart in the lung, including sheets and irregular nests of cells with scant cytoplasm, large hyperchromatic nuclei with molding, and inconspicuous nucleoli.

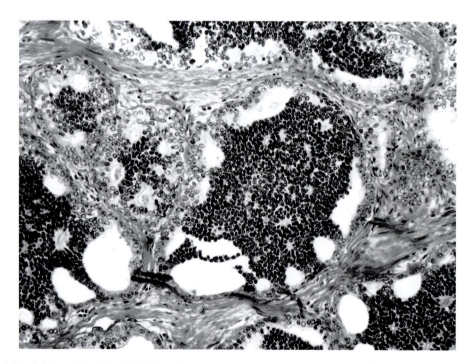

Figure 9.8   Adenocarcinoma with intra-acinar small-cell carcinoma forming rosette-like pattern. This pattern is extremely rare in our experience (Source: case courtesy of Robert H. Young, Boston, MA.)

Farrow, 1992). The same cells may express peptide hormones and PSA and PAP, but pure small-cell carcinoma does not usually display immunoreactivity for PSA. Serotonin, chromo-granin and synaptophysin are the most useful markers of neuroendocrine cells in formalin-fixed sections of prostate (Abrahamsson *et al.*, 1986; Di Sant' Agnese, 1992; Bostwick *et al.*, 1994).

Ultrastructurally, small-cell carcinoma and carcinoid tumor of the prostate contain a variable number of round, regular, membrane-bound neurosecretory granules (Di Sant' Agnese and de Mesy Jensen, 1984). Well-defined cytoplasmic processes are usually present which contain neurosecretory granules. The cells are small, with dispersed chromatin and small inconspicuous nucleoli.

The differential diagnosis of neuroendocrine carcinoma of the prostate includes metastases from other sites. High-grade carcinoma from the bladder which invades the prostate may be mistaken for neuroendocrine carcinoma. Other rare tumors such as peripheral neuro-ectodermal tumor (PNET), desmoplastic small round cell tumor and malignant lymphoma may be mistaken for prostatic neuroendocrine carcinoma, particularly in extraprostatic sites, but these are rare and often have unique clinical features.

9.6 SQUAMOUS CELL AND ADENOSQUAMOUS CARCINOMA

Squamous cell carcinoma is very rare in the prostate (Gray and Marshall, 1975; Mott, 1979; Al Adani, 1985; Moyana, 1987; Wernert *et al.*, 1990; Sarma, Weilbaecher and Moon, 1991; Little *et al.*, 1993; Moskovitz *et al.*, 1993; Miller, Reuter and Scher, 1995). Adenosquamous carcinoma refers to the combination of squamous cell carcinoma and typical acinar carcinoma, and is also rare (Figures 9.9 and 9 10) (Saito, Davis and Ollipally, 1984; Devaney, Dorman and Leader, 1991; Gattuso *et al.*, 1995).

Presenting signs and symptoms are similar to those of typical prostatic adenocarcinoma, although there is often a history of hormonal therapy or radiation therapy (Miller, Reuter and Scher, 1995). Squamous cell carcinoma of the prostate may also arise in patients with *Schistosoma haematobium* (Al Adani, 1985). Serum PSA and PAP concentration is usually normal, even with metastases, and bone metastases are typically osteolytic rather than osteoblastic (Mott, 1979; Sarma, Weilbaecher and Moon, 1991; Moskovitz *et al.*, 1993). The prognosis is poor, with a mean survival of 14 months regardless of therapy (Mott, 1979). These tumors appear to be unresponsive to androgen deprivation therapy.

Squamous cell carcinoma of the prostate is histopathologically similar to its counterpart in other organs, consisting of irregular nests and cords of malignant cells with keratinization and squamous differentiation, rarely with squamous pearls. Keratinizing squamous cell carcinoma of the prostate usually arises in the periurethral ducts, and is very rare; otherwise, the site of origin of squamous cell carcinoma is unknown (Moskovitz *et al.*, 1993). Mott required an absence of acinar differentiation for the diagnosis of squamous cell carcinoma, as well as a lack of bladder involvement; mixed tumors are best classified simply as adeno-squamous carcinoma (Mott, 1979). He also required no prior estrogen therapy, but we consider this exclusion unnecessary. Metastases may consist of adenosquamous carcinoma in cases without a squamous component in the primary tumor, perhaps due to sampling error.

Saito and coworkers identified PAP immunoreactivity in the acinar and squamous components of their case of adenosquamous carcinoma (Saito, Davis and Ollipally, 1984). Conversely, Gattuso and colleagues found staining only in the acinar component of their case; interestingly, they noted immunoreactivity in the squamous component for high-molecular-weight keratin AE-3, but not in the acinar component (Gattuso *et al.*, 1995). The adenosquamous carcinoma reported by Devaney and coworkers showed PSA and PAP immunoreactivity in the acinar component but

177

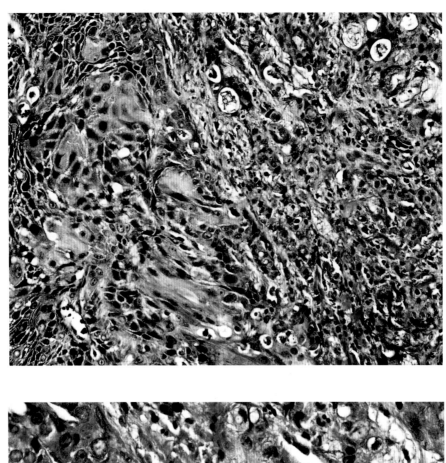

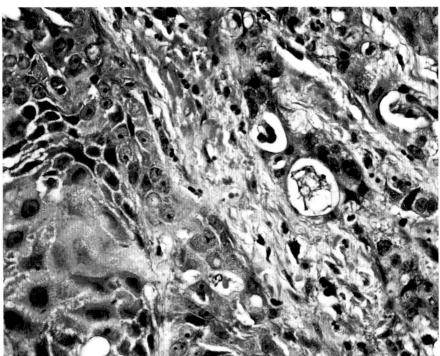

Figure 9.9 Adenosquamous carcinoma of the prostate. **(a)** The malignant squamous component comprised a minority of the tumor and occurred only after the patient had received radiation therapy and androgen deprivation therapy. **(b)** The nuclei in the squamous component are larger than those in the adenocarcinoma, which is adjacent.

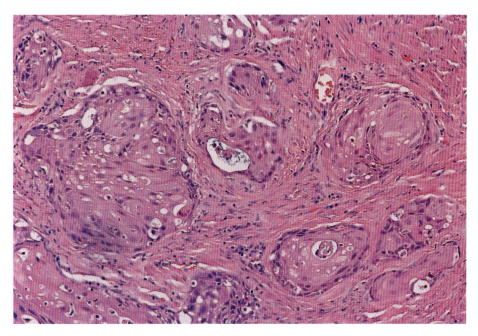

Figure 9.10 Adenosquamous cell carcinoma of the prostate. This tumor was identified many years after radiation therapy and androgen deprivation therapy for typical acinar adenocarcinoma (Source: case courtesy of Dr Manuel Doria, Chicago, IL.)

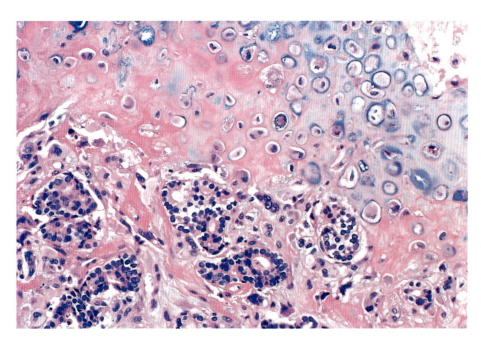

Figure 9.11 Sarcomatoid carcinoma with heterologous elements (carcinosarcoma). There is an intimate admixture of adenocarcinoma and malignant cartilage (chondroblastic osteosarcoma).

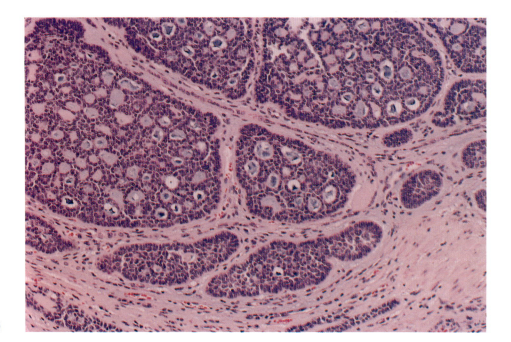

(a)

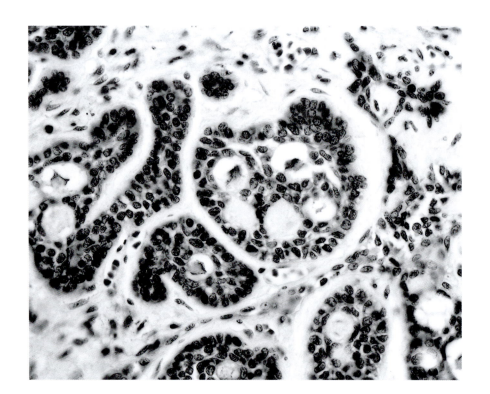

(b)

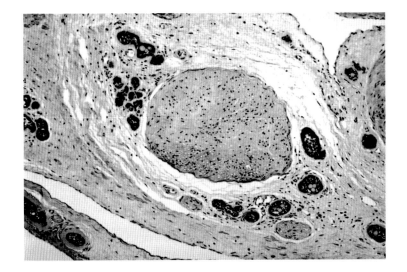

(c)

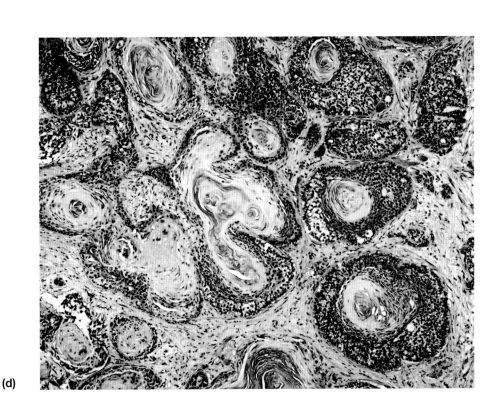

(d)

Figure 9.12 Adenoid cystic/basal cell carcinoma. **(a)** At low magnification, the circumscribed tumor nests of varying size are punctuated by predominantly round fenestrations containing mucin and collagenous stroma. **(b)** At high magnification, the tumor cells contain uniform cells with small round to oval basaloid nuclei. **(c)** Same case as **(a)** and **(b)**, showing prominent perineural invasion. **(d)** Another case with extensive keratinizing squamous metaplasia centrally within tumor cell nests.

181

not in the squamous component; both components were diploid (Devaney, Dorman and Leader, 1991). PSA immunoreactivity was identified by Al Adani in two Iraqi patients with squamous cell carcinoma arising in association with schistosomiasis; PAP was negative (Al Adani, 1985).

The differential diagnosis of squamous cell carcinoma of the prostate includes squamous cell carcinoma of the bladder with prostatic invasion, squamous metaplasia due to infarction, radiation therapy and hormonal therapy, and prostatic adenocarcinoma with benign squamous metaplasia.

9.7 SARCOMATOID CARCINOMA (CARCINOSARCOMA; METAPLASTIC CARCINOMA)

Sarcomatoid carcinoma is considered by many to be synonymous with carcinosarcoma (Figure 9.11) (Wick *et al.*, 1989; Shannon *et al.*, 1992; Lauwers *et al.*, 1993; Dundore *et al.*, 1995). Authors who separate these tumors define sarcomatoid carcinoma as an epithelial tumor showing spindle cell (mesenchymal) differentiation and carcinosarcoma as adenocarcinoma intimately admixed with heterologous malignant soft tissue elements (Figure 9.11). Regardless of terminology, these tumors are rare.

Patients tend to be older men who present with symptoms of urinary outlet obstruction, similar to typical adenocarcinoma. Serum PSA concentration may be normal at the time of diagnosis (Dundore *et al.*, 1995). About half of patients have a prior history of typical acinar adenocarcinoma treated by radiation therapy or androgen deprivation therapy. Treatment is variable, and has no apparent influence on the poor prognosis.

Pathologically, the distinction between sarcomatoid carcinoma and carcinosarcoma is often difficult, and of no apparent clinical significance. However, metastases may consist of carcinoma and/or sarcoma, so careful search of the primary tumor is useful to identify a component of carcinoma. Coexistent adenocarcinoma is almost always high-grade (Gleason score 9 or 10). According to Dundore *et al.*, the most common soft tissue elements are osteosarcoma, with or without cartilaginous differentiation, and leiomyosarcoma (Dundore *et al.*, 1995). The epithelial component displays cytoplasmic immunoreactivity for keratin, PSA and PAP, similar to typical prostatic adenocarcinoma. The soft tissue component usually displays immunoreactivity for vimentin, with variable staining for desmin, actin and S-100 protein. Ultrastructurally, tumor cells within the sarcomatoid areas occasionally display desmosomes and filaments which apparently represent cytokeratin.

The differential diagnosis includes sarcoma, and this distinction may be difficult and clinically unimportant, although immunohistochemical stains and electron microscopy are helpful. Keratin immunoreactivity has been identified in some cases of leiomyosarcoma, so this finding alone may not be sufficient to determine epithelial differentiation (Chapter 12).

9.8 ADENOID CYSTIC CARCINOMA/BASAL CELL CARCINOMA

Adenoid cystic carcinoma/basal cell carcinoma (basal cell carcinoma; basaloid carcinoma; adenoid cystic carcinoma; adenoid cystic-like tumor; adenoid basal cell tumor) consists of basal cell nests of varying size infiltrating the stroma (Figure 9.12).

The malignant potential of adenoid cystic carcinoma/basal cell carcinoma is uncertain because of the small number of reported cases and limited follow-up, but some cases are malignant with extraprostatic extension and distant metastases. At present, adenoid cystic/basal cell carinoma is probably best considered a tumor of low malignant potential (Young *et al.*, 1988; Cohen *et al.*, 1993).

There are two architectural patterns of adenoid cystic carcinoma/basal cell carcinoma: adenoid cystic (Frankel, 1974;

Tannenbaum, 1975b; Kramer, Bredael and Krueger, 1978; Shond-San and Walters, 1984; Gilmour and Bell, 1986; Young *et al.*, 1988) and basaloid (Denholm *et al.*, 1992). The adenoid cystic pattern consists of irregular clusters of crowded basal cells punctated by rounded fenestrations, many of which contain mucinous material resembling salivary gland adenoid cystic carcinoma. The basaloid pattern consists of variably sized, rounded basaloid cell nests with prominent peripheral palisading. These patterns frequently coexist, although pure forms have been described.

Both patterns are histologically similar to basal cell hyperplasia and basal cell adenoma, but the tumor involves large areas of the prostate with little or no circumscription and often displays perineural invasion (Grignon *et al.*,1988; Deveraj and Bostwick, 1993). The basal cell nests are large and irregular, separated by benign myxoid stroma, and the tumor cells are predominately elongate, with narrow tapering nuclei. Cell crowding is prominent and the basal cell masses frequently display multiple lumens, some of which are round, sharply circumscribed and punched-out. Nucleoli are usually small and inconspicuous, similar to basal cell hyperplasia. Pale yellow amorphous material is present within the lumens in hematoxylin-and-eosin-stained sections. In limited samples such as TURP specimens, it may be difficult to separate basal cell adenomatosis and adenoid cystic carcinoma/basal cell carcinoma.

Adenoid cystic carcinoma/basal cell carcinoma displays variable immunoreactivity with keratin 34βE12; there may be luminal cell staining or peripheral basal cell staining (Grignon *et al.*, 1988; Deveraj and Bostwick, 1993). Rare scattered cells show PSA and PAP immunoreactivity, but these may represent entrapped residual secretory luminal cells (Kuhajda and Mann, 1984); other cells may show chromogranin staining. S-100 protein and NSE stains are negative. The amorphous luminal material is negative with all stains.

9.9 LYMPHOEPITHELIOMA-LIKE CARCINOMA

Carcinoma accompanied by a dense lymphocytic infiltrate is referred to as lymphoepithelioma-like carcinoma or medullary carcinoma (Figure 9.13).

This histologically distinctive tumor is most common in the head and neck region, although rare cases have been described in the breast, bladder and other sites. One case arising in the prostate was large and contained typical acinar and cribriform adenocarcinoma (Bostwick and Adlakha, 1994); about 50% was composed of nests of undifferentiated carcinoma surrounded by sheets of mature lymphocytes. The malignant cells had enlarged, vesicular, pleomorphic nuclei with prominent nucleoli; mitotic figures were numerous. The cytoplasm was eosinophilic with indistinct margins. Focal areas of necrosis and comedocarcinoma areas were present. The lymphocytic infiltrate was composed chiefly of T cells, like the lymphocytic response in lymphepithelioma-like carcinoma at other sites. No atypical lymphocytes were observed, and there were no features of malignant lymphoma or leukemia. There was extensive perineural and lymphatic invasion. The clinical significance of prostatic lymphoepithelioma-like carcinoma is uncertain.

9.10 CARCINOMA WITH ONCOCYTIC FEATURES

Prostatic adenocarcinoma rarely has diffuse oncocytic change, consisting of tumor cells with abundant eosinophilic granular cytoplasm which reflects the presence of abundant mitochondria (Beer, Occhionero and Welsch, 1990; Ordonez, Ro and Ayala, 1992; Pinto, Gonzalez and Granadillo, 1994). Tumor cells display PSA immunoreactivity. The clinical behavior appears to be the same as typical acinar adenocarcinoma. The differential diagnosis includes prostatic nodular hyperplasia with oncocytic change, neuroendocrine carcinoma and rhabdoid tumor.

183

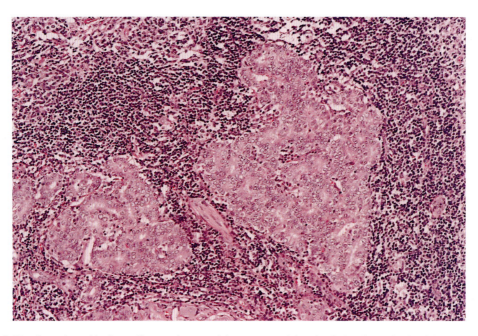

Figure 9.13 Lymphoepithelioma-like carcinoma of the prostate. Islands of closely packed acini are surrounded by a dense uniform infiltrate of mature lymphocytes. Epstein–Barr virus was not found.

9.11 COMEDOCARCINOMA

Comedocarcinoma is characterized by luminal necrosis within ducts expanded by malignant cells, similar to comedocarcinoma of the breast. This morphological variant of adenocarcinoma is included in the Gleason grading system as poorly differentiated (grade 5) carcinoma based on the degree of acinar differentiation. There is a high frequency of aneuploidy in comedocarcinoma, suggesting aggressiveness (Currin, Lee and Walther, 1988). PSA and PAP are present in the majority of tumor cells. Comedocarcinoma is invariably found in association with other patterns of adenocarcinoma, and probably does not warrant separation as a clinicopathological entity.

9.12 CRIBRIFORM CARCINOMA

The cribriform pattern is a histologically distinct variant of Gleason grade 3 carcinoma

which is characterized by large intraductal epithelial cell masses punctuated by multiple small lumens. Unlike cribriform PIN, cribriform carcinoma does not have a basal cell layer at the periphery of acini (McNeal *et al.*, 1986; Bostwick *et al.*, 1993; Montironi *et al.*, 1993; Amin, Schultz and Zarbo, 1994). In a series of 23 prostatectomies for cancer that contained cribriform acini, 55% of these acini were cribriform PIN rather than cribriform adenocarcinoma (Amin, Schultz and Zarbo, 1994). These results are similar to those of McNeal *et al.*, who found that up to 70% of cribriform masses were intraductal; however, they described this as 'cribriform carcinoma' and suggested that the cribriform pattern has the same biological behavior as Gleason pattern 4 adenocarcinoma (McNeal *et al.*, 1986). The association of cribriform PIN and Gleason pattern 4 carcinoma was not confirmed in another study of 60 totally sectioned prostatectomies (Bostwick *et al.*, 1993). The term 'cribriform carcinoma' is most commonly used as a descriptive term, if it is used at all, and does not refer to a specific histogenetic category of prostatic adenocarcinoma. The cribriform pattern is invariably found in association with other patterns of adenocarcinoma.

REFERENCES

Abbas, F., Civantos, F., Benedetto, P. and Soloway, M. S. (1995) Small cell carcinoma of the bladder and prostate. *Urology*, **46**, 617–630.

Abrahamsson, P. A., Wadstrom, L. B., Alumets, J. *et al.* (1986) Peptide-hormone- and serotonin-immunoreactive cells in normal and hyperplastic prostate glands. *Pathol. Res. Pract.*, **181**, 675–683.

Abrahamsson, P. A., Wadstrom, L. B., Alumets, J. *et al.* (1987) Peptide-hormone- and serotonin-immunoreactive tumour cells in carcinoma of the prostate. *Pathol. Res. Pract.*, **182**, 298–307.

Abrahamsson, P-A., Ptak, A., Nakada, S. Y. *et al.* (1993) Immunohistochemical localization of the androgen receptor in neuroendocrine cells in human prostatic tissue and prostatic carcinoma. *Mod. Pathol.*, **6**, 54A.

Adlakha, H. and Bostwick, D. G. (1994) Paneth cell-like change in prostatic adenocarcinoma represents neuroendocrine differentiation: report of 30 cases. *Hum. Pathol.*, **25**, 135–139.

Al Adani, M. S. (1985) Schistosomiasis, metaplasia and squamous cell carcinoma of the prostate: histogenesis of the squamous cells determined by localization of specific markers. *Neoplasma*, **32**, 613–622.

Alguacil-Garcia, A. (1986) Artifactual changes mimicking signet ring cell carcinoma in transurethral prostatectomy specimens. *Am. J. Surg. Pathol.*, **10**, 795–800.

Alline, K. M. and Cohen, M. B. (1992) Signet-ring cell carcinoma of the prostate. *Arch. Pathol. Lab. Med.*, **116**, 99–102.

Almagro, U. A., Tieu, T. M., Remeniuk, E. *et al.* (1986) Argyrophilic 'carcinoid-like' prostatic carcinoma. *Arch. Pathol. Lab. Med.*, **110**, 916–919.

Amin, M. B., Schultz, D. S. and Zarbo, R. J. (1994) Analysis of cribriform morphology in prostate neoplasia using antibody to high molecular weight cytokeratins. *Arch. Pathol. Lab. Med.*, **118**, 260–264.

Ansari, M. A., Pintozzi, R. L., Choi, Y. S. *et al.* (1981) Diagnosis of carcinoid-like metastatic prostatic carcinoma by an immunoperoxidase method. *Am. J. Clin. Pathol.*, **76**, 94–99.

Aprikian, A. G., Cordon-Cardo, C., Fair, W. R. and Reuter, V. E. (1993) Characterization of neuroendocrine differentiation in human benign prostate and prostatic adenocarcinoma. *Cancer*, **71**, 3952–3965.

August, C. Z. and Oyasu, R. (1983) Adenocarcinoma of the prostate gland. A spectrum of differentiation. *Arch. Pathol. Lab. Med.*, **107**, 501–502.

Aydin, F. (1993) Endometrioid adenocarcinoma of prostatic urethra presenting with anterior urethral implantation. *Urology*, **41**, 91–95.

Azumi, N., Shibuya, H. and Ishikura, M. (1984) Primary prostatic carcinoid tumor with intracytoplasmic prostatic acid phosphatase and prostate-specific antigen. *Am. J. Surg. Pathol.*, **8**, 545–551.

Barkin, J., Crassweller, P. O., Roncari, D. A. K. and Onrot, J. (1984) Hypercalcemia associated with cancer of prostate without any metastases. *Urology*, **24**, 368–379.

Beer, M., Occhionero, F., Welsch, U. (1990) Oncocytoma of the prostate: a case report with ultrastructural and immunohistochemical evaluation. *Histopathology*, **17**, 370–372.

Berner, A., Nesland, J. M., Waehre, H. *et al.* (1993) Hormone resistant prostatic adenocarcinoma. An evaluation of prognostic factors in pre- and post-treatment specimens. *Br. J. Cancer*, **68**, 380–384.

Bonkhoff, H., Wernert, N., Dhom, G. and Remberger, K. (1991) Relation of endocrine-paracrine cells to cell proliferation in normal, hyperplastic and neoplastic human prostate. *Prostate*, **19**, 91–98.

Bostwick, D. G. and Adlakha, K. (1994) Lympho-epithelioma-like carcinoma of the prostate. *J. Urol. Pathol.*, **2**, 319–325.

Bostwick, D. G., Kindrachuk, R. W. and Rouse, R. V. (1985) Prostatic adenocarcinoma with endometrioid features. *Am. J. Surg. Pathol.*, **9**, 595–609.

Bostwick, D. G., Wollan, P. and Adlakha, K. (1995) Collagenous micronodules in prostate cancer. A specific but infrequent diagnostic finding. *Arch. Pathol. Lab. Med.*, **119**, 444–447.

Bostwick, D. G., Amin, M. B., Dundore, P. *et al.* (1993) Architectural patterns of high grade prostatic intraepithelial neoplasia. *Hum. Pathol.*, **24**, 298–310.

Bostwick, D. G., Dousa, M. K., Crawford, B. G. and Wollan, P. C. (1994) Neuroendocrine differentiation in prostatic intraepithelial neoplasia and adenocarcinoma. *Am. J. Surg. Pathol.*, **18**, 1240–1246.

Cantrell, B. B., Leifer, G., DeKlerk, D. P. and Eggleston, J. C. (1981) Papillary adenocarcinoma of the prostatic urethra with clear-cell appearance. *Cancer*, **48**, 2661–2667.

Capella, C., Usellini, L. Buffa, R. *et al.* (1981) The endocrine component of prostatic carcinomas, mixed adenocarcinoma-carcinoid tumours of the prostate: histochemical and ultrastructural identification of the endocrine cells. *Histopathology*, **5**, 175–192.

Catton, P. A., Hartwick, R. W. J. and Srigley, J. R. (1992) Prostate cancer presenting with malignant ascites. Signet-ring cell variant of prostatic adenocarcinoma. *Urology*, **39**, 495–497.

Christenson, W. N., Steinberg, C., Walsh, P. C. and Epstein, J. I. (1991) Prostatic duct adenocarcinoma: findings at radical prostatectomy. *Cancer*, **67**, 2118–2124.

Cohen, R. J., Glezerson, G. and Haffejee, Z. (1991) Neuroendocrine cells. A new prognostic parameter in prostate cancer. *Br. J. Urol.*, **68**, 258–262.

Cohen, R. J., Glezerson, G. and Haffejee, Z. (1992) Prostate specific antigen and prostate specific acid phosphatase in neuroendocrine cells of prostate cancer. *Arch. Pathol. Lab. Med.*, **116**, 65–66.

Cohen, R. J., Glezerson, G., Haffejee, Z. and Afrika, D. (1990) Prostatic carcinoma: histological and immunohistological factors affecting prognosis. *Br. J. Urol.*, **66**, 405–410.

Cohen, R. J., Goldberg, R. D., Verhaart, M. J. and Cohen, M. (1993) Adenoid cyst-like carcinoma of the prostate. *Arch. Pathol. Lab. Med.*, **117**, 799–801.

Currin, S. M., Lee, S. E. and Walther, P. J. (1988) Flow cytometric analysis of comedocarcinoma of the prostate: an uncommon histopathological variant of prostatic adenocarcinoma. *J. Urol.*, **140**, 96–100.

Denholm, S. W., Webb, J. N., Howard, G. C. W. and Chisholm, G. D. (1992) Basaloid carcinoma of the prostate gland: histogenesis and review of the literature. *Histopathology*, **20**, 151–155.

Devaney, D. M., Dorman, A. and Leader, M. (1991) Adenosquamous carcinoma of the prostate: a case report. *Hum. Pathol.*, **22**, 1046–1050.

Devaraj, L. T. and Bostwick, D. G. (1993) Atypical basal cell hyperplasia of the prostate. Immunophenotypic profile and proposed classification of basal cell proliferations. *Am. J. Surg. Pathol.*, **17**, 645–659.

Di Sant' Agnese, P. A. (1992) Neuroendocrine differentiation in carcinoma of the prostate. Diagnostic, prognostic, and therapeutic implications. *Cancer*, **70**, 254–268.

Di Sant' Agnese, P. A. and de Mesy Jensen, K. L. (1984) Endocrine–paracrine cells of the prostate and prostatic urethra: an ultrastructural study. *Hum. Pathol.*, **15**, 1034–1041.

Dundore, P. A., Nascimento, A. G., Cheville, J. C. *et al.* (1995) Carcinosarcoma of the prostate. Report of 22 cases. *Cancer*, **76**, 1035–1042.

Efros, M. D., Fischer, J., Mallouh, C. *et al.* (1992) Unusual primary prostatic malignancies. *Urology*, **39**, 407–411.

Egan, A. J., Youngkin, T. P., Bostwick, D. G. (1996) Mixed carcinoid-adenocarcinoma of the prostate with spindle cell carcinoid: The spectrum of neuroendocrine differentiation in prostatic neoplasia. *Pathol. Case Rev.*, (in press).

Elbadawi, A., Graig, W., Linke, C. A. *et al.* (1979) Prostatic mucinous carcinoma. *Urology*, **13**, 658–659.

Epstein, J. I. and Fynheer, J. (1992) Acid mucin in the prostate: can it differentiate adenosis from adenocarcinoma? *Hum. Pathol.*, **23**, 1321–1325.

Epstein, J. I. and Lieberman, P. H. (1985) Mucinous adenocarcinoma of the prostate gland. *Am. J. Surg. Pathol.*, **9**, 299–308.

Epstein, J. I. and Woodruff, J. M. (1986) Adenocarcinoma of the prostate with endometrioid features: a light microscopic and immunohistochemical study of ten cases. *Cancer*, **57**, 111–119.

Ferguson, J. K., Sebo, T. A., Husmann, D. A. *et al.* (1995) Androgen receptor expression predicts survival in small cell carcinoma of the prostate. *J. Urol.*, **153**, 483A.

Frankel, K. C. Jr (1974) Adenoid cystic carcinoma of the prostate. Report of a case. *Am. J. Clin. Pathol.*, **62**, 639–645.

Franks, L. M., O'Shea, D. D. and Thompson, A. E. R. (1964) Mucin in the prostate. A histochemical study in normal glands, latent, clinical, and colloid carcinoma. *Cancer*, **17**, 983–991.

Frydman, C. P., Bleiweiss, I. J., Unger, P. D. *et al.* (1992) Paneth cell-like metaplasia of the prostate gland. *Arch. Pathol. Lab. Med.*, **116**, 274–276.

Gattuso, P., Carson, H. J., Candel, A. and Castelli, M. J. (1995) Adenosquamous carcinoma of the prostate. *Hum. Pathol.*, **26**, 123–126.

Ghali, V. S. and Gargia, R. L. (1984) Prostatic adenocarcinoma with carcinoidal features producing adrenocorticotropic syndrome. *Cancer*, **54**, 1042–1048.

Ghandur-Mnaynmah, L., Satterfield, S. and Block, N. L. (1986) Small cell carcinoma of the prostate gland with inappropriate antidiuretic hormone secretion: morphological, immunohistochemical, and clinical expressions. *J. Urol.*, **135**, 1263–1266.

Gilmour, A. M. and Bell, T. J. (1986) Adenoid cystic carcinoma of the prostate. *Br. J. Urol.*, **58**, 105–106.

Giltman, L. I. (1981) Signet ring cell adenocarcinoma of the prostate. *J. Urol.*, **126**, 134–135.

Goldstein, N., Qian, J. and Bostwick, D. G. (1995) Mucin expression in atypical adenomatous hyperplasia of the prostate. *Hum. Pathol.*, **26**, 887–891.

Gray, G. F. Jr and Marshall, V. F. (1975) Squamous carcinoma of the prostate. *J. Urol.*, **113**, 736–738.

Greene, L. F., Farrow, G. M., Ravits, J. M. and Tomera, K. M. (1979) Prostatic adenocarcinoma of ductal origin. *J. Urol.*, **121**, 303–305.

Grignon, D. J. and O'Malley, F. P. (1993) Mucinous metaplasia in the prostate gland. *Am. J. Surg. Pathol.*, **17**, 287–290.

Grignon, D. J., Ro, J. Y., Ordonez, N. G. *et al.* (1988) Basal cell hyperplasia, adenoid basal cell tumor, and adenoid cystic carcinoma of the prostate gland: an immunohistochemical study. *Hum. Pathol.*, **19**, 1425–1433.

Guerin, D., Hasan, N. and Keen, C. E. (1993) Signet ring cell differentiation in adenocarcinoma of the prostate: a study of five cases. *Histopathology*, **22**, 367–371.

Haratake, J., Akio, H. and Kenji, I. (1987) Argyrophilic adenocarcinoma of the prostate with Paneth cell-like granules. *Acta Pathol. Jpn.*, **37**, 831–836.

Hejka, A. G. and England, D. M. (1989) Signet ring cell carcinoma of prostate: immunohistochemical and ultrastructural study of a case. *Urology*, **24**, 155–158.

Hukill, P. B. and Vidone, R. A. (1967) Histochemistry of mucus and other polysaccharides in tumors II. Carcinoma of the prostate. *Lab. Invest.*, **16**, 395–406.

Humphrey, P. A. (1991) Mucin in severe dysplasia in the prostate. *Surg. Pathol.*, **4**, 137–143.

Ishizu, K., Yoshihiro, S., Joko, K. *et al.* (1991) Mucinous adenocarcinoma of the prostate with good response to hormonal therapy: a case report. *Acta Urol. Jpn.*, **37**, 1057–1059.

Kramer, S. A., Bredael, J. J. and Krueger, R. P. (1978) Adenoid cystic carcinoma of the prostate: report of a case. *J. Urol.*, **120**, 383–384.

Krogh, J. and Lund, P. G. (1988) Mucinous adenocarcinoma of the prostate presenting as a retrovesical cyst. *Scand. J. Urol. Nephrol.*, **22**, 235–236.

Kuhajda, F. P., Gipson, T. and Mendelsohn, G. (1984) Papillary adenocarcinomas of the prostate: an immunohistochemical study. *Cancer*, **54**, 1328–1332.

Kuhajda, F. P. and Mann, R. G. (1984) Adenoid cystic carcinoma of the prostate. A case report with immunoperoxidase staining for prostate-specific acid phosphatase and prostate-specific antigen. *Am. J. Clin. Pathol.*, **81**, 257–260.

Kums, J. J. and van Helsdingen, P. J. (1985) Signet-ring cell carcinoma of the bladder and the prostate. Report of 4 cases. *Urol. Int.*, **40**, 116–121.

Lauwers, G. Y., Schevchuk, M., Armenakas, N. and Reuter, V. E. (1993) Carcinosarcoma of the prostate. *Am. J. Surg. Pathol.*, **17**, 342–349.

Lee, S. S. (1994) Endometrioid adenocarcinoma of the prostate. A clinicopathologic and immunohistochemical study. *J. Surg. Oncol.*, **55**, 235–238.

Little, N. A., Wiener, J. S., Walther, P. J. *et al.* (1993) Squamous cell carcinoma of the prostate: 2 cases of a rare malignancy and review of the literature. *J. Urol.*, **149**, 137–139.

McNeal, J. E., Reese, J. H., Redwine, E. A. *et al.* (1986) Cribriform adenocarcinoma of the prostate. *Cancer*, **58**, 1714–1719.

McNeal, J. E., Alroy, J., Villers, A. *et al.* (1991) Mucinous differentiation in prostatic adenocarcinoma. *Hum. Pathol.*, **22**, 979–988.

Mahadevia, P. S., Ramaswamy, A., Greenwald, E. S. *et al.* (1983) Hypercalcemia in prostatic carcinoma. Report of eight cases. *Arch. Intern. Med.*, **143**, 1339–1342.

Melicow, M. M. and Pachter, M. R. (1967) Endometrial carcinoma of prostatic utricle (uterus masculinus). *Cancer*, **20**, 1715–1721.

Miller, V. A., Reuter, V. and Scher, H. I. (1995) Primary squamous cell carcinoma of the prostate after radiation seed implantation for adenocarcinoma. *Urology*, **46**, 111–113.

Montironi, R., Santinelli, A., Galluzzi, C. M. and Giannulis, I. (1993) Proliferating cell nuclear antigen (PCNA) evaluation in the diagnostic quantitative pathology of cribriform adenocarcinoma of the prostate. *In Vivo*, **7**, 343–346.

Moore, S. R., Reinberg, Y. and Zhang, G. (1992) Small cell carcinoma of prostate: effectiveness of hormonal versus chemotherapy. *Urology*, **39**, 411–416.

Moskovitz, N., Munichor, M., Bolkier, M. and Livne, P. M. (1993) Squamous cell carcinoma of the prostate. *Urol. Int.*, **51**, 181–183.

Mott, L. J. M. (1979) Squamous cell carcinoma of the prostate. Report of 2 cases and review of the literature. *J. Urol.*, **121**, 833–836.

Moyana, T. N. (1987) Adenosquamous carcinoma of the prostate. *Am. J. Surg. Pathol.*, **11**, 402–407.

Odom, D. G., Donatucci, C. F. and Dedshon, G. E. (1986) Mucinous adenocarcinoma of the prostate. *Hum. Pathol.*, **17**, 863–868.

Oesterling, J. E., Hauzear, C. G. and Farrow, G. M. (1992) Small cell anaplastic carcinoma of the prostate: a clinical, pathological and immunohistological study of 27 patients. *J. Urol.*, **147**, 804–809.

Ordonez, N. G., Ro, J. Y. and Ayala, A. G. (1992) Metastatic prostatic carcinoma presenting as an oncocytic tumor. *Am. J. Surg. Pathol.*, **16**, 1007–1012.

Pinder, S. E. and McMahon, R. F. T. (1990) Mucins in prostatic carcinoma. *Histopathology*, **16**, 43–46.

Pinto, J. A., Gonzalez, J. E. and Granadillo, M. A. (1994) Primary carcinoma of the prostate with diffuse oncocytic changes. *Histopathology*, **25**, 286–288.

187

Proia, A. D., McCarty, S. and Woodard, B. H. (1981) Prostatic mucinous adenocarcinoma. *Am. J. Surg. Pathol.*, **5**, 701–706.

Remmele, W., Weber, A. and Harding, P. (1988) Primary signet-ring cell carcinoma of the prostate. *Hum. Pathol.*, **19**, 478–480.

Ro, J. Y., Tetu, B., Ayala, A. G. *et al.* (1987a) Small cell carcinoma of the prostate: immunohistochemical and electron microscopic studies of 18 cases. *Cancer* **59**, 977–984.

Ro, J. Y., Tetu, B., Ayala, A. G. *et al.* (1987b) Small cell carcinoma of the prostate: II. Immunohistochemical and electron microscopic studies of 18 cases. *Cancer*, **59**, 977–982.

Ro, J. Y., Ayala, A. G., Wishow, K. I. *et al.* (1988a) Prostatic duct adenocarcinoma with endometrioid features: immunohistochemical and electron microscopic study. *Sem. Diag. Pathol.*, **5**, 301–311.

Ro, J. Y., El-Naggar, A., Ayala, A. G. *et al.* (1988b) Signet-ring-cell carcinoma of the prostate. *Am. J. Surg. Pathol.*, **12**, 453–460.

Ro, J. Y., Grignon, D. J., Troncoso, P. and Ayala, A. G. (1988c) Mucin in prostatic adenocarcinoma. *Sem. Diag. Pathol.*, **5**, 273–283.

Ro, J. Y., Grignon, D. J., Ayala, A. G. *et al.* (1989) Mucinous adenocarcinoma of the prostate gland. *J. Urol.*, **141**, 1447–1451.

Ro, J. Y., Grignon, D. J., Ayala, A. G. *et al.* (1990) Mucinous adenocarcinoma of the prostate: histochemical and immunohistochemical studies. *Hum. Pathol.*, **21**, 593–600.

Saito, R., Davis, B. K. and Ollipally, E. P. (1984) Adenosquamous carcinoma of the prostate. *Hum. Pathol.*, **15**, 87–89.

Sarma, D. P., Weilbaecher, T. G. and Moon, T. D. (1991) Squamous cell carcinoma of prostate. *Urology*, **37**, 260–262.

Schron, D. S., Gipson, T. and Mendelsohn, G. (1984) The histogenesis of small cell carcinoma of the prostate. *Cancer*, **53**, 2478–2480.

Segawa, T. and Kakehi, Y. (1993) Primary signet ring cell adenocarcinoma of the prostate: a case report and literature review. *Acta Urol. Jpn.*, **39**, 565–568.

Shannon, R. L., Ro, J. Y., Grignon, D. J. *et al.* (1992) Sarcomatoid carcinoma of the prostate. A clinicopathologic study of 12 cases. *Cancer*, **69**, 2676–2682.

Sharma, S. K., Malik, K. A. K. and Bapna, B. C. (1980) Squamous cell carcinoma of prostate. *Indian J. Cancer*, **17**, 134–135.

Shond-San, C. and Walters, M. N. I. (1984) Adenoid cystic carcinoma of prostate. Report of a case. *Pathology*, **16**, 337–338.

Smith, C., Feddersen, R. M., Dressler, L. *et al.* (1994) Signet ring cell adenocarcinoma of prostate. *Urology*, **43**, 397–400.

Stratton, M., Evans, D. J. and Lampert, I. A. (1986) Prostatic adenocarcinoma evolving into carcinoid: selective effect of hormonal treatment? *J. Clin. Pathol.*, **39**, 750–756.

Sufrin, G., Gaeta, J., Staubitz, W. J. *et al.* (1986) Endometrial carcinoma of prostate. *Urology*, **27**, 18–23.

Tannenbaum, M. (1975a) Endometrial tumors and or associated carcinomas of prostate. *Urology*, **6**, 372–375.

Tannenbaum, M. (1975b) Adenoid cystic or 'salivary gland' carcinomas of prostate. *Urology*, **6**, 2338–2339.

Taylor, N. S. (1979) Histochemistry in the diagnosis of early prostatic carcinoma. *Hum. Pathol.*, **10**, 513–520.

Teichman, J. M. H., Shabaik, A. and Demby, A. M. (1994) Mucinous adenocarcinoma of the prostate and hormone sensitivity. *J. Urol.*, **151**, 701–702.

Tetu, B., Ro, J. Y., Ayala, A. G. *et al.* (1987) Small cell carcinoma of the prostate. I. A clinicopathologic study of 20 cases. *Cancer*, **59**, 1803–1809.

Tetu, B., Ro, J. Y., Ayala, A. G. *et al.* (1989) Small cell carcinoma of prostate associated with myasthenic (Eaton–Lambert) syndrome. *Urology*, **33**, 148–152.

Turbat-Herrera, E. A., Herrera, G. A., Gore, I. *et al.* (1988) Neuroendocrine differentiation in prostatic carcinomas: a retrospective autopsy study. *Arch. Pathol. Lab. Med.*, **112**, 1100–1106.

Uchijima, Y., Ito, H., Takahashi, M. and Yamashina, M. (1990) Prostate mucinous adenocarcinoma with signet ring cell. *Urology*, **36**, 267–268.

Van de Voorde, W., Poppel, H. V., Haustermans, K. *et al.* (1994) Mucin-secreting adenocarcinoma of the prostate with neuroendocrine differentiation and paneth-like cells. *Am. J. Surg. Pathol.*, **18**, 200–207.

Walter, A. N., Mills, S. E., Fechner, R. E. and Perry, J. M. (1982) 'Endometrial' adenocarcinoma of the prostatic urethra arising in a villous polyp. A light microscopic and immunoperoxidase study. *Arch. Pathol. Lab. Med.*, **106**, 624–627.

Walther, M. M., Massar, V., Harruff, H. C. *et al.* (1985) Endometrial carcinoma of the prostatic utricle: a tumor of prostatic origin. *J. Urol.*, **134**, 769–773.

Wasserstein, P. W. and Goldman, R. L. (1979) Primary carcinoid of prostate. *Urology*, **13**, 318–320.

Weaver, M. G., Fadi, W. and Abdul-Karim Srigley, J. R. (1992) Paneth cell-like change and small cell carcinoma of the prostate. Two divergent forms of prostatic neuroendocrine differentiation. *Am. J. Surg. Pathol.*, **16**, 1013–1106.

Weaver, M. G., Fadi, W., Abdul-Karim Srigley, J. *et al.* (1992) Paneth cell-like change of the prostate gland: a histological immunohistochemical and electron microscopic study. *Am. J. Surg. Pathol.*, **16**, 62–68.

Wenk, R. E., Bhagavan, B. S., Levy, R. *et al.* (1977) Ectopic ACTH, prostatic oat cell carcinoma, and marked hypernatremia. *Cancer*, **40**, 773–778.

Wernert, N., Luchtrath, H., Seeliger, H. *et al.* (1987) Papillary carcinoma of the prostate, location, morphology, and immunohistochemistry: the histogenesis and entity of so-called endometrioid carcinoma. *Prostate*, **10**, 123–132.

Wernert, N., Goebbels, R., Bonkhoff, H. and Dhom, G. (1990) Squamous cell carcinoma of the prostate. *Histopathology*, **17**, 339–344.

Wick, M. R., Young, R. H., Malvesta, R. *et al.* (1989) Prostatic carcinosarcomas: clinical, histologic, and immunohistochemical data on two cases, with a review of the literature. *Am. J. Clin. Pathol.*, **92**, 131–139.

Witters, S., Moerman, P., Bussche, L. V. *et al.* (1986) Papillary adenocarcinoma of the prostatic urethra. *Eur. Urol.*, **12**, 143–146.

Wright, C., Grignon, D., Shum, D. and Porter, A. (1992) Neuroendocrine differentiation in prostatic adenocarcinoma is not an independent prognostic indicator. *Mod. Pathol.*, **5**, 61A.

Young, R. H., Frierson, H. F., Mills, S. E. *et al.* (1988) Adenoid cystic-like tumor of the prostate gland. A report of two cases and review of the literature on 'adenoid cystic carcinoma' of the prostate. *Am. J. Clin. Pathol.*, **89**, 49–56.

Zaloudek, C., Williams, J. W. and Kempson, R. L. (1976) 'Endometrial' adenocarcinoma of the prostate. A distinctive tumor of probable prostatic duct origin. *Cancer*, **37**, 2255–2262.

10

TREATMENT EFFECTS

The histological changes in adenocarcinoma following therapy such as androgen deprivation or radiation therapy often present a significant diagnostic challenge, particularly in biopsy specimens. The clinical history is invaluable in such cases.

10.1 ANDROGEN DEPRIVATION THERAPY

The use of androgen deprivation therapy for prostate cancer is expected to increase with the recent introduction of new agents such as the 5-alpha-reductase inhibitor finasteride and bicalutamide; other approved agents continue to be popular for selected patients, including estrogen (diethylstilbesterol), leuprolide and flutamide. Androgen deprivation is used for preoperative tumor shrinkage and treatment of prostatic hyperplasia, and may be effective for cancer prophylaxis, although this remains speculative. Androgen deprivation of normal, hyperplastic and dysplastic epithelial cells causes acceleration of programmed cell death of single cells (apoptosis), with fragmentation of tumor DNA, emergence of apoptotic bodies and inhibition of cell growth (Kyprianou, English and Isaacs, 1990).

Characteristic involutional changes occur in the prostate after androgen deprivation therapy (Figures 10.1 and 10.2; Table 10.1).

Benign acini show marked lobular and acinar atrophy, epithelial vacuolation, basal cell hyperplasia, squamous metaplasia, transitional metaplasia and acinar rupture with extravasation of secretions (Tetu *et al.*, 1991). Androgen deprivation therapy also causes a marked reduction in the presence and extent of high-grade prostatic intraepithelial neoplasia (Ferguson *et al.*, 1994). Cancer shows an increase in Gleason grade and a substantial reduction in nuclear and nucleolar size, accompanied by prominent cytoplasmic clearing (Schmeller *et al.*, 1986; Böcking and Auffermann, 1987; Murphy, Soloway and Barrows, 1991; Tetu *et al.*, 1991; Ellison *et al.*, 1996; Hellström *et al.*, 1993; Armas *et al.*, 1994; Montironi *et al.*, 1994; Smith and Murphy, 1994; Civantos *et al.*, 1995). These changes are rarely seen in benign acini and untreated carcinoma, and the combination of features following therapy is sufficiently distinctive to allow recognition of this morphological change. It is important to be aware of these changes because of the reliance typically placed on nuclear and nucleolar size in the diagnosis of prostatic adenocarcinoma, particularly in small specimens and lymph node metastases. The mechanism of action varies among the different androgen deprivation agents, so comparative studies are needed to assess subtle differences beyond those recognized to date and to define the biological significance of these changes.

Androgen deprivation therapy causes an apparent increase in the Gleason grade of the tumor, which is accompanied by nuclear size reduction, loss of recognizable nucleoli, chromatin condensation, nuclear pyknosis and cytoplasmic vacuolation ('nucleolus-poor clear cell adenocarcinoma') (Schmeller *et al.*, 1986; Böcking and Auffermann, 1987; Murphy, Soloway and Barrows, 1991; Tetu *et al.*, 1991; Ellison *et al.*, 1996; Hellström *et al.*, 1993; Armas *et al.*, 1994; Smith and Murphy, 1994; Montironi *et al.*, 1994; Civantos *et al.*, 1995). This 'uncoupling' of the architectural and cytological pattern is vexing on account of the presence of small shrunken nuclei within malignant acini particularly in lymph nodes submitted for frozen section evaluation. One expert has dubbed androgen-deprivation changes in prostate cancer 'the new nightmare' in biopsy interpretation (D. Grignon, personal communication, 1994). Grading systems have been proposed for therapy-induced adenocarcinoma regression, chiefly by German investigators, but have not been adopted by others (Schmeller *et al.*, 1986; Böcking *et al.*, 1987). Armas *et al.* consider grading after therapy to be potentially misleading and recommend against it (Armas *et al.*, 1994).

Immunohistochemical studies for PSA, PAP and basal-cell-specific keratin 34βE12 are useful in identifying carcinoma following therapy. PSA and PAP are retained in tumor cells after therapy and keratin 34βE12 remains negative, indicating an absent basal cell layer. No differences are found in expression of neuroendocrine differentiation markers such as chromogranin, neuron-specific enolase,

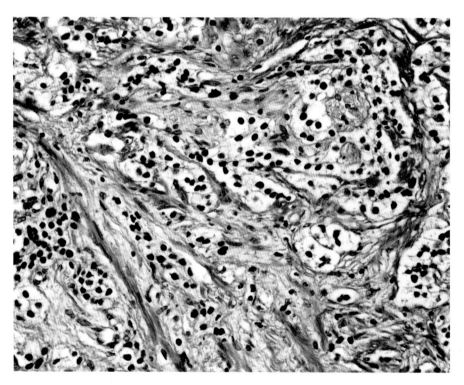

(a)

Figure 10.1 Androgen deprivation effect. **(a)** Irregular linear arrays of malignant acini contain cells with abundant clear cytoplasm and shrunken hyperchromatic nuclei.

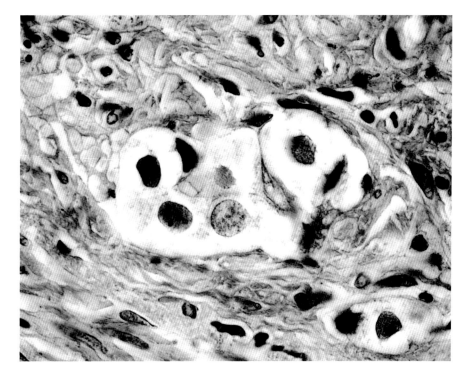

(b)

Figure 10.1   **(b)** Tumor cell nuclei often lack nucleolomegaly and distinct cell margins, apparently floating in abundant clear cytoplasm.

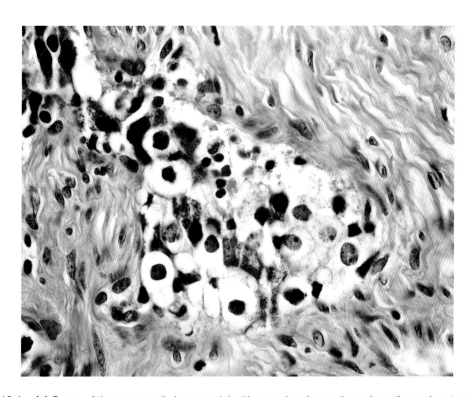

(c)

Figure 10.1   **(c)** Some of the tumor cells have nuclei with granular chromatin and small prominent nucleoli.

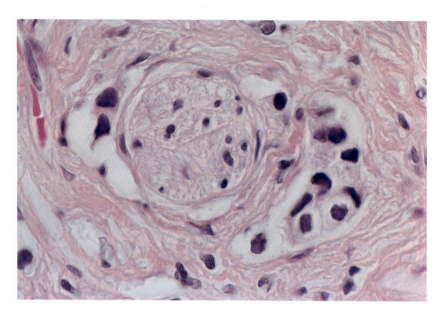

(d)

Figure 10.1   **(d)** Perineural invasion may be mistaken for stromal lymphocytes or myocytes.

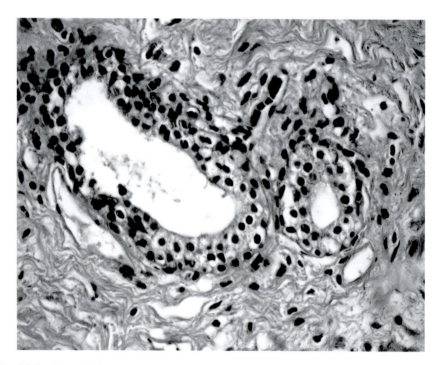

(e)

Figure 10.1   **(e)** Benign acini have cytological changes similar to malignant acini, including nuclear shrinkage and small dark nuclei.

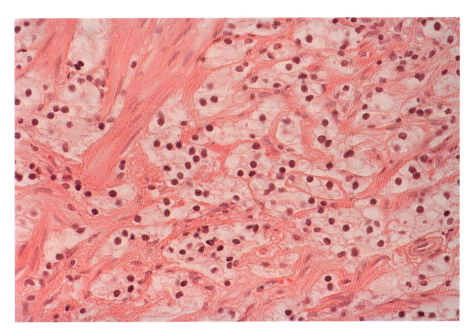

Figure 10.2 Androgen deprivation therapy in prostatic adenocarcinoma reveals prominent cytoplasmic clearing and small hyperchromatic nuclei.

Table 10.1 Androgen deprivation therapy: histological features in the prostate (these changes affect benign, hyperplastic, and neoplastic epithelium; there is some variability depending on the method of therapy)

Architecture
- Prominent acinar atrophy
- Decreased ratio of acini to stroma
- Basal cell hyperplasia in benign epithelium
- Foci of epithelial hyperplasia
- Stromal edema in early stages; fibrosis in late stages
- Squamous metaplasia
- Decrease in extent of PIN

Cytology
- Prominent clear cell change
- Nuclear shrinkage
- Nuclear hyperchromasia
- Nucleolar shrinkage

B-hCG and serotonin. Proliferative activity according to proliferating cell nuclear antigen (PCNA) immunoreactivity falls after androgen deprivation therapy (Armas *et al.*, 1994).

The differential diagnosis of carcinoma following androgen deprivation therapy includes a variety of atrophic and hyperplastic changes in benign acini, including clear cell cribriform hyperplasia, sclerosing adenosis, acinar atrophy, atypical adenomatous hyperplasia and atypical basal cell hyperplasia (Table 10.2).

Significant difficulty may also be encountered in separating minute clusters and single file ribbons of tumor cells after androgen deprivation from lymphocytes, myocytes and fibroblasts. Low-power scanning may fail to identify tumor because of the deceptively benign-appearing cytoplasm and nuclei after therapy.

10.2 RADIATION THERAPY

For about 12 months after irradiation, needle biopsy is of limited value because of the delayed manifestation of tumor cell death (Table 10.3) (Bostwick, Egbert and Fajardo, 1982).

195

Table 10.2 Adenocarcinoma following androgen deprivation therapy: differential diagnosis and distinguishing features

	Lobular configuration	Large nucleoli	Clear cell change in benign glands	Keratin 34βE12 immunoreactivity	Other features
Adenocarcinoma following androgen deprivation therapy	-	±	+	-	History of androgen deprivation therapy; usually Gleason primary grade 4
Clear cell cribriform hyperplasia	+	-	+	±	Occurs in transition zone with nodular hyperplasia; benign
Atypical basal cell hyperplasia	+	+	-	+	Occurs in transition zone with nodular hyperplasia; benign
Sclerosing adenosis	+	-	-	+	Occurs in transition zone with nodular hyperplasia; S-100-protein-and actin-positive; benign
Glandular atrophy	+	-	-	+	Occurs in all zones; benign
Atypical adenomatous hyperplasia (AAH)	+	±	±	±*	Occurs in transition zone with nodular hyperplasia; considered benign
Clear cell adenocarcinoma of transition zone	-	+	-	-	Occurs in transition zone with nodular hyperplasia; usually Gleason primary pattern 1, 2, or 3

± may or may not be present

* basal cell layer is fragmented and discontinuous

After this period, however, biopsy is the best method for assessing local tumor control, with a low level of sampling error that is minimized by obtaining multiple specimens (Bostwick, Egbert and Fajardo, 1982; Brawer and Bostwick, 1990; Dugan *et al.*, 1991; Helpap and Koch, 1991; Kabalin, 1992; Siders and Lee, 1992; Wheeler, Zagars and Ayala, 1993). Histopathological changes of radiation injury in the prostate include acinar atrophy, shrinkage, and distortion, marked cytological abnormalities of the epithelium, basal cell hyperplasia, stromal fibrosis and decreased ratio of acini to stroma (Figures 10.3 and 10.4). Vascular sclerosis is also prominent, and may involve small and large vessels.

No definitive method exists for assessment of tumor viability after irradiation. PAP expression usually persists, suggesting to one author that tumor cells capable of protein production probably retain the potential for cell division and consequent metastatic spread (Mahon *et al.*, 1980). PSA and keratin 34βE12 expression also persist after radiation therapy

and are often of value in separating treated adenocarcinoma and some of its mimics. Other reports claim that if prostatic carcinoma is not histologically ablated by radiotherapy after 12 months it is probably biologically active (Bostwick, Egbert and Fajardo, 1982; Helpap and Koch, 1991; Siders and Lee, 1992).

Cancer grading after radiation therapy has yielded conflicting results, with some observers noting no difference from pretherapy grade and others finding a substantial increase in grade (Bostwick, Egbert and Fajardo, 1982; Siders and Lee, 1992; Wheeler *et al.*, 1993). There may also be a shift toward aneuploid DNA content in up to 31% of pretreatment diploid tumors, indicating increasing histological and biological tumor aggressiveness (Siders and Lee, 1992). Despite conflicting results, some investigators recommend grading of specimens after therapy, recognizing that the biological significance of grade may be different than in untreated cancer.

Table 10.3 Radiation therapy: histological features

Architecture
- Prominent acinar atrophy and distortion
- Decrease in ratio of acini to stroma
- Basal cell hyperplasia in benign epithelium
- Squamous and squamoid metaplasia
- Foci of epithelial hyperplasia
- Stromal fibrosis with smooth muscle atrophy
- Decrease in extent of PIN

Cytology
- Nuclear hyperchromasia
- Marked variation in nuclear size and shape
- High nucleus:cytoplasmic ratio
- Variable nucleolar enlargement
- Decreased secretory activity of cells

Other
- Vascular myointimal proliferation
- Phlebosclerosis
- Seminal vesicle atrophy and fibrosis (pigment persists)
- Acute and chronic inflammation which regresses

10.3 ULTRASOUND HYPERTHERMIA, MICROWAVE HYPERTHERMIA AND LASER THERAPY

All forms of hyperthermia for nodular hyperplasia result in sharply circumscribed hemorrhagic coagulative necrosis that soon organizes with granulation tissue; the pattern and extent of injury is determined by the method of thermocoagulation employed, the duration of treatment, tissue perfusion factors and the ratio of epithelium to stroma in the tissue being treated (Figures 10.5 and 10.6) (Susani *et al.*, 1993; Orihuela *et al.*, 1995). Transurethral methods may be safer and more effective than transrectal methods because they appear to avoid injury to the rectal mucosa.

When delivered transurethrally, laser thermocoagulation and microwave hyperthermia do not usually involve the peripheral zone or neighboring structures, presumably

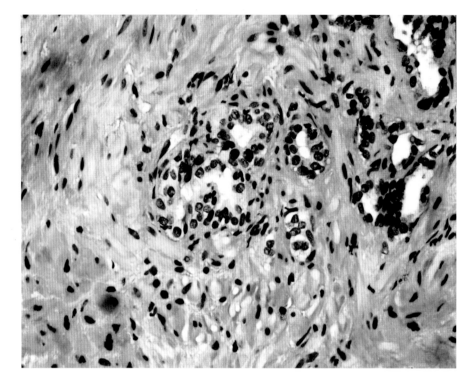

(a)

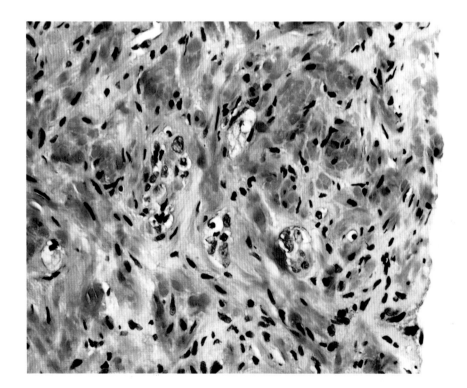

(b)

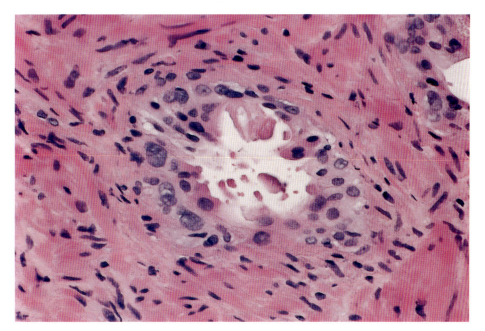

(c)

Figure 10.3 Radiation effect. **(a)** Benign acini with moderate changes of radiation, including acinar distortion, atrophy and nuclear shrinkage and hyperchromasia. **(b)** Benign acini 18 months after external beam radiation therapy, consisting of small irregular pale-staining cellular aggregates without lumens which were initially mistaken for adenocarcinoma; immunohistochemical stains for high-molecular-weight keratin revealed an intact basal cell layer (not shown). **(c)** Benign acinus with marked variation in size, shape and spacing of nuclei, often with prominent nucleoli, which may be mistaken for malignancy.

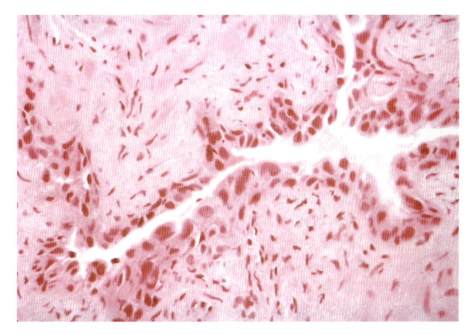

Figure 10.4 Radiation change of the prostatic epithelium mimicking high-grade PIN. There are marked nuclear abnormalities, including variation in size and shape and hyperchromasia.

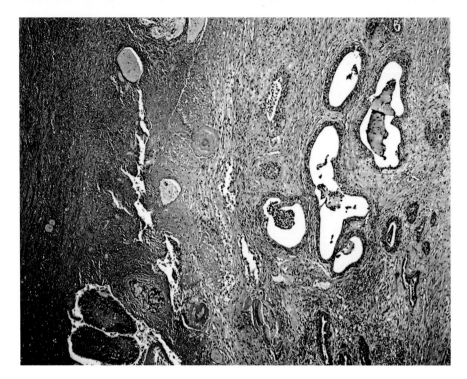

Figure 10.5 Laser treatment effect. The boundary is narrow between devitalized tissue with hemorrhagic necrosis (left) and viable but acutely inflamed tissue (right). These changes are identical to those seen at the edge of treatment effect with all forms of hyperthermia or cryotherapy.

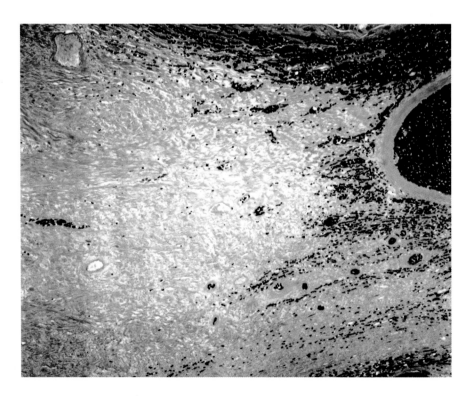

(a)

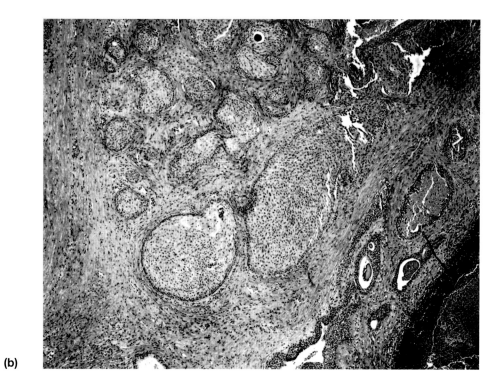

(b)

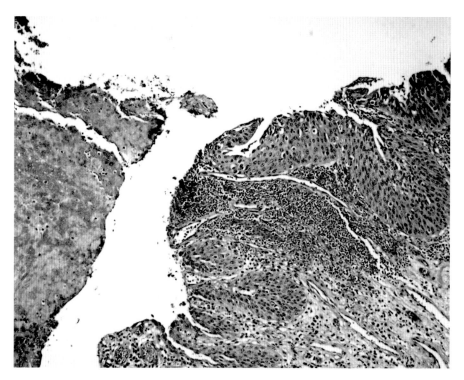

(c)

Figure 10.6 Transurethral microwave hyperthermia treatment effect. **(a)** Devitalized tissue persists as shadows of mummified pale cells; note red blood cells on edge which indicate hemorrhagic necrosis. **(b)** Basal cell hyperplasia in viable tissue after hyperthermia treatment. **(c)** The prostatic urothelium is partially preserved but inflamed (right); note necrotic tissue (left).

because of differences in tissue perfusion (Bostwick and Larson, 1995; Orihuela *et al.*, 1995). Coagulation necrosis is greater in areas of predominantly epithelial nodular hyperplasia than in predominantly stromal hyperplasia and the dense fibromuscular tissue of the bladder neck. Confluent coagulation necrosis occurs when multiple laser lesions are created in a single transverse plane.

10.4 CRYOABLATION THERAPY (CRYOSURGERY)

Cryosurgical ablation refers to freezing of the prostate. Multiple cryoprobe needles filled with circulating liquid nitrogen transform the prostate into an iceball, resulting in substantial tissue destruction and death of benign and malignant cells. The flow of liquid nitrogen through the probes is adjusted to create the desired freezing pattern and extent of tissue destruction in the prostate; no liquid nitrogen comes in contact with the tissue. Preliminary results with cryoablation for prostate cancer are encouraging, but the method is still considered difficult, experimental and of unproven value.

Following cryosurgery, the prostate shows typical features of repair, including marked stromal fibrosis and hyalinization, basal cell hyperplasia with ductal and acinar regeneration, squamous metaplasia, and stromal hemorrhage and hemosiderin deposition (Hansen and Wanstrup, 1973; Petersen *et al.*, 1978;

Table 10.4 Cryoablation therapy: histological features (source: data from Shabiak *et al.*, 1995)

- Stromal fibrosis and hyalinization
- Basal cell hyperplasia
- Squamous metaplasia
- Stromal hemorrhage
- Hemosiderin deposition
- Chronic inflammation
- Focal coagulative necrosis
- Dystrophic calcification
- Residual or recurrent carcinoma (grade unchanged)

Shabaik *et al.*, 1995; Borokowski *et al.*, 1996) (Table 10.4).

Coagulative necrosis is present between 6 and 30 weeks of therapy, but patchy chronic inflammation is more common. Focal granulomatous inflammation is associated with epithelial disruption due to corpora amylacea. Dystrophic calcification is infrequent, and usually appears in areas with the greatest reparative response. Atypia and PIN are not seen in areas that otherwise show changes of postcryoablation therapy. Biopsy after cryosurgery may reveal no evidence of recurrent or residual carcinoma; in other cases, the tumor appears unchanged, with no change in grade or definite evidence of immune response.

10.5 PHYTOTHERAPY

Phytotherapy refers to the use of plant extracts for treatment of nodular hyperplasia. This therapy is popular in Germany and other countries, and has been shown to improve micturition and urinary flow rate. The use of *Sabal* extract, one type of phytotherapy, reduces stromal edema, mucoid degeneration and intraglandular congestion in the setting of nodular hyperplasia but has no influence on benign or neoplastic epithelium (Helpap *et al.*, 1995).

REFERENCES

Armas, O. A., Aprikian, A. G., Melamed, J. *et al.* (1994) Clinical and pathobiological effects of neoadjuvant total androgen ablation therapy on clinically localized prostatic adenocarcinoma. *Am. J. Surg. Pathol.*, **18**, 979–991.

Böcking, A. and Auffermann, W. (1987) Cytological grading of therapy-induced tumor regression in prostatic carcinoma: proposal of a new system. *Diag. Cytopathol.*, **3**, 108–111.

Borkowski, P., Robinson, M. J., Poppiti, R. J., Jr and Nash, S. C. (1996) Histologic findings in postcryosurgical prostatic biopsies. *Mod. Pathol.*, **9**, 807–811.

Bostwick, D. G., Egbert, B. M. and Fajardo, L. F. (1982) Radiation injury of the normal and neoplastic prostate. *Am. J. Surg. Pathol*, **6**, 541–548.

Bostwick, D. G. and Larson, T. (1995) Transurethral microwave thermal therapy: pathologic findings in the canine prostate. *Prostate*, **26**, 116–122.

Brawer, M. K. and Bostwick, D. G. (1990) Interpretation of postradiation prostate biopsies, in *Pathology of the Prostate*, (ed. D. G. Bostwick), Churchill Livingstone, New York, pp. 193–205.

Civantos, F., Marcial, M. A., Banks, E. R. *et al.* (1995) Pathology of androgen deprivation therapy in prostatic carcinoma. A comparative study of 173 patients. *Cancer*, **75**, 1634–1641.

Dugan, T. C., Shipley, W. U., Young, R. H. *et al.* (1991) Biopsy after external beam radiation therapy for adenocarcinoma of the prostate: correlation with original histological grade and current prostate specific antigens levels. *J. Urol.*, **146**, 1313–1316.

Ellison, E., Chuang, S.-S., Zincke, H. *et al.* (1996) Prostate adenocarcinoma after androgen deprivation therapy: a comparative study of morphology, morphometry, immunohistochemistry, and DNA ploidy. *Pathol. Case Rev.*, (in press).

Ferguson, J., Zincke, H., Ellison, E. *et al.* (1994) Decrease of prostatic intraepithelial neoplasia (PIN) following androgen deprivation therapy in patients with stage T3 carcinoma treated by radical prostatectomy. *Urology*, **44**, 91–95.

Hansen, R. I. and Wanstrup, J. (1973) Cryoprostatectomy. Histological changes elucidated by serial biopsies. *Scand. J. Urol. Nephrol.*, **7**, 100–104.

Hellström, M., Häggman, M., Brändstedt, S. *et al.* (1993) Histopathological changes in androgen-deprived localized prostatic cancer. A study in total prostatectomy specimens. *Eur. Urol.*, **24**, 461–465.

Helpap, B. and Koch, V. (1991) Histological and immunohistochemical findings of prostatic carcinoma after external or interstitial radiotherapy. *J. Cancer Res. Clin. Oncol.*, **117**, 608–614.

Helpap, B., Oehler, U., Weisser, H. *et al.* (1995) Morphology of benign prostatic hyperplasia after treatment with Sabal Extract IDS89 or placebo. Results of a prospective, randomized, double-blind trial. *J. Urol. Pathol.*, **3**, 175–182.

Kabalin, J. N. (1992) Biopsy after external beam radiation therapy for adenocarcinoma of the prostate: correlation with original histological grade and current prostate specific antigen levels. *J. Urol.*, **148**, 1565–1566.

Kyprianou, N., English, H. and Isaacs, J. T. (1990) Programmed cell death during regression of

PC-82 human prostate cancer following androgen ablation. *Cancer Res.*, **50**, 3748–3753.

Mahan, D. E., Bruce, A. W., Manley, P. N. and Franchi. L. (1980) Immunohistochemical evaluation of prostatic carcinoma before and after radiotherapy. *J. Urol.*, **124**, 488–492.

Montironi, R., Magi Galluzzi, C., Muzzonigro, G. *et al.* (1994) Effects of combination endocrine treatment on normal prostate, prostatic intraepithelial neoplasia, and prostatic adenocarcinoma. *J. Clin. Pathol.*, **47**, 906–913.

Murphy, W. M., Soloway, M. S. and Barrows, G. H. (1991) Pathologic changes associated with androgen deprivation therapy for prostate cancer. *Cancer* **68**, 821–828.

Orihuela, E., Motamedi, M., Pow-Sang, M. *et al.* (1995) Histopathological evaluation of laser thermocoagulation in the human prostate: optimization of laser irradiation for benign prostatic hyperplasia. *J. Urol.*, **153**, 1531–1536.

Petersen, D. S., Milleman, L. A., Rose, E. F. *et al.* (1986) Biopsy and clinical course after cryosurgery for prostatic cancer. *J. Urol.*, **120**, 308–311.

Schmeller, N. T., Jocham, D., Staehler, G. *et al.* (1986) Cytological regression grading of hormone-treated prostatic cancer. *Prostate*, **9**, 1–7.

Shabaik, A., Wilson, S., Bidair, M. *et al.* (1995) Pathologic changes in prostate biopsies following cryoablation therapy of prostate carcinoma. *J. Urol. Pathol.*, **3**, 183–194.

Siders, D. B. and Lee, F. (1992) Histologic changes of irradiated prostatic carcinoma diagnosed by transrectal ultrasound. *Hum. Pathol.*, **23**, 344–351.

Smith, D. M. and Murphy, W. M. (1994) Histologic changes in prostate carcinomas treated with leuprolide (luteinizing hormone-releasing hormone effect). Distinction from poor tumor differentiation. *Cancer*, **73**, 1472–1474.

Susani, M., Maderbacher, S., Kratzik, C. and Vingers, L. (1993) Morphology of tissue destruction induced by focused ultrasound. *Eur. Urol.*, **23** (Suppl 1), 34–38.

Tetu, B., Srigley, J. R., Boivin, J. *et al.* (1991) Effect of combination endocrine therapy (LHRH agonist and flutamide) on normal prostate and prostatic adenocarcinoma. *Am. J. Surg. Pathol.*, **15**, 111–120.

Wheeler, J. A., Zagars, G, K. and Ayala, A. G. (1993) Dedifferentiation of locally recurrent prostate cancer after radiation therapy. *Cancer*, **71**, 3783–3787.

11

UROTHELIAL CARCINOMA

Urothelial carcinoma (transitional cell carcinoma) of the prostate is rarely primary, accounting for less than 4% of tumors originating in the prostate, and usually represents synchronous or metachronous spread from carcinoma in the bladder and urethra

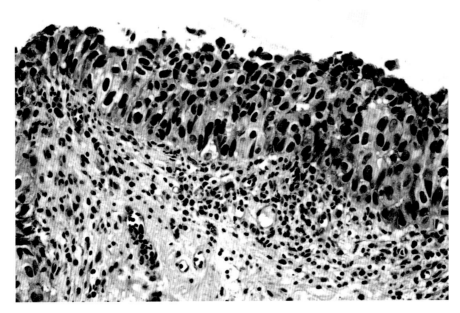

Figure 11.1   Urothelial carcinoma *in situ* of the prostatic urethra; the patient also had bladder involvement. There is full thickness dysplasia with loss of polarity and prominent cytological changes.

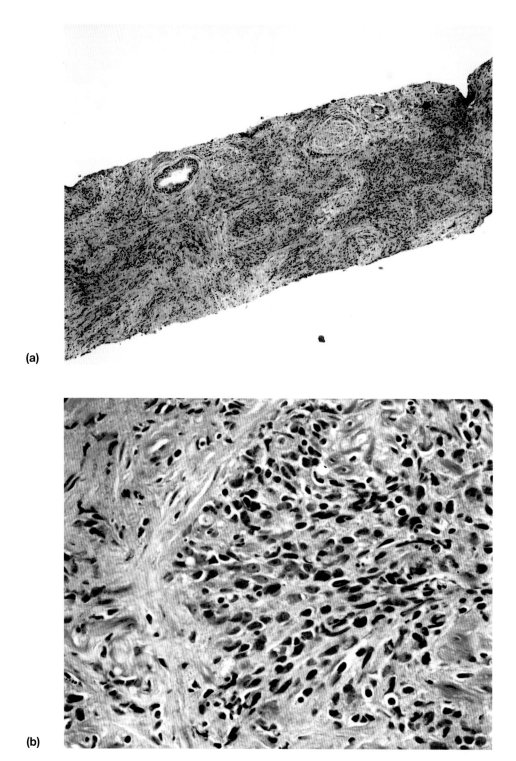

Figure 11.2 Urothelial carcinoma replacing a needle biopsy of the prostate. **(a)** At low magnification, it is difficult to determine the nature of the cellular process, although there is a suggestion that the ductules and acini are filled and expanded. Compare with **(b)**, which shows the characteristic cytological abnormalities of urothelial carcinoma; the tumor was present within ductules and acini as well as in the stroma. The patient had a previous history of invasive papillary grade 3 (of 3) urothelial carcinoma of the bladder.

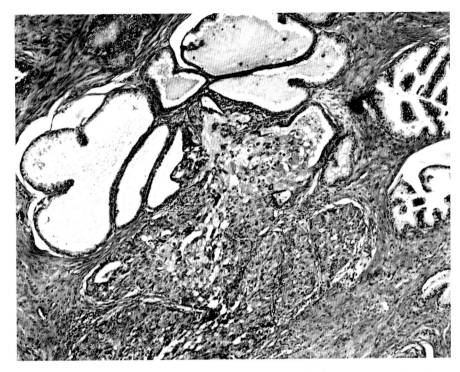

Figure 11.3 Urothelial carcinoma *in situ* spreading through the prostatic ducts. Despite extensive spread, there was no evidence of stromal invasion in this transurethral resection specimen.

(Schellhammer, Bean and Whitmore, 1977; Wendelken *et al.*, 1979; Taylor and Blom, 1983; Mahadevia, Koss and Tar, 1986; Hardeman and Soloway, 1988; Wishnow and Ro, 1988; Babaian *et al.*,1989; Wood *et al.*, 1989; Takashi *et al.*, 1990; Frazier *et al.*, 1993). It involves the prostate and urethra in about 40% of radical cystoprostatectomy specimens for bladder carcinoma (Mahadevia, Koss and Tar, 1986; Babaian *et al.*, 1989; Wood *et al.*, 1989).

11.1 CLINICAL FEATURES

Patients usually present with symptoms of hematuria, urinary obstruction, or prostatitis. Serum PSA and PAP concentrations are not elevated. Clinically, it may be mistaken for prostatitis or nodular hyperplasia.

11.2 PATHOLOGY

Urothelial carcinoma of the prostate involves the periurethral prostatic ducts and acini (Figures 11.1–11.5).

Diagnostic criteria are identical to those for urothelial cancer of the bladder and urethra; most cancers are moderately differentiated and usually associated with prominent chronic inflammation. Squamous metaplasia is infrequent.

Carcinoma *in situ* (high-grade urothelial dysplasia, or urothelial intraepithelial neoplasia) is often overlooked in specimens submitted for histological examination. It is usually multifocal, with bladder and urethral involvement; the prevalence varies from 4% to 32% in cystoprostatectomies for bladder cancer (Bryan *et al.*, 1993).

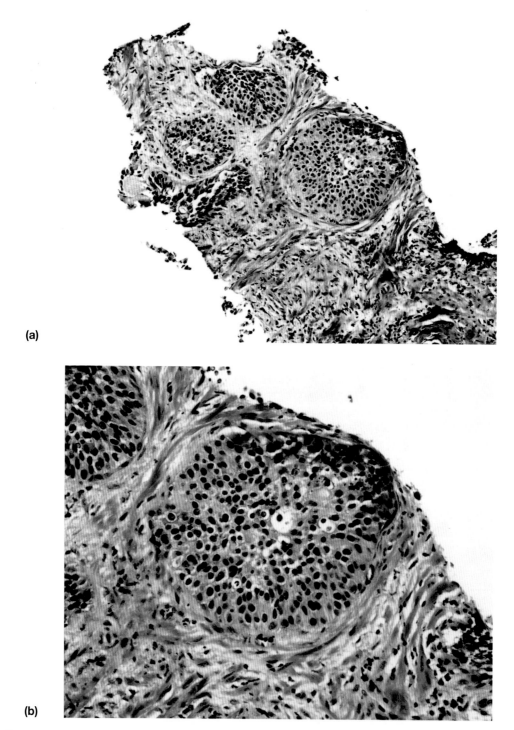

(a)

(b)

Figure 11.4 Low-grade urothelial carcinoma involving prostatic ductules. **(a)** Numerous ductules and acini are expanded by this epithelial proliferation, but there is no stromal invasion. **(b)** At high magnification there are low-grade cytological abnormalities. This is one of the most difficult problems in prostate biopsy interpretation, recognizing that normal urothelium can mimic low-grade carcinoma; clinical history is necessary. This patient had a previous history of bladder and urethral involvement by low-grade papillary urothelial carcinoma.

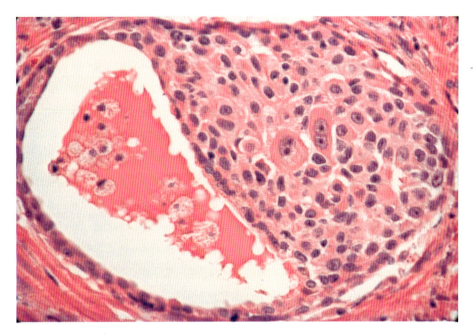

Figure 11.5 Urothelial carcinoma showing pagetoid spread through this periurethral prostatic duct.

11.3 TREATMENT AND OUTCOME

Radical cystoprostatectomy is the treatment of choice for urothelial carcinoma of the prostate and urethra (Babaian *et al.*, 1989; Takahi *et al.*, 1990; Frazier *et al.*, 1993). In a study of 21 patients by Hardeman and Soloway, radical surgery was found to be the most useful therapy (Hardeman and Soloway, 1988). These authors also noted that bladder cancer extending into the prostate can easily be missed cystoscopically, and random biopsies of the prostate were recommended.

11.4 DIFFERENTIAL DIAGNOSIS

The distinction from prostatic adenocarcinoma is important due to the estrogen unresponsiveness of urothelial carcinoma; these tumors often coincidentally coexist. High-grade adenocarcinoma may be mistaken for urothelial carcinoma with pseudoacinar pattern. Immunohistochemical stains for PSA and PAP often distinguish these tumors, with immunoreactivity exclusively in adenocarcinoma.

REFERENCES

Babaian, R. J., Troncoso, P., Ayala, A. G. *et al.* (1989) Involvement of prostatic urethra and prostatic ducts by transitional cell carcinoma in patients with bladder cancer. *J. Urol.*, **141**, 1415.

Bryan, R. L., Newman, J., Suarex, V. *et al.* (1993) The significance of urothelial dysplasia. *Histopathology*, **22**, 501–503.

Frazier, H. A., Robertson, J. E., Dodge, R. K. and Paulson, D. F. (1993) The value of pathologic factors in predicting cancer-specific survival among patients treated with radical cystectomy for transitional cell carcinoma of the bladder and prostate. *Cancer*, **71**, 3993–4001.

Hardeman, S. W. and Soloway, M. S. (1988) Transitional cell carcinoma of the prostate: diagnosis, staging and management. *Urology*, **6**, 170–174.

Mahadevia, P. S., Koss, L. G. and Tar, I. J. (1986) Prostatic involvement in bladder cancer. *Cancer*, **58**, 2096–2102.

Schellhammer, P. F., Bean, M. A. and Whitmore, W. F. Jr (1977) Prostatic involvement by transitional cell carcinoma: pathogenesis, patterns and prognosis. *J. Urol.*, **118**, 399–403.

Takashi, M., Sakata, T., Nagai, T. *et al.* (1990) Primary transitional cell carcinoma of prostate: case with lymph node metastasis eradicated by neoadjuvant methotrexate, vinblastine, doxorubicin, and cisplatin (M-VAC) therapy. *Urology*, **36**, 96–99.

Taylor, H. G. and Blom, J. (1983) Transitional cell carcinoma of the prostate. *Cancer*, **51**, 1800–1802.

Wendelken, J. R., Schellhammer, P. F., Ladaga, L. E. and El-Mahdi, A. M. (1979) Transitional cell carcinoma: cause of refractory cancer of the prostate. *Urology*, **13**, 557–560.

Wishnow, K. I. and Ro, J. Y. (1988) Importance of early treatment of transitional cell carcinoma of prostatic ducts. *Urology*, **32**, 11–12.

Wood, D. P. Jr, Montie, J. E., Pontes, J. E. *et al.* (1989) Transitional cell carcinoma of the prostate in cystoprostatectomy specimens removed for bladder cancer. *J. Urol.*, **141**, 346–349.

12

SOFT TISSUE TUMORS

Interpretation of small prostatic biopsy specimens containing soft tissue proliferations is often difficult because of the potential for sampling error. Patient age and clinical history are essential in this setting. The serum PSA concentration is usually not significantly elevated. A classification of soft tissue tumors of the prostate is shown in Table 12.1.

12.1 BENIGN SOFT TISSUE TUMORS

12.1.1 Leiomyoma and fibroma

These benign soft tissue tumors are often confused with nodular hyperplasia and the distinction may be impossible in biopsies or transurethral resection specimens. Leiomyoma is defined as a circumscribed solitary smooth muscle nodule greater than 1 cm in diameter (Persaud and Douglas, 1982; Regan, Barrett and Wold, 1987; Karolyi *et al.*, 1988; Leonard *et al.*, 1988). It is histologically identical to leiomyoma occurring in the uterus and other sites, consisting of a proliferation of benign smooth muscle cells with a variable amount of collagen. Fibroma is a similar nodule composed of collagen with few fibroblasts; fibroma may be indistinguishable from a pure stromal nodule of nodular hyperplasia. Some authors have questioned the existence of these tumors, preferring to consider them within the spectrum of nodular hyperplasia.

Variants of leiomyoma include cellular leiomyoma, atypical leiomyoma and leiomyoblastoma (Persaud and Douglas, 1982). The cellular variant is distinguished by increased density of cells; although some cases have been reported as having occasional mitotic figures, these are usually absent. The atypical (symplastic; bizarre) variant contains multinucleated giant cells with smudged nuclear detail, probably representing degenerative changes. Mitotic figures are rare or absent.

The differential diagnostic considerations are leiomyosarcoma and stromal hyperplasia with atypia. The small number of published cases limits conclusions regarding the behavior of the variants of leiomyoma, but they appear to be benign. There are no strict morphological criteria that separate atypical leiomyoma from stromal hyperplasia with atypia.

12.1.2 Postoperative spindle cell nodule (postsurgical inflammatory myofibroblastic tumor)

This rare benign reparative process occurs within months of surgery and consists of

Table 12.1 Classification of soft tissue tumors and tumor-like proliferations of the prostate

Benign
- Tumor-like proliferations
  - Granulomatous prostatis
  - Postoperative spindle cell nodule
  - Inflammatory myofibroblastic tumor
  - Blue nevus
  - Stromal hyperplasia with atypia

- Tumors
  - Leiomyoma
  - Fibroma
  - Paraganglia/pheochromocytoma
  - Hemangiopericytoma
  - Hemangioma
  - Neurilemmoma
  - Chondroma
  - Fibroadenoma
  - Fibromyxoid tumor

Tumors of uncertain malignant potential
- Low-grade phyllodes tumor

Malignant
- Rhabdomyosarcoma
- Leiomyosarcoma
- Intermediate or high-grade phyllodes tumor
- Other (fibrosarcoma, osteosarcoma, angiosarcoma, chondrosarcoma, neurofibrosarcoma, liposarcoma, malignant fibrous histiocytoma)
- Carcinosarcoma (sarcomatoid carcinoma)
- Mixed mesenchymal tumor
- Rhabdoid tumor
- Neuroblastoma
- Malignant lymphoma and leukemia*

* Although not soft tissue tumors, these are included for historical reasons ('lymphosarcoma') and to complete the differential diagnosis of tumor-like proliferations of the prostrate.

nodules of spindle cells arranged in fasicles with occasional or numerous mitotic figures (up to 25 mitotic figures/10 high-power fields) (Proppe, Scully and Rosai, 1984; Huang *et al.*, 1990). The cells have central elongate to ovoid nuclei, small prominent nucleoli and abundant cytoplasm. Necrosis may be present but is usually not a prominent feature.

The main differential diagnostic consideration is sarcoma, but postoperative spindle cell nodule is distinguished by the small size of the nodules, the presence of chronic inflammation, plexiform pattern of blood vessels, lack of significant nuclear pleomorphism and atypical mitotic figures, and lack of recurrence after conservative excision (Table 12.2). Clinical history is useful in distinguishing postoperative spindle cell tumor and inflammatory pseudotumor with no prior operation.

12.1.3 Inflammatory myofibroblastic tumor (inflammatory pseudotumor; myofibroblastoma; low-grade inflammatory fibrosarcoma; spindle cell proliferation with no prior operation; pseudosarcoma; nodular fasciitis; pseudosarcomatous fibromyxoid tumor)

This rare benign pathological entity of unknown etiology occurs in the bladder, prostate, urethra and other sites without a history of prior surgery (Hafiz, Toker and Sutula, 1984; Young and Scully, 1987; Tetu *et al.*, 1988; Sahin *et al.*, 1991; Ro *et al.*, 1993). The Panel on Soft Tissue Tumors of the World Health Organization recommends the term inflammatory myofibroblastic tumor to refer to these neoplasms.

Patients range in age from 16 to 73 years (mean 41 years), with a slight female predilection in the bladder. Mean tumor size is 3.6 cm, but it can measure up to 8 cm in diameter. The stroma is loose, edematous and myxoid, with abundant small slit-like blood vessels resembling granulation tissue (Figure 12.1).

Mitotic figures are infrequent, with less than 3 per 10 high-power fields; none are atypical. Ulceration and focal necrosis are present in most cases, but is not prominent.

The myxoid stromal cells contain abundant non-sulfated acid mucopolysaccharides, with strong staining for alcian blue at pH 2.7 but not at pH 0.9; There is strong vimentin immunoreactivity and rare immunoreactivity for smooth muscle actin, desmin and keratin; S-100 protein and myoglobin are negative. Ultrastructural studies may reveal myofibroblastic

Table 12.2 Myxoid lesions of the prostate: differential diagnosis (± = Variably positive; + = positive; - = negative)

	Inflammatory myofibroblastic tumor* (inflammatory pseudotumor)	Postoperative spindle cell nodule	Carcinosarcoma (sarcomatoid carcinoma)	Myxoid leiomyosarcoma	Myxoid rhabdomyosarcoma	Myxoid MFH
Light-microscopic findings						
Cellularity	Variable, often low	Variable, often low	High	Variable	Variable	Variable
Growth pattern	Tissue-culture-like	Tissue-culture-like	Biphasic	Intersecting fascicles	Subepithelial condensation	Storiform
Pleomorphism	+	-	+++	±	++	+++
Vessels	Slit-like	Unremarkable	Unremarkable	Unremarkable	Unremarkable	Unremarkable
Necrosis	+	+	++	++	+	++
Mitotic figures	+	++	++	+ (variable)	++	+++
Atypical mitotic figures	-	-	+	+	+	+
Ultrastructural findings	Fibroblasts and myofibroblasts	Fibroblasts and myofibroblasts	Epithelial ± mesenchymal	Smooth muscle	Striated muscle	Fibroblasts and myofibroblasts
Immunohistochemical findings						
Cytokeratin	- (rarely +)	- (rarely +)	+	- (rarely +)	- (rarely +)	- (rarely +)
Vimentin	+	+	+	+	+	+
Epithelial membrane antigen (EMA)	-	-	±	-	-	-
Desmin	±	±	±	+	+	- (rarely +)
Smooth muscle actin	+	±	±	+	+	-
Muscle-specific actin	+	+	±	+	+	- (rarely +)
S-100 protein	-	-	±	-	-	-

* Also referred to as spindle cell proliferation with no prior operation
Note: Myxoid rhabdomyosarcoma is a subset of embyronal rhabdomyosarcoma.

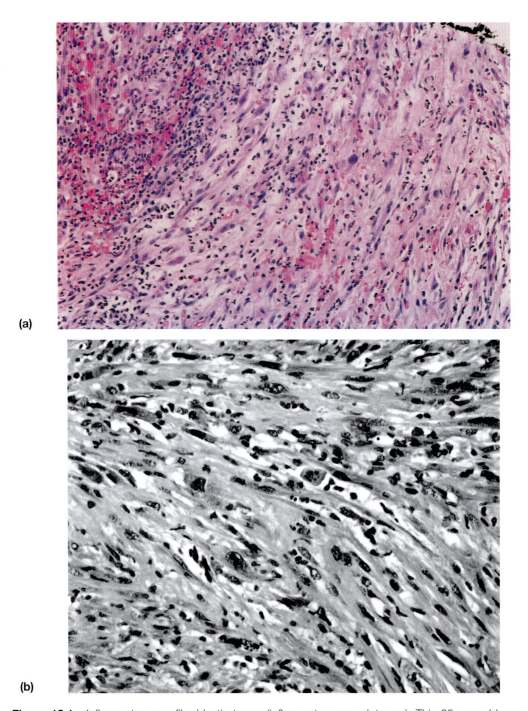

(a)

(b)

Figure 12.1 Inflammatory myofibroblastic tumor (inflammatory pseudotumor). This 65-year-old man with a history of prostatitis underwent transurethral resection of a mass in the prostate protruding into the urethral lumen. **(a)** The biopsy core was replaced by a mixture of spindle cells and focally dense chronic inflammation. **(b)** At high magnification, the spindle cells show moderate nuclear abnormalities. The patient had no history of infection, calculous disease or instrumentation of the urinary tract.

differentiation, including cytoplasmic microfil-aments and dense bodies; no epithelial dif-ferentiation is evident. Tumors are usually diploid, with a low S-phase fraction.

The differential diagnosis is the same as postoperative spindle cell nodule, including leiomyoma, aggressive angiomyxoma, phyl-lodes tumor, leiomyosarcoma and sarcomatoid carcinoma (Table 12.2). Differentiation from leiomyosarcoma may be especially difficult, as the tumor cells may show actin immunoreac-tivity. Inflammatory myofibroblastic tumor is similar to postoperative spindle cell nodule, although the tumor nodule tends to be larger. The pseudosarcomatous stromal reaction occasionally present with urothelial carcinoma may mimic inflammatory pseudotumor. Caution is warranted when making this diag-nosis in small biopsy specimens (Ro *et al.*, 1993).

Follow-up as long as 13 years indicates that inflammatory myofibroblastic tumor is a benign tumor even with conservative excision or biopsy, with no cases of metastasis or death from tumor; some bulky tumors require wide excision.

12.1.4 Hemangiopericytoma

Fewer than 10 cases of prostatic hemangio-pericytoma have been reported (Reyes *et al.*, 1977; Wunsch and Muller, 1982; Chen, 1987), and the diagnostic features are similar to those at other sites. Of three cases with follow-up, one patient was free of tumor 3 years after diagnosis and two had recurrences, including one with metastases to the bone and skin.

12.1.5 Paraganglia and pheochromocytoma

Paraganglia are present in about 10% of radical prostatectomy specimens, usually appearing as small lobular or diffuse clusters of uniform cells with abundant cytoplasm and indistinct cell margins (Freedman and Goldman, 1975; Nielson, Skovgaard and Kvist, 1987; Rode,

Bentley and Parkinson, 1990; Ostrowski and Wheeler, 1994. They are usually present in the periprostatic soft tissues near the neurovascu-lar bundles or seminal vesicles, although rare cases are found in the prostatic stroma (Cohen and Nixon, 1995). Small nerve twigs may be in close proximity, but ganglion cells are absent. Immunohistochemical stains for chromo-granin, synaptophysin and neuron-specific enolase are usually positive. The main differ-ential diagnostic considerations are hyper-nephroid pattern of adenocarcinoma, adrenal rest and xanthoma.

Pheochromocytoma of the prostate is rare (Mehta *et al.*, 1979; Dennis *et al.*, 1989; Voges *et al.*, 1990). Patients usually have hypertension and the tumor is likely to secrete noradrena-line. Surgical manipulation may precipitate hypertensive crisis and precautions must be taken to avoid this.

12.1.6 Other benign soft tissue tumors

Other benign tumors arise in the prostate, including hemangioma, lymphangioma, neurofibroma, neurilemoma, chrondroma and others.

12.2 MALIGNANT SOFT TISSUE TUMORS

Sarcoma of the prostate accounts for less than 0.1% of prostatic neoplasms. One-third occur in children and most of these are rhabdo-myosarcoma; leiomyosarcoma is most common in adults. Symptoms include prosta-tism and pelvic pain. Tumors may be 15 cm or more in diameter and are usually soft with focal necrosis. The lung is the most common site of metastases, although rhabdomyosar-coma often involves regional lymph nodes (Waring and Newland, 1992).

12.2.1 Rhabdomyosarcoma

Rhabdomyosarcoma has a peak incidence between birth and 6 years of age, but sporadic

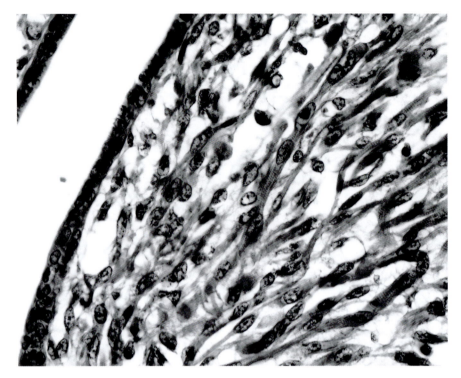

Figure 12.2 Rhabdomyosarcoma of the prostate and bladder in a 2-year-old boy. Subtle cytoplasmic cross-striations were observed within spindle cells and there was intense immunoreactivity for desmin (data not shown).

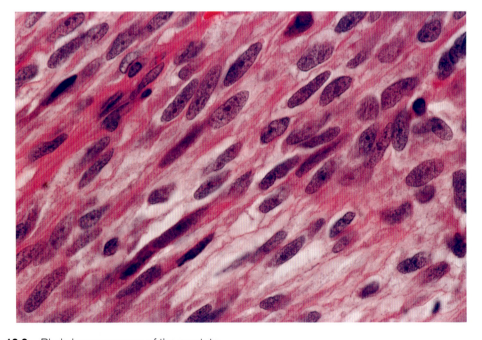

Figure 12.3 Rhabdomyosarcoma of the prostate.

cases have been reported in men as old as 80 years (Ghavimi *et al.*, 1984). The prostate, bladder and vagina account for 21% of cases in children, second only to head and neck origin. Serum PSA and PAP concentration is normal. Three adults had hypercalcemia due to bone metastases (Waring and Newland, 1992).

The tumor is usually large and bulky, with a mean diameter up to 9 cm. It usually involves the prostate, bladder and periurethral, perirectal and perivesicular soft tissues. Urethral involvement may not be apparent cytoscopically (Loughlin *et al.*, 1989). Symptoms include acute or chronic urethral obstruction, bladder displacement and rectal compression. The prostate may be palpably normal, although large tumors often fill the pelvis and can be palpated suprapubically.

Most are embryonal rhabdomyosarcoma and the remainder are alveolar, botryoid and spindle cell subtypes (Asmar *et al.*, 1994). Tumor cells are arranged in sheets of immature round to spindle cells set in a myxoid stroma (Figures 12.2 and 12.3).

Polypoid tumor fragments ('botryoid pattern') may fill the urethral lumen, covered by intact urothelium with condensed underlying tumor cells creating a distinctive cambium layer. Nuclei are usually pleomorphic and darkly staining. Scattered rhabdomyoblasts may be present, with eosinophilic cytoplasmic processes containing cross-striations.

Tumor cells display immunoreactivity for myoglobin, desmin and vimentin, but are negative for PSA and PAP. Ultrastructural study reveals two cell types, as in rhabdomyosarcoma at other sites: large oval or elongate tumor cells contain segments of sarcomere with abundant glycogen, and smaller round cells contain abundant cytoplasmic organelles but lack myofibrils. All tumors appear to be aneuploid by flow cytometry (Boyle *et al.*, 1988; Moroz, Crespo and de las Morenas, 1995).

Combination chemotherapy in combination with surgery and radiotherapy results in 3-year survival rate of over 70%, according to the Intergroup Rhabdomyosarcoma Study (Raney *et al.*, 1990); long-term survival has been reported (Verga and Parigi, 1993).

The differential diagnosis includes other small cell neoplasms, including lymphoma, acute leukemia, neuroblastoma, neuroendocrine carcinoma, poorly differentiated carcinoma, primitive neuroectodermal tumor (PNET), rhabdoid tumor and other high-grade sarcomas. The botryoid pattern may be mistaken for benign fibroepithelial polyp.

12.2.2 Leiomyosarcoma

Leiomyosarcoma presents as a large bulky mass which replaces the prostate and periprostatic tissues. It is the most common sarcoma in adults and accounts for 26% of all prostatic sarcomas. Patients range in age from 40 to 71 years (mean 59 years), with sporadic reports in younger patients (Witherow *et al.*, 1980; Cheville *et al.*, 1995).

In a recent series of 23 cases from the Mayo Clinic, tumors ranged in size from 3.3 to 21 cm (mean 9). No tumors were grade 1, seven were grade 2, 10 were grade 3, and six were grade 4 (Cheville *et al.*, 1995). The tumors were histologically similar to leiomyosarcoma at other sites. Prominent sclerotic stroma was noted in two cases. Five tumors had epithelioid features and one had a focal area reminiscent of neurilemoma. Necrosis may be extensive. Although the criteria for separating leiomyoma from low-grade leiomyosarcoma have not been precisely defined in the prostate, they are probably similar to those in other organs, including degree of cellularity, cytological anaplasia, number of mitotic figures, amount of necrosis, vascular invasion and size.

Tumor cells usually display intense cytoplasmic immunoreactivity for smooth-muscle-specific actin and vimentin, and weak desmin immunoreactivity. Most are negative for cytokeratin (AE1/AE3) and S-100 protein, but exceptions have been described, particularly in those with epithelioid features in which keratin immunoreactivity may be seen (Witherow *et al.*, 1980; Ramos *et al.*, 1993; Cheville *et al.*, 1995).

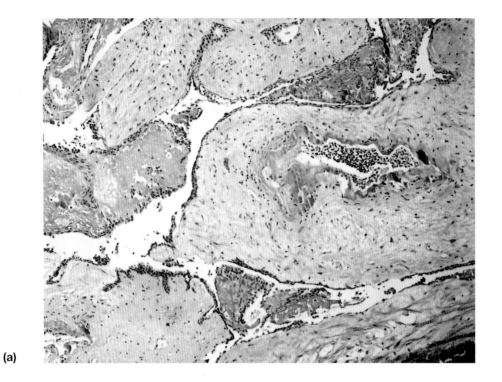

(a)

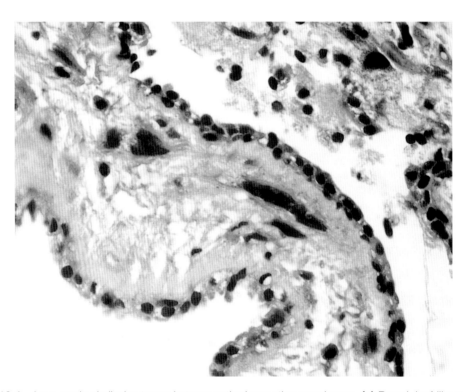

(b)

Figure 12.4 Low-grade phyllodes tumor in transurethral resection specimens. **(a)** Broad, leaf-like masses of epithelium-lined stroma protrude into cleft and slit-like spaces of variable size. There is no necrosis. **(b)** At high magnification there is focal marked enlargement of smudged hyperchromatic nuclei without mitotic figures.

Local recurrence and distant metastasis are frequent, and the prognosis is poor. Mean survival after diagnosis was less than 3 years in one series (range 0.2–6.5 years), and most patients died from tumor (Ramos *et al.*, 1993; Cheville *et al.*, 1995). Rare long-term survivors have been reported. Radical surgery is the preferred treatment, although limited data are available (Witherow *et al.*, 1980; Ramos *et al.*, 1993; Cheville *et al.*, 1995).

12.2.3 Phyllodes tumor (cystic epithelial–stromal tumor; phyllodes type of atypical hyperplasia; cystadenoleiomyofibroma; cystosarcoma phyllodes)

Phyllodes tumor of the prostate is a rare lesion which should be considered a neoplasm rather than atypical hyperplasia due to the frequent early recurrences, infiltrative growth and potential for extraprostatic spread in some cases (Figures 12.4 and 12.5) (Attah and Nkposong, 1976; Kafandaris and Polyzonis,

1983; Yokota *et al.*, 1984; Kendall *et al.*, 1986; Manivel *et al.*, 1986; Reese *et al.*, 1987; Ito *et al.*, 1989; Lopez-Beltran *et al.*, 1990; Mishina *et al.*, 1990; Maluf *et al.*, 1991; Viskens *et al.*, 1991; Yum, Miller and Agrawal, 1991; Kerley, Pierce and Thomas, 1992; Young, Jensen and Wiley, 1992; Kevwitch *et al.*, 1993; Bostwick *et al.*, 1997).

Dedifferentiation with multiple recurrences in some cases is further evidence of the potentially aggressive nature of this tumor (Mishina *et al.*, 1990; Bostwick *et al.*, 1996). Although a benign clinical course has been emphasized in some reports (Reese *et al.*, 1987), the cumulative evidence in the literature indicates that some patients develop local recurrence (Mishina *et al.*, 1990; Bostwick *et al.*, 1997).

Patients with prostatic phyllodes tumor typically present with urinary obstruction, hematuria and dysuria. There may be severe urinary obstruction, often occurring at a younger age than expected for typical prostatic hyperplasia. Most tumors range in size from 4 to 25 cm, with one report of a 58 cm tumor

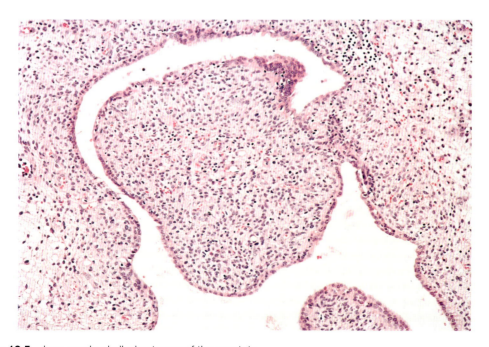

Figure 12.5 Low-grade phyllodes tumor of the prostate.

weighing 11.2 kg (Maluf *et al.*, 1991; Kerley, Pierce and Thomas, 1992). At the time of transurethral resection, the urologist may note an unusual spongy or cystic texture of the involved prostate.

The diagnosis of phyllodes tumor is usually made on resected tissue, and it may be overlooked on needle biopsy, in which it is difficult to appreciate the pattern of the tumor. Important diagnostic clues include diffuse infiltration, variably cellular stroma surrounding cysts and compressed, elongated channels, which often have a leaf-like configuration.

Prostatic phyllodes tumor exhibits a spectrum of histological features similar to its counterpart in the breast (Figure 12.4). It may be subdivided into low-grade, intermediate grade, and high-grade groups, but even low-grade tumors may recur (Table 12.3) (Bostwick *et al.*, 1997).

High-grade prostatic phyllodes tumor has a high stromal–epithelial ratio, prominent stromal cellularity and overgrowth, marked cytological atypia and increased mitotic activity. A sarcomatous component may arise within a low-grade tumor over time, invariably after multiple recurrences over many years (Yum, Miller and Agrawal, 1991; Bostwick *et al.*, 1997). One reported case consisted of phyllodes tumor containing an incidental focus of well-differentiated adenocarcinoma (Kerley, Pierce and Thomas, 1992).

Immunohistochemical studies reveal intense cytoplasmic immunoreactivity in most stromal cells for vimentin and actin, in luminal epithelial cells for PSA, PAP, and keratin AE1/AE3 and in basal epithelial cells for high-molecular-weight keratin 34βE12; no staining was observed for desmin and S-100 protein.

The histogenesis is uncertain, but is not considered müllerian for the following reasons:

- Müllerian remnants are rare in the adult prostate; the müllerian epithelium in the prostatic utricle is replaced by the urogenital sinus early in life;
- PSA and PAP are present in the epithelium of the adult utricle, indicating the endodermal (prostate-like) nature of this tissue;
- PSA is present in the epithelium of prostate phyllodes tumors (Manivel *et al.*, 1986; Mishina *et al.*, 1990; Young, Jensen and Wiley, 1992; Bostwick *et al.*, 1996).

Phyllodes tumor must be considered potentially aggressive and an individualized approach to complete excision of the tumor is needed. Low-grade tumors may be treated conservatively, recognizing that recurrences may be higher-grade and require complete excision (Bostwick *et al.*, 1997). Rarely, tumors with overtly malignant stroma give rise to lung, bone and abdominal wall metastases of sarcoma. Lymph node metastases have not been observed.

The differential diagnosis of phyllodes tumor includes stromal hyperplasia with atypical nuclei, giant multilocular prostatic cystadenoma, hyperplasia with cystic acini, and cysts such as müllerian duct cyst and congenital and acquired seminal vesicle cyst. Phyllodes tumor may also arise in the seminal vesicle as a supraprostatic retrovesicular mass but is separated from its prostatic counterpart by the absence of PSA and PAP immunoreactivity in the epithelium. Stromal hyperplasia with atypical nuclei is a cellular lesion with enlarged hyperchromatic degenerative-appearing nuclei occurring in the stroma adjacent to typical hyperplastic acini or within

Table 12.3 Prostatic phyllodes tumor: grading

Grade	Stromal cellularity	Cytological atypia	Mitotic figures	Stromal:epithelial ratio
Low	Low to moderate	Low to moderate	Rare (< 1 per 10 high power fields)	Low
Intermediate	Moderate to high	Moderate to high	Uncommon	Low to high
High	Moderate to high	High	Common	High

nodular hyperplasia. Giant multilocular cystadenoma of the prostate is a solitary tumor with cysts lined by prostatic epithelium surrounded by dense fibrous stroma. Cystic adenoma of the prostate has also been described, consisting of complex inward growth of papillary epithelial fronds with scant stroma. Nodular hyperplasia commonly contains small cystic acini within hyperplastic nodules, and infrequently small fibroadenoma-like foci may be misinterpreted as phyllodes tumor. Müllerian duct cyst (typically midline) and seminal vesicle cyst (typically lateral) are usually unilocular and lack the prostatic epithelial lining and stromal cellularity of phyllodes tumor. Primary sarcoma of the prostate such as leiomyosarcoma is also a diagnostic consideration, but this tumor consists of a monophasic densely cellular proliferation of spindle cells that lacks the epithelial component of phyllodes tumor. Sarcomatoid carcinoma is a concern when an overtly malignant spindle cell component is present, but is distinguished by the presence of a malignant epithelial component or evidence of epithelial differentiation within the neoplastic spindle cells.

12.2.4 Other sarcomas

Other sarcomas reported in the prostate include fibrosarcoma, osteosarcoma, malignant fibrous histiocytoma (Bain et al., 1985; Chin, Fay and Ortega, 1986), angiosarcoma (Smith et al., 1986), chondrosarcoma, neurofibrosarcoma and liposarcoma. Sarcomatoid carcinoma (carcinosarcoma), although not truly or exclusively mesenchymal, must be included in the differential diagnoses of pleomorphic spindle cell neoplasms with necrosis and numerous mitotic figures. Recognition of epithelial elements is useful, as metastases may contain only epithelial elements (Dundore et al., 1995). Sarcoma of the prostate is occasionally unclassifiable, and we diagnose this as undifferentiated sarcoma. Regardless of classification, the prognosis of most adult prostatic sarcomas is poor.

REFERENCES

Asmar, L., Gehan, E. A., Newton, W. A. et al. (1994) Agreement among and within groups of pathologists in the classification of rhabdomyosarcoma and related childhood sarcomas. Report of an international study of four pathology classifications. Cancer, **74**, 2579–2588.

Attah, E. B. and Nkposong, E. O. (1976) Phyllodes type of atypical prostatic hyperplasia. J. Urol., **115**, 762–764.

Bain, G. O., Jewell, L. D., Danyluk Manickavel, V. and Shnitka, T. K. (1985) Malignant fibrous histiocytoma of prostate gland. Urology, **26**, 89–91.

Bostwick, D. G., Halling, A. C., Jones, E. C. et al. (1997) Prostatic phyllodes tumor: proposed grading system based on clinicopathologic study of seven cases and review of the literature. (submitted).

Boyle, E. T. Jr, Reiman, H. M., Kramer, S. A. et al. (1988) Embryonal rhabdomyosarcoma of bladder and prostate: nuclear DNA patterns studied by flow cytometry. J. Urol., **140**, 1119–1121.

Chen, K. T. K. (1987) Hemangiopericytoma of the prostate. J. Surg. Oncol., **35**, 42–45.

Cheville, J., Bostwick, D. G., Dundore, P. A. et al. (1995) Leiomyosarcoma of the prostate: report of 23 cases. Cancer, **76**, 1035–1042.

Chin, W., Fay, R. and Ortega, P. (1986) Malignant fibrous histiocytoma of prostate. Urology, **27**, 363–365.

Cohen R. J. and Nixon, J. M. (1995) Intraprostatic ganglia (letter). Hum. Pathol., **26**, 807–808.

Dennis, P. J., Lewandowski, A. E., Rohner, T. J. Jr et al. (1989) Pheochromocytoma of the prostate: an unusual location. J. Urol., **141**, 130–132.

Dundore, P. A., Nascimento, A. G., Cheville, J. C. et al. (1995) Carcinosarcoma of the prostate. Report of 22 cases. Cancer, **76**, 1035–1042.

Freedman, S. R. and Goldman, R. L. (1975) Normal paraganglia in the human prostate. J. Urol., **113**, 874–875.

Ghavimi, F., Herr, H., Jereb, B. and Exelby, P. R. (1984) Treatment of genitourinary rhabdomyosarcoma in children. J. Urol., **132**, 313.

Hafiz, M. A., Toker, C. and Sutula, M. (1984) An atypical fibromyxoid tumor of the prostate. Cancer, **54**, 2500–2504.

Huang, W. L., Ro, J. Y., Grignon, D. J. *et al.* (1990) Postoperative spindle cell nodule of the prostate and bladder. *J. Urol.*, **143**, 824–826.

Ito, H., Ito, M., Nitsuhata, N. and Tahara, E. (1989) Phyllodes tumor of the prostate. A case report. *Jpn. J. Clin. Oncol.*, **19**, 299–304.

Kafandaris, P. M. and Polyzonis, M. B. (1983) Fibroadenoma-like foci in human prostatic nodular hyperplasia. *Prostate*, **4**, 33–36.

Karolyi, P., Endes, P., Krasznai, G. and Tonkol, I. (1988) Bizarre leiomyoma of the prostate. *Virchows Arch. Pathol. Anat. Histol.*, **412**, 383–387.

Kendall, A. R., Stein, B. S., Shea, F. J. *et al.* (1986) Cystic pelvic mass. *J. Urol.*, **135**, 550–553.

Kerley, S. W., Pierce, P. and Thomas, J. (1992) Giant cystosarcoma phyllodes of the prostate associated with adenocarcinoma. *Arch. Pathol. Lab. Med.*, **116**,195–197.

Kevwitch, M. K., Walloch, J. L., Waters, W. B. and Flanigan, R. C. (1993) Prostatic cystic epithelial-stromal tumors: a report of 2 new cases. *J. Urol.*, **149**, 860–864.

Leonard, A., Baert, L., Van Praet, F. *et al.* (1988) Solitary leiomyoma of the prostate. *Br. J. Urol.*, **60**,184–187.

Lopez-Beltran, A., Gaeta, J. F., Huben, R. and Croghan, G. A. (1990) Malignant phyllodes tumor of the prostate. *Urology*, **35**,164–167.

Loughlin, K. R., Retik, A. B., Weinstein, H. J. *et al.* (1989) Genitourinary rhabdomyosarcoma in children. *Cancer*, **63**, 1600–1606.

Maluf, H. M., King, M. E., DeLuca, F. R. *et al.* (1991) Giant multilocular prostatic cystadenoma: a distinctive lesion of the retroperitoneum in men. *Am. J. Surg. Pathol.*, **15**, 131–135.

Manivel, C., Shenoy, B. V., Wick, M. R. and Dehner, L. P. (1986) Cystosarcoma phyllodes of the prostate: a pathologic and immunohistochemical study. *Arch. Pathol. Lab. Med.*, **110**, 534–538.

Mehta, M., Nadel, N. S., Lonn, Y. and Al, I. (1979) Malignant paraganglioma of the prostate and retroperitoneum. *J. Urol.*, **121**, 376–378.

Mishina, T., Shimada, N., Toki, J. and Ikehara, S. (1990) A case report of phyllodes tumor of the prostate: review of the literature and analysis of bizarre giant cell origin. *Acta Urol. Jpn.*, **36**, 1185–1188.

Moroz, K., Crespo, P. and de las Morenas, A. (1995). Fine needle aspiration of prostatic rhabdomyosarcoma. A case report demonstrating the value of DNA ploidy. *Acta Cytol.*, **39**, 785–790.

Nielson, V. M., Skovgaard, N. and Kvist, N. (1987) Phaeochromocytoma of the prostate. *Br. J. Urol.*, **59**, 478–479.

Ostrowski, M. L. and Wheeler T. M. (1994) Paraganglia of the prostate. Location, frequency, and differentiation from prostatic adenocarcinoma. *Am. J. Surg. Pathol.*, **18**, 412–420.

Persaud, V. and Douglas, L. L. (1982) Bizarre (atypical) leiomyoma of the prostate gland. *W. Indian Med. J.*, **31**, 217–220.

Proppe, K. H., Scully, R. E. and Rosai, J. (1984) Postoperative spindle cell nodules of genitourinary tract resembling sarcomas: a report of eight cases. *Am. J. Surg. Pathol.*, **8**, 101–108.

Ramos, A., Davis, C., Sesterhenn, I. and Mostofi, F. (1993) Preliminary findings in 20 prostatic leiomyosarcomas. *Mod. Pathol.*, **6**, 67A.

Raney, R. B. Jr, Gehan, E. A., Hays, D. M. *et al.* (1990) Primary chemotherapy with or without radiation therapy and/or surgery for children with localized sarcoma of the bladder, prostate, vagina, uterus, and cervix. A comparison of the results in Intergroup Rhabdomyosarcoma Studies I and II. *Cancer*, **66**, 2072–2081.

Reese, J. H., Lombard, C. M., Krone, K. and Stamey, T. A. (1987) Phyllodes type of atypical prostatic hyperplasia: a report of 3 new cases. *J. Urol.*, **138**, 623–626.

Regan, J. B., Barrett, D. M. and Wold, L. E. (1987) Giant leiomyoma of the prostate. *Arch. Pathol. Lab. Med.*, **111**, 381–383.

Reyes, J. W., Shinozuka, H., Garry, P. *et al.* (1977) A light and electron microscopic study of a hemangiopericytoma of the prostate with local extension. *Cancer*, **40**, 1122–1127.

Ro, J. Y., El-Naggar, A. K., Amin, M. B. *et al.* (1993) Pseudosarcomatous fibromyxoid tumor of the urinary bladder and prostate. Immunohistochemical, ultrastructural, and DNA flow cytometric analyses of nine cases. *Hum. Pathol.*, **24**, 1203–1210.

Rode, J., Bentley, A. and Parkinson, C. (1990) Paraganglial cells of urinary bladder and prostate: potential diagnostic problem. *J. Clin. Pathol.*, **43**, 13–16.

Sahin, A. A., Ro, J. Y., El-Naggar, A. K. *et al.* (1991) Pseudosarcomatous fibromyxoid tumor of the prostate. *Am. J. Clin. Pathol.*, **96**, 253–258.

Smith, D. M., Manivel, C., Kapps, D. and Uecker, J. (1986) Angiosarcoma of the prostate: report of 2 cases and review of the literature. *J. Urol.*, **135**, 382–384.

Tetu, B., Ro, J. Y., Ayala, A. G. *et al.* (1988) Atypical spindle cell lesions of the prostate. *Sem. Diag. Pathol.*, **5**, 284–293.

Verga, G. and Parigi, G. B. (1993) Conservative surgery of bladder–prostate rhabdomyosarcoma in children: results after long-term follow-up. *J. Pediatr. Surg.*, **28**, 1016–1018.

Viskens, D., Van Hove, C., Fransen, G. and Bermans, G. (1991) Phyllodes type of atypical prostatic hyperplasia. *Acta Chirurg. Belg.*, **91**, 22–26.

Voges, G. E., Wippermann, F., Duber, C. and Hohenfellner, R. (1990) Pheochromocytomas in the pediatric age group: the prostate an unusual location. *J. Urol.*, **144**, 1219–1221.

Waring, P. M. and Newland, R. C. (1992) Prostatic embryonal rhabdomyosarcoma in adults. A clinicopathologic review. *Cancer*, **69**, 755–762.

Witherow, R., Molland, E., Oliver, T. and Hind, C. (1980) Leiomyosarcoma of prostate and superficial soft tissue. *Urology*, **15**, 513.

Wunsch, P. H. and Muller, H. A. (1982) Hemangiopericytoma of the prostate: a light microscopic study of an unusual tumor. *Pathol. Res. Pract.*, **172**, 334–336.

Yokota, T., Yamashita, Y., Okuzono, Y. *et al.* (1984) Malignant cystosarcoma phyllodes of prostate. *Acta Pathol. Jpn.*, **34**, 663–668.

Young, J. F., Jensen, P. E. and Wiley, C. A. (1992) Malignant phyllodes tumor of the prostate: a case report with immunohistochemical and ultrastructural findings. *Arch. Pathol. Lab. Med.*, **116**, 296–299.

Young, R. H. and Scully, R. E. (1987) Pseudosarcomatous lesions of the urinary bladder, prostate gland, and urethra: a report of three cases and review of the literature. *Arch. Pathol. Lab. Med.*, **111**, 354–358.

Yum, M., Miller, J. C. and Agrawal, B. L. (1991) Leiomyosarcoma arising in atypical fibromuscular hyperplasia (phyllodes tumor) of the prostate with distant metastasis. *Cancer*, **68**, 910–915.

13

OTHER RARE MALIGNANT TUMORS

13.1 MALIGNANT LYMPHOMA AND LEUKEMIA

Hematological malignancies, including primary involvement or secondary spread from nodal lymphoma, leukemia or myeloma, are rare in the prostate.

13.1.1 Malignant lymphoma

Patients with malignant lymphoma involving the prostate are usually older men (mean age 61 years), presenting with urinary obstructive symptoms, including urgency, frequency, acute urinary retention, urinary tract infections and hematuria (Bostwick and Mann, 1985; Ben-Ezra *et al.*, 1986; Fell, O'Connor and Smith, 1987; Banerjee and Harris, 1988; Suzuki *et al.*, 1991). Systemic symptoms, including fever, chills, night sweats and weight loss, are infrequent and only occur in patients with widespread lymphoma. The prostate gland with malignant lymphoma is diffusely enlarged, non-tender and firm or rubbery. Serum PSA concentration is usually not elevated.

Secondary spread to the prostate by malignant lymphoma is much more frequent than primary lymphoma. The prevalence of primary prostatic lymphoma at autopsy is 0.2% of extranodal lymphomas (Fell, O'Connor and Smith, 1987). Diagnostic criteria for primary lymphoma include symptoms attributable to prostatic enlargement, lymphoma chiefly involving the prostate with or without involvement of adjacent tissues, and lack of liver, spleen, lymph nodes and peripheral blood involvement within 1 month of diagnosis (Bostwick and Mann, 1985).

Microscopically, prostatic lymphoma is diffuse or patchy within the stroma, with characteristic preservation of acini (Figure 13.1).

The infiltrate is usually extensive, but may be irregular and patchy, often extending into the extraprostatic soft tissues. Tumor cell infiltration into the acinar epithelium is uncommon and rarely includes aggregates in the lumens. The most frequent lymphoma involving the prostate is diffuse non-Hodgkin's lymphoma, including small-cleaved-cell, large-cell and mixed-cell types; Hodgkin's disease is very rare, with fewer than five documented cases (Bostwick and Mann, 1985). Angiotropic lymphoma has also been described, including one case with spurious immunoreactivity for PAP (PSA was negative), presumably due to tumor cell absorption from the phosphatase-rich vessel contents (Figure 13.2) (Ben-Ezra *et al.*, 1986; Banerjee and Harris, 1988). Rare cases have coincident adenocarcinoma.

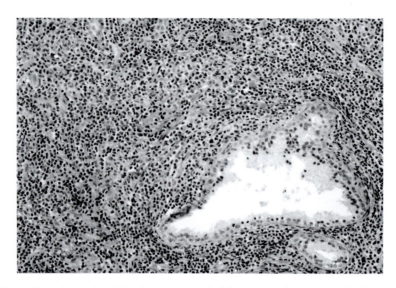

Figure 13.1 Malignant lymphoma involving the prostate. Acini are intact but surrounded by a dense stromal infiltrate. The lymphoma was classified as diffuse mixed small- and large-cell, B-cell immunophenotype.

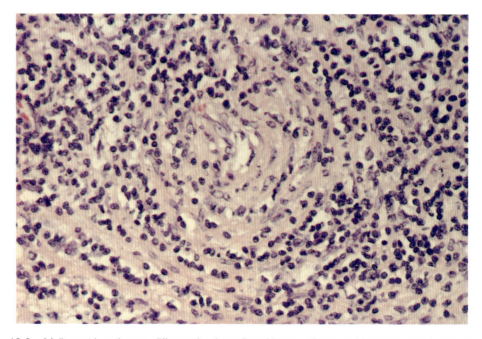

Figure 13.2 Malignant lymphoma, diffuse mixed small and large cell type, with prominent angiotropism.

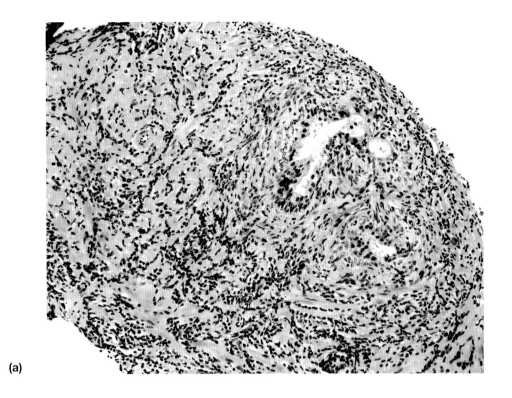

(a)

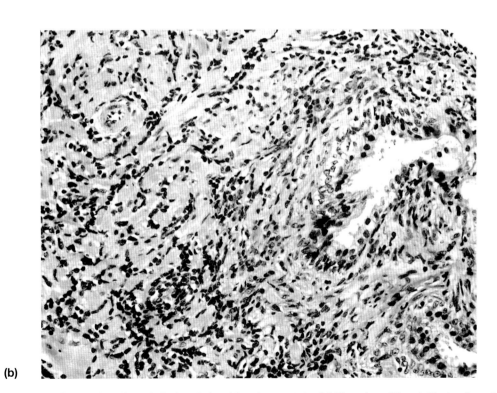

(b)

Figure 13.3 Chronic lymphocytic leukemia involving the prostate. **(a)** There is a diffuse infiltrate of small mature lymphocytes. Compare with **(b)**, showing preservation of acini. The patient had a history of CLL.

The prognosis of lymphoma involving the prostate is usually poor, regardless of patient age, stage of the tumor, histological classification, type of involvement (primary or secondary) or type of therapy. In one series, 12 of 13 patients reported died within 2 years of diagnosis, but most of these were treated before modern methods of chemotherapy and radiation therapy were available (Bostwick and Mann, 1985). Surgery is used chiefly for symptomatic relief of urinary obstruction.

The differential diagnosis of lymphoma includes leukemia, granulocytic sarcoma, granulomatous prostatitis, chronic prostatitis with follicular hyperplasia and neuroendocrine carcinoma. Unlike lymphoma, granulomatous prostatitis causes acinar destruction. Prostatic pseudolymphoma was described by Peison et al. (1977), occurring in a 68-year-old man with no prior history of lymphoma who presented with acute urinary obstruction and normal blood count. Histologically, there was prominent lymphoid hyperplasia in the transurethral resection specimen without evidence of malignancy. Long-term follow-up was not available. Humphrey and Vollmer described extramedullary hematopoiesis of the prostate in a 75-year-old man with a history of myelofibrosis and progressive outlet obstruction (Humphrey and Vollmer, 1991). The transurethral resection specimen revealed a diffuse stromal infiltrate of atypical megakaryocytes, immature myeloid elements and normoblasts; the epithelium was preserved. Chloroacetate esterase stain was useful in confirming the myeloid nature of the infiltrate.

13.1.2 Leukemia

Chronic lymphocytic leukemia is the most common leukemia involving the prostate, with more than 100 reported cases (Viadana, Bross and Pickren, 1978; Sridhar and Woodhouse, 1983; Cachia et al., 1987; Thalhammer et al., 1994). The autopsy prevalence of prostatic involvement is about 20% of cases of leukemia (Viadana, Bross and Pickren, 1978). The clinical symptoms and histological patterns in the prostate are similar to malignant lymphoma, but are distinguished from lymphoma by the presence of blood involvement (Figures 13.3 and 13.4). Bladder neck obstruction in patients with leukemia may respond to surgery if chemotherapy is ineffective; radiation therapy is recommended for granulocytic sarcoma (Frame et al., 1987).

13.1.3 Multiple myeloma

Multiple myeloma involving the prostate is rare, with fewer than 10 reported cases (Yasuda, Ohmori and Usui, 1994). Most are diagnosed at autopsy. IgD and IgA myeloma have been described and may rarely cause urinary obstructive symptoms. The incidence of prostatic involvement by myeloma is unknown.

13.2 GERM CELL TUMOR

Germ cell tumor rarely arises in the prostate, invariably with metastases and massive prostatic involvement. This tumor may arise from sequestration of germ cells during migration, usually occurring in the midline, accounting for germ cell tumor in the vagina, mediastinum, retroperitoneum and liver.

Two patients with yolk sac tumor of the prostate, aged 29 years and 51 years, died 10 months after diagnosis despite radical surgery and chemotherapy (Benson, Segura and Carney, 1978; Dalla Palma et al., 1988). A patient with coexistent retroperitoneal and prostatic seminoma was described by Arai et al. (1988). Michel et al. reported a 40-year-old with mixed germ cell tumor (embryonal carcinoma and teratoma) who was alive 2 years after treatment (Michel et al., 1986). Choriocarcinoma of the prostate has also been described in older reports (Prym, 1927; Dvoracek, 1949).

The main differential diagnostic considerations include metastases from testicular or retroperitoneal primary, sarcomatoid carcinoma (carcinosarcoma), mucinous carcinoma, typical acinar adenocarcinoma and ductal carcinoma. The diagnosis of primary

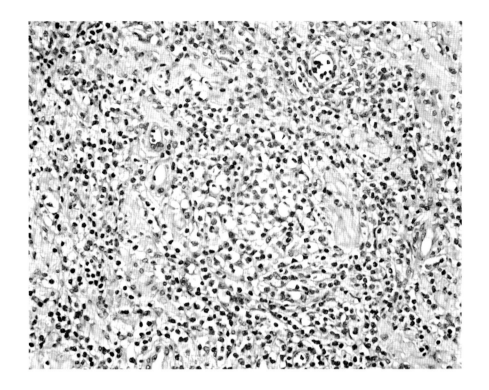

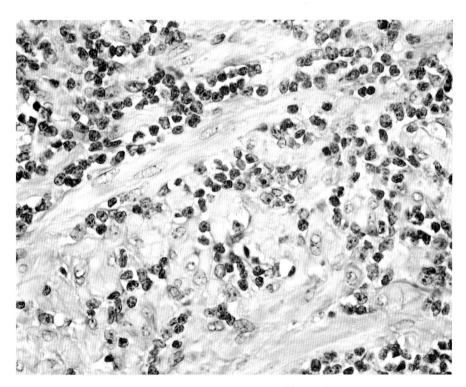

Figure 13.4 Chronic lymphocytic leukemia of the prostate initially mistaken for Gleason pattern 5 adenocarcinoma. **(a)** There are sheets of cells with small hyperchromatic nuclei and focally vacuolated cytoplasm, suggesting carcinoma with focal signet-ring-cell pattern. **(b)** There is some nuclear variability and rare cells have prominent punctate nucleoli.

germ cell tumor of the prostate should only be considered after all other possibilities are excluded. The usual histological features of germ cell tumor at other sites are present. For yolk sac tumor, these include Schiller–Duval bodies, hyaline PAS-positive globules and elevated serum AFP concentration; PSA and PAP are negative (Dalla Palma et al., 1988).

13.3 METASTASES TO THE PROSTATE

The prostate is occasionally involved by tumors arising in other organs, usually due to contiguous spread. Metastases are extremely rare, with involvement at autopsy in 0.5–2.2% of men dying of malignancies (Johnson, Chalbaud and Ayala, 1974; Zein et al., 1985). The most common is squamous cell carcinoma of the bronchus, accounting for almost half of all prostatic metastases (Johnson, Chalbaud and Ayala, 1974; Zein et al., 1985). Malignant melanoma accounts for about 27% of metastases, with an incidence of 1.1% of patients with malignant melanoma at autopsy (Berry and Reese, 1953; Thompson, Albers and Broders, 1953; Albers and Stephenson, 1962; Dowd, 1964; Johnson et al., 1974; Stein and Kendall, 1984; Zein et al., 1985; Grignon, Ro and Ayala, 1989; Parr, Grigor and Ritchie, 1992). Grignon and coworkers described an unusual case of tumor-to-tumor metastasis of malignant melanoma to prostatic adenocarcinoma (Grignon, Ro and Ayala, 1989). Other metastases to the prostate arise from a variety of sites (Thompson, Albers and Broders, 1953; Dowd, 1964), including pancreatic carcinoma (Dowd, 1964) and goblet cell carcinoid of the appendix (Parr, Grigor and Ritchie, 1992).

13.4 OTHER

13.4.1 Wilms tumor

A case of primary Wilms tumor of the prostate was reported in a 32-year-old man with hematospermia and obstructive symptoms (Casiraghi et al., 1991). The characteristic triphasic pattern was observed, including blastema, epithelial tubules and spindled stroma. The patient developed pulmonary metastases 1 year after presentation. Extrarenal Wilms tumor is thought to arise from embryonic rests of metanephric blastema, explaining the occurrence of this tumor in other urogenital areas such as the scrotum, spermatic cord and an ovotestis. The differential diagnosis includes sarcoma such as rhabomyosarcoma, sarcomatoid carcinoma and teratoma.

13.4.2 Rhabdoid tumor

Rhabdoid tumor is a poorly differentiated malignant neoplasm, with light-microscopic features of rhadomyosarcoma, which displays epithelial differentiation, including intense cytoplasmic immunoreactivity for keratin protein and epithelial membrane antigen, rare cell junctions, occasional intracytoplasmic lumens and distinctive paranuclear aggregates of intermediate filaments. Most cases occur in the kidney but extrarenal tumors have been identified, including rare cases in the prostate (Ekfors, Aho and Kekomaki, 1985).

13.4.3 Neuroblastoma

A single case of neuroblastoma has been reported in the prostate (Mostofi and Price, 1973).

REFERENCES

Albers, D. D. and Stephenson, P. L. (1962) Metastatic carcinoma of the prostate from silent carcinoma of the stomach. A case report. J. Okla. Med. Assn, 55, 78.

Arai, Y., Watanabe, J., Kounami, T. et al. (1988) Retroperitoneal seminoma with simultaneous occurrence in the prostate. J. Urol., 139, 382–385.

Banerjee, S. S. and Harris, M. (1988) Angiotropic lymphoma presenting in the prostate. *Histopathology*, **12**, 667–683.

Ben-Ezra, J., Sheibani, K., Kendrick, F. E. *et al.* (1986) Angiotropic large cell lymphoma of the prostate gland: an immunohistochemical study. *Hum. Pathol.*, **17**, 964–966.

Benson, R. C. Jr, Segura, J. W. and Carney, J. A. (1978) Primary yolk-sac (endodermal sinus) tumor of the prostate. *Cancer*, **41**, 1395–1398.

Berry, N. E. and Reese, L. (1953) Malignant melanoma which had its first clinical manifestations in the prostate gland. *J. Urol.*, **69**, 286–287.

Bostwick, D. G. and Mann, R. B. (1985) Malignant lymphomas involving the prostate. A study of 13 cases. *Cancer*, **56**, 2932–2938.

Cachia, P. G., McIntyre, M. A., Dewar, A. E. and Stockdill, G. (1987) Prostatic infiltration in chronic lymphatic leukaemia. *J. Clin. Pathol.*, **40**, 342–345.

Casiraghi, O., Martinez-Madrigal, F., Mostofi, F. K. *et al.* (1991) Primary prostatic Wilms' tumor. *Am. J. Surg. Pathol.*, **15**, 885–890.

Dalla Palma, P., Dante, S., Guazzieri, S. and Sperandio, P. (1988) Primary endodermal sinus tumor of the prostate: report of a case. *Prostate*, **12**, 255–261.

Dowd, J. B. (1964) Carcinoma of the pancreas presenting as obstructing cancer of the prostate. *Lahey Clin. Bull.*, **13**, 214–215.

Dvoracek, C. (1949) Primarni chorionepitheliom prostaty s gynekomastii. *Cas. Lak. Cesk.*, **88**, 198–202.

Ekfors, T. O., Aho, H. J. and Kekomaki, M. (1985) Malignant rhabdoid tumor of the prostatic region. Immunohistological and ultrastructural evidence for epithelial origin. *Virchows Arch. Pathol. Anat. Histol.*, **406**, 381–388.

Fell, P., O'Connor, M. and Smith, J. M. (1987) Primary lymphoma of prostate presenting as bladder outflow obstruction. *Urology*, **29**, 555–559.

Frame, R., Head, D., Lee, R. *et al.* (1987) Granulocytic sarcoma of the prostate. Two cases causing urinary obstruction. *Cancer*, **59**, 142–146.

Grignon, D. J., Ro, J. Y. and Ayala, A. G. (1989) Malignant melanoma with metastasis to adenocarcinoma of the prostate. *Cancer*, **63**, 196–198.

Humphrey, P. A. and Vollmer, R. T. (1991) Extramedullary hematopoiesis in the prostate. *Am. J. Surg. Pathol.*, **15**, 186–190.

Johnson, D. E., Chalbaud, R. and Ayala, A. G. (1974) Secondary tumors of the prostate. *J. Urol.*, **112**, 507–508.

Michel, F., Gattengo, B., Roland, J. *et al.* (1986) Primary nonseminomatous germ cell tumor of the prostate. *J. Urol.*, **135**, 597–599.

Mostofi, F. K. and Price, E. B. Jr (1973) *Tumors of the Male Genital System, Atlas of Tumor Pathology*, fascicle 8, second series, Armed Forces Institute of Pathology, Washington, DC, pp. 244–245.

Parr, N. J., Grigor, K. M. and Ritchie, A. W. S. (1992) Metastatic carcinoid tumour involving the prostate. *Br. J. Urol.*, **70**, 103–104.

Peison, B., Benisch, B., Nicora, B. and Lind, E. (1977) Acute urinary obstruction secondary to pseudolymphoma of prostate. *Urology*, **10**, 478–479.

Prym, P. (1927) Spontanheilung eines bosartigen, wahrscheinlich chorionepitheliomatosen Gewachses im Hodem. *Virchows Arch. Pathol. Anat.*, **265**, 239–244

Sridhar, K. N. and Woodhouse, C. R. J. (1983) Prostatic infiltration in leukaemia and lymphoma. *Eur. Urol.*, **9**, 153–156.

Stein, B. S. and Kendall, A. R. (1984) Malignant melanoma of the genitourinary tract. *J. Urol.*, **132**, 956–961.

Suzuki, H., Nakada, T., Iijima, Y. *et al.* (1991) Malignant lymphoma of the prostate. Report of a case. *Urol. Int.*, **47**, 172–175.

Thalhammer, F., Gisslinger, H., Chott, A. *et al.* (1994) Granulocytic sarcoma of the prostate as the first manifestation of a late relapse of acute myelogenous leukemia. *Ann. Hematol.*, **68**, 97–99.

Thompson, G. J., Albers, D. D. and Broders, A. C. (1953) Unusual carcinomas involving the prostate gland. *J. Urol.*, **69**, 416–418.

Viadana, E., Bross, I. D. J. and Pickren, J. W. (1978) An autopsy study of the metastatic patterns of human leukaemias. *Oncology*, **35**, 87–96.

Yasuda, N., Ohmori, S-I. and Usui, T. (1994) IgD myelomas involving the prostate. *Am. J. Hematol.*, **47**, 65–66.

Zein, T. A., Huben, R., Lane, W. *et al.* (1985) Secondary tumors of the prostate. *J. Urol.*, **133**, 615–616.

14

SEMINAL VESICLES

Atypical nuclear changes that occur in the aging seminal vesicles are discussed in Chapter 1.

14.1 AMYLOIDOSIS (SENILE SEMINAL VESICLE AMYLOIDOSIS)

Localized amyloidosis of the seminal vesicles increases in frequency with patient age, present in up to 8% of men younger than 60 years and 34% over 75 years (Pitkanen *et al.*, 1983; Seidman *et al.*, 1989; Cornwell *et al.*, 1992; Kaji *et al.*, 1992; Khan *et al.*, 1992; Coyne and Kealy, 1993; Ramchandani *et al.*, 1993). It often extends bilaterally along the ejaculatory ducts, forming linear or massive nodular subepithelial deposits of amorphous eosinophilic fibrillar material. Basement membrane thickening is observed and deposits may be seen within the vesicular lumens, occasionally causing significant luminal narrowing. Rare cases are associated with calcification or florid foreign body giant cell reaction (Khan *et al.*, 1992). By contrast, systemic amyloidosis infrequently affects the seminal vesicles, involving vascular walls, smooth muscle and stroma. Vesicular amyloidosis is usually asymptomatic, but may cause hematospermia or chronic perineal pain, or mimic seminal vesiculitis. It cannot be visualized by imaging studies except for pelvic MRI, and may mimic tumor invasion from bladder or prostate cancer. Localized and systemic amyloidosis may coexist (Coyne and Kealy, 1993).

14.2 SEMINAL VESICULITIS

Seminal vesiculitis is an uncommon disorder associated with infection and inflammation of adjacent organs, including the prostate, bladder, ejaculatory ducts, vas deferens and epididymis (Krishnan and Heal, 1991). Acute vesiculitis is usually caused by retrograde infection with or without indwelling catheter, ureteral or ejaculatory duct stenosis or anatomic anomaly, calculi or surgical trauma. Antibiotic therapy is usually effective, employing the same agents used for acute prostatitis; biopsies are rarely obtained in such cases and may be contraindicated due to complications of abscess formation and stricture. Protracted acute and chronic seminal vesiculitis result in atrophy and ejaculatory duct stricture.

Chronic vesiculitis is associated with chronic prostatitis and both respond poorly to antibiotic therapy. Prior to the antibiotic era, the most common cause was tuberculosis, which resulted in perineal fistula, fibrous adhesions, ejaculatory duct stricture and massive circumferential calcification of the walls of the seminal vesicles at the site of previous necrotizing granulomas. Schistosomiasis, usually secondary to *S. haematobium* infection of the bladder, involves the seminal vesicles more commonly than the prostate. Viruses, fungi, and parasites are rare causes of seminal vesiculitis. Echinococcal cyst of the seminal vesicles and prostate has been reported (DeKlotz, 1976).

14.3 CALCIFICATION

Calcification often follows seminal vesiculitis, particularly with tuberculosis. Patients with long histories of diabetes mellitus or uremia also develop dystrophic calcification of the seminal vesicles and other mesonephric derivatives. Most foci of calcification are idiopathic and asymptomatic, and imaging studies of the pelvis may detect them incidentally. Calcification may be unilateral or bilateral, and usually coexists with calcification of the vas deferens (Silber and McDonald, 1971). The cal-

cification is present in the muscular wall, often forming concentric rings; the mucosa is rarely involved. Osseous metaplasia is also rarely observed in the wall.

Calculi are more frequent in the seminal vesicles than in the vas deferens, appearing as brown stones of variable number up to 1 cm in diameter. They usually consist of phosphate and carbonate salts. The mechanism of formation is uncertain, but may be due to reflux of urine up the ejaculatory ducts (Li, 1991; Wilkinson, 1993).

14.4 SEMINAL VESICLE CYSTS

Seminal vesicle cysts are rare and may be congenital or acquired. Congenital cyst is associated with ipsilateral renal agenesis in 80% of cases, and commonly with ureteral ectopia, ureteral agenesis (Zinner's syndrome) (King *et al.*, 1991; Rappe, Meuleman and Debruyne, 1993), and ipsilateral absence of the testis (Das and Amar, 1980) or hemivertebra (Sheih *et al.*, 1993). The cyst is usually unilateral and unilocular, lateral to the midline, and up to three

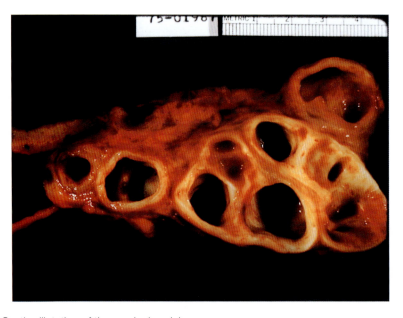

Figure 14.1 Cystic dilatation of the seminal vesicles.

times larger than the normal seminal vesicle, considerably smaller than müllerian duct cyst (Figure 14.1).

Enlargement is due to insufficient drainage with accumulation of seminal fluid. This unilocular cyst contains viscous, pale/white fluid, similar to the usual secretions of the seminal vesicles, and is lined by a cuboidal or flattened epithelium with a fibrous wall of variable thickness. Massive enlargement is referred to as hydrocele or hydrops. Bilateral congenital cysts are rare and may be associated with absent vasa deferentia (Ornstein and Kershaw, 1985).

Acquired cyst is usually associated with inflammation and obstruction of the ejaculatory ducts and seminal vesicles. This fluctuant cyst may be palpable on digital rectal examination and often contains red cells, white cells and spermatozoa. The epithelial lining is inflamed or sloughed, depending on the duration and severity of inflammation. Echinococcal (hydatid) cyst can occur in the retrovesicular region, invariably in association with infection in another organ (DeKlotz, 1976). Megavesicles consist of massive dilatation of the seminal vesicles.

The differential diagnosis of seminal vesicle cyst includes prostatic cyst, ejaculatory duct diverticulum and cystic dilatation of wolffian and müllerian duct remnants.

14.5 RADIATION CHANGES

Radiation therapy for prostatic carcinoma causes atrophy and fibrosis of the seminal vesicles and perivesicular fat in 89% of patients (Bostwick, Egbert and Fajardo, 1982; Chan and Kressel, 1991). The golden-brown lipochrome pigment characteristic of the seminal vesicle epithelium is retained.

14.6 TUMORS

The seminal vesicles are frequently involved by tumors originating elsewhere, particularly prostatic carcinoma. Primary neoplasms of the seminal vesicles are rare, and pathological documentation of some reported cases is incomplete.

14.6.1 Adenocarcinoma

Adenocarcinoma is the most common primary malignancy of the seminal vesicles but is extremely rare (Benson, Clark and Farrow, 1984; Tanaka et al., 1987; Chinoy and Kulkarni, 1993; Ohmori et al., 1994). Mean patient age is 62 years (range 17–90 years) and presenting symptoms include urinary obstruction and hematospermia. The diagnosis of seminal vesicle adenocarcinoma requires the following:

- tumor located primarily in the seminal vesicles;
- no evidence of carcinoma in the prostate, bladder or colon;
- architectural features of adenocarcinoma, usually with papillary or sheet-like growth and mucinous differentiation;
- *in situ* adenocarcinoma in the seminal vesicle epithelium;
- cytoplasmic immunoreactivity for carcinoembryonic antigen (CEA) and absence of staining for PSA and PAP.

With high-stage, poorly differentiated adenocarcinoma the precise site of origin may be impossible to determine. Tumor cells may be hobnail, columnar or polygonal, with clear cytoplasm and rarely lipofuscin. Radical surgery and external beam radiation therapy have been employed, but the prognosis is poor. Androgen deprivation therapy may also be of value (Okada et al., 1992; Gohji, Kamidono and Okada, 1993).

14.6.2 Metastasis and contiguous spread

Seminal vesicle involvement by prostatic adenocarcinoma is common, observed in about 12% of radical prostatectomy specimens

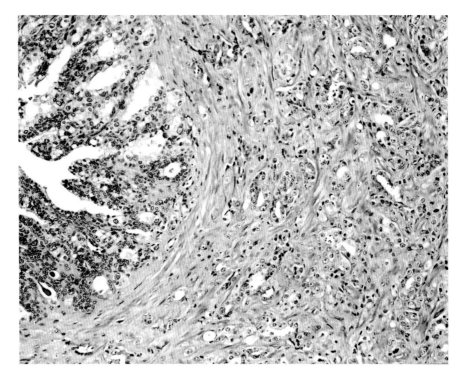

Figure 14.2 Prostatic adenocarcinoma with extensive involvement of the muscular wall of the seminal vesicles and sparing of the epithelium.

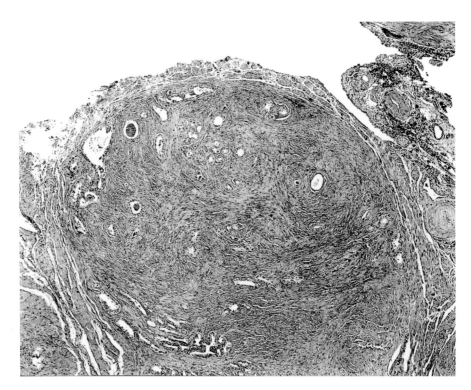

Figure 14.3 Smooth muscle nodular hyperplasia of the seminal vesicles. Note entrapped benign acini.

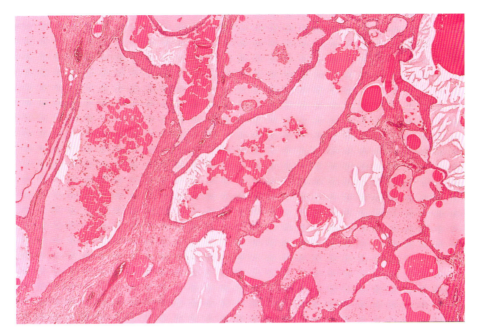

Figure 14.4 Benign cystadenoma of the seminal vesicles. The patient had no recurrence of this 12 cm diameter tumor of the seminal vesicles after 27 years, and died of unrelated cause.

(Figure 14.2) (Terris, McNeal and Stamey, 1990).

There are three patterns of seminal vesicle invasion:

- direct spread along the ejaculatory duct complex into the seminal vesicles;
- prostatic capsular perforation followed by extension into the periprostatic soft tissues and spread into the seminal vesicles;
- isolated deposits of cancer in the seminal vesicles (Mukamel *et al.*, 1987; Villers *et al.*, 1990; Epstein, Carmichael and Walsh, 1993; Ohori *et al.*, 1993).

Bulky urothelial carcinoma of the bladder may also invade the seminal vesicles by direct extension or mucosal spread (Ro *et al.*, 1987). Mucosal involvement by *in situ* urothelial carcinoma is rare, present in only 1% of cases. It spreads along the mucosa of the prostatic urethra, the prostatic and ejaculatory ducts and seminal vesicles by intraepithelial replacement and pagetoid spread along the basement membrane. Rectal adenocarcinoma occasionally invades the seminal vesicles and prostate and may cause diagnostic difficulty.

14.6.3 Soft tissue tumors and other tumors

A variety of benign and malignant soft tissue tumors have been described in the seminal vesicles, including cystadenoma (Soule and Dockerty, 1951; Damjanov and Apic, 1974; Mazzucchelli, Studer and Zimmermann, 1992; Lagalla *et al.*, 1993), phyllodes tumor (Mazur, Myers and Maddox, 1987; Laurila *et al.*, 1992; Fain *et al.*, 1993), leiomyoma (Figure 14.3) (Gentile *et al.*, 1994), fibroma, adenomyosis (Fujisawa *et al.*, 1993), mesonephric hamartoma (Kinas and Kuhn, 1987) and sarcoma (Chiou, Limas and Lane, 1985; Schned, Ledbetter and Selikowitz, 1986; Lamont *et al.*, 1991; Amirkhan *et al.*, 1994).

Cystadenoma is a rare benign tumor composed of cysts lined by a simple columnar epithelium with chronically inflamed loose fibrous stroma or fibromuscular stroma. The cysts are grossly multilocular, ranging in size from 5 to 15 cm in diameter (Figure 14.4).

Phyllodes tumor consists of a mixture of variably cellular stroma and acinar elements. The density and cytological features of the stroma determine whether the tumor is a fibroadenoma, low-grade phyllodes tumor or high-grade phyllodes tumor (cytosarcoma phyllodes). Features predictive of malignancy include infiltrating margins, stromal atypia, high numbers of mitotic figures and overgrowth of acini by stroma.

Sarcoma of the seminal vesicle is rare, and usually grows locally and compresses adjacent pelvic organs such as the prostate, bladder and rectum. Carcinosarcoma may also arise in the seminal vesicles (Zenklusen et al., 1990).

Rare primary germ cell tumors have been reported in the seminal vesicles, presumably due to midline entrapment of embryonic germ cells, including choriocarcinoma and seminoma (Adachi et al., 1991; Fairey et al., 1993). Primary carcinoid tumor has also been reported (Soyer et al., 1991).

REFERENCES

Adachi, Y., Rokujyo, M., Kojima, H. and Nagashima, K. (1991) Primary seminoma of the seminal vesicle: report of a case. *J. Urol.*, **146**, 857–859.

Amirkhan, R. H., Mohlberg, K. H., Wiley, E. L. *et al.* (1994) Primary leiomyosarcoma of the seminal vesicle. *Urology*, **44**, 132–135.

Benson, R. C. Jr, Clark, W. R. and Farrow, G. M. (1984) Carcinoma of the seminal vesicle. *J. Urol.*, **132**, 483–485.

Bostwick, D. G., Egbert, B. M. and Fajardo, J. L. (1982) Radiation injury of the normal and neoplastic prostate. *Am. J. Surg. Pathol.*, **6**, 541–551.

Chan, T. W. and Kressel, H. Y. (1991) Prostate and seminal vesicles after irradiation: MR appearance. *J. M. R. I.*, **1**, 503–511.

Chinoy, R. F. and Kulkarni, J. N. (1993) Primary papillary adenocarcinoma of the seminal vesicle. *Indian J. Cancer*, **30**, 82–84.

Chiou, R. K., Limas, C. and Lange, P. H. (1985) Hemangiosarcoma of the seminal vesicle: case report and literature review. *J. Urol.*, **134**, 371–373.

Cornwell, G. G. III, Westermark, G. T., Pitkanen, P. and Westermark, P. (1992) Seminal vesicle amyloid: the first example of exocrine cell origin of an amyloid fibril precursor. *J. Pathol.*, **167**, 297–303.

Coyne, J. D. and Kealy, W. F. (1993) Seminal vesicle amyloidosis: morphological, histochemical and immunohistochemical observations. *Histopathology*, **22**, 173–176.

Damanjov, I. and Apic, R. (1974) Cystadenoma of seminal vesicles. *J. Urol.*, **111**, 808–809.

Das, S. and Amar, A. D. (1980) Ureteral ectopia into cystic seminal vesicle with ipsilateral dysgenesis and monorchia. *J. Urol.*, **124**, 574–575.

DeKlotz, R. J. (1976) Echinococcal cyst involving the prostate and seminal vesicles. A case report. *J. Urol.*, **115**, 116–117.

Epstein, J. I., Carmichael, M. and Walsh, P. C. (1993) Adenocarcinoma of the prostate invading the seminal vesicle. Definition and relation of tumor volume, grade, and margins of resection to prognosis. *J. Urol.*, **149**, 1040–1045.

Fain, J. S., Cosnow, I., King, B. F. *et al.* (1993) Cystosarcoma phyllodes of the seminal vesicle. *Cancer*, **71**, 2055–2061.

Fairey, A. E., Mead, G. M., Murphy, D. and Theaker, J. (1993) Primary seminal vesicle choriocarcinoma. *Br. J. Urol.*, **71**, 756–757.

Fujisawa, M., Ishigami, J., Kamidono, S. and Yamanaka, N. (1993) Adenomyosis of the seminal vesicle with hematospermia. *Hinyokika Kiyo Acta Urol. Jpn.*, **39**, 73–76.

Gentile, A. T., Moseley, H. S., Quinn, S. F *et al.* (1994) Leiomyoma of the seminal vesicle. *J. Urol.*, **151**, 1027–1029.

Gohji, K., Kamidono, S. and Okada, S. (1993) Primary adenocarcinoma of the seminal vesicle. *Br. J. Urol.*, **72**, 514–515.

Kaji, Y., Sugimura, K., Nagaoka, S. and Ishida, T. (1992) Amyloid deposition in seminal vesicles mimicking tumor invasion from bladder cancer: MR findings. *J. Comp. Assist. Tomog.*, **16**, 989–991.

Khan, S. M., Birch, P. J., Bass, P. S. *et al.* (1992) Localized amyloidosis of the lower genitourinary tract. A clinicopathological and immunohistochemical study of nine cases. *Histopathology*, **21**, 143–147.

Kinas, H. and Kuhn, M. (1987) Mesonephric hamartoma of the seminal vesicle: a rare cause of a retrovesical mass. *NY State J. Med.*, **87**, 48–49.

King, B. F., Hattery, R. R., Lieber, M. M. *et al.* (1991) Congenital cystic disease of the seminal vesicle. *Radiology*, **178**, 207–211.

Krishnan, R. and Heal, M R (1991) Study of seminal vesicles in acute epididymitis. *Br. J. Urol.*, **67**, 632–637.

Lagalla, R., Zappasodi, F., Lo Casto, A. and Zenico, T. (1993) Cystadenoma of the seminal vesicle. US and CT findings. *Abdom. Imaging*, **18**, 298–300.

Lamont, J. S., Hesketh, P. J., De Las Morenas, A. and Babayan, R. K. (1991) Primary angiosarcoma of the seminal vesicle. *J. Urol.*, **146**, 165–167.

Laurila, P., Leivo, I., Makisalo, H. *et al.* (1992) Müllerian adenosarcomalike tumor of the seminal vesicle. A case report with immunohistochemical and ultrastructural observations. *Arch. Pathol. Lab. Med.*, **116**, 1072–1076.

Li, Y. K. (1991) Diagnosis and management of large seminal vesicle stones. *Br. J. Urol.*, **68**, 322–323.

Mazur, M. T., Myers, J. L. and Maddox, W. A. (1987) Cystic epithelium–stromal tumor of the seminal vesicle. *Am. J. Surg. Pathol.*, **11**, 210–217.

Mazzucchelli, L., Studer, U. E. and Zimmermann, A. (1992) Cystadenoma of the seminal vesicle: case report and literature review. *J. Urol.*, **147**, 1621–1624.

Mukamel, E., DeKernion, J. B., Hannah, J. *et al.* (1987) The incidence and significance of seminal vesicle invasion in patients with adenocarcinoma of the prostate. *Cancer*, **59**, 1535–1538.

Ohmori, T., Okada, K., Tabei, R. *et al.* (1994) CA125-producing adenocarcinoma of the seminal vesicle. *Pathol. Int.*, **44**, 333–337.

Ohori, M., Scardino, P. T., Lapin, S. L. *et al.* (1993) The mechanisms and prognostic significance of seminal vesicle involvement by prostate cancer. *Am. J. Surg. Pathol.*, **17**, 1252–1261.

Okada, Y., Tanaka, H., Takeuchi, H. and Yoshida, O. (1992) Papillary adenocarcinoma in a seminal vesicle cyst associated with ipsilateral renal agenesis: a case report. *J. Urol.*, **148**, 1543–1545.

Ornstein, M. H. and Kershaw, D. R. (1985) Cysts of the seminal vesicle are Müllerian in origin. *J. Roy. Soc. Med.*, **78**, 1050–1051.

Pitkanen, P., Westermark, P., Cornwell, G. G. III and Murdoch, W. (1983) Amyloid of the seminal vesicles: a distinctive and common localized form of senile amyloidosis. *Am. J. Pathol.*, **110**, 64–69.

Ramchandani, P., Schnall, M. D., LiVolsi, V. A. *et al.* (1993) Senile amyloidosis of the seminal vesicles mimicking metastatic spread of prostatic carcinoma on MR images. *Am. J. Roentgenol.*, **161**, 99–100.

Rappe, B. J. M., Meuleman, E. J. H. and Debruyne, F. M. J. (1993) Seminal vesicle cyst with ipsilateral renal agenesis. *Urol. Int.*, **50**, 54–56.

Ro, J. Y., Ayala, A. G., El-Nagger, A. and Wishnow, K. I. (1987) Seminal vesicle involvement by in situ and invasive transition cell carcinoma of the bladder. *Am. J. Surg. Pathol.*, **11**, 951–958.

Schned, A. R., Ledbetter, J. S. and Selikowitz, S. M. (1986) Primary leiomyosarcoma of the seminal vesicle. *Cancer*, **57**, 2202–2206.

Seidman, J. D., Shmookler, B. M., Connolly, B. and Lack, E. E. (1989) Localized amyloidosis of seminal vesicles: report of three cases in surgically obtained material. *Mod. Pathol.*, **2**, 671–675.

Sheih, C-P., Liao, Y-J., Li, Y-W. and Yang, L-Y. (1993) Seminal vesicle cyst associated with ipsilateral renal malformation and hemivertebra. Report of 2 cases. *J. Urol.*, **150**, 1214–1215.

Silber, S. J. and McDonald, F. D. (1971) Calcification of the seminal vesicles and vas deferens in a uremic patient. *J. Urol.*, **105**, 542–544.

Soule, E. H. and Dockerty, M. B. (1951) Cystadenoma of the seminal vesicle, a pathologic curiosity. Report of a case and review of the literature concerning benign tumors of the seminal vesicle. *Mayo Clinic Proc.*, **26**, 406–414.

Soyer, P., Rougier, P., Gad, M. and Roche, A. (1991) Primary carcinoid tumor of the seminal vesicles: CT and MR findings. *J. Belg. Radiol.*, **74**, 117–119.

Tanaka, T., Takeuchi, T., Oguchi, K. *et al.* (1987) Primary adenocarcinoma of the seminal vesicle. *Hum. Pathol.*, **18**, 200–202.

Terris, M. K., McNeal, J. E. and Stamey, T. A. (1990) Invasion of the seminal vesicles by prostatic cancer: detection with transrectal sonography. *Am. J. Roentgenol.*, **155**, 811–815.

Villers, A. A., McNeal, J. E., Redwine, E. A. *et al.* (1990) Pathogenesis and biological significance of seminal vesicle invasion in prostatic adenocarcinoma. *J. Urol.*, **143**, 1183–1187.

Wilkinson, A. G. (1993) Case report: calculus in the seminal vesicle. *Pediat. Radiol.*, **23**, 327.

Zenklusen, H. R., Weymuth, G., Rist, M. and Mihatsch, M. J. (1990) Carcinosarcoma of the prostate in combination with adenocarcinoma of the prostate and adenocarcinoma of the seminal vesicles. A case report with immunocytochemical analysis and review of the literature. *Cancer*, **66**, 998–1001.

15

PROSTATIC URETHRA

The prostatic urethra extends from the internal urethral orifice at the bladder neck to the prostatic apex. This 3–4 cm long tube is lined by a smooth urothelium punctuated by the openings of the periurethral glands, the prostatic ducts and the ejaculatory ducts on either side of the utricle at the verumontanum. The membranous urethra, distal to the prostatic urethra, is lined by pseudostratified columnar epithelium and contains the small, paired bulbourethral Cowper glands embedded within the musculature of the urogenital diaphragm. The male accessory sex glands often express prostate-specific markers such as PSA and PAP

Table 15.1 Urothelial abnormalities of the urethra and bladder (excluding dysplasia and carcinoma)

- Von Brunn's nests
- Cystitis cystica
- Glandular (intestinal) metaplasia
- Nephrogenic metaplasia
- Squamous metaplasia
- Papillary (polypoid) urethritis
- Papillary hyperplasia
- Diffuse papillomatosis
- Condyloma acuminatum
- Fibroepithelial polyp
- Prostatic-type polyp
- Hamartoma

(Frazier *et al.*, 1992; Elgamel *et al.*, 1994).

Delicate circumferential slings of skeletal muscle at the bladder neck and prostatic urethra act as sphincters, which control micturition. Loss of skeletal muscle at the apex is the usual cause of incontinence following prostatectomy. To preserve this muscular tissue during transurethral resection of the prostate, urologists limit their procedure to the portion of the prostate and prostatic urethra proximal to the verumontanum.

15.1 INFLAMMATION AND METAPLASIA

A variety of inflammatory conditions affect the urethra, often in association with cystitis and prostatitis (Table 15.1). Long-standing chronic inflammation usually results in metaplasia.

15.1.1 Urethritis

Men with urethritis may present with discharge or dysuria, but many have no symptoms. Causative agents include the entire spectrum of sexually transmitted diseases, including *Chlamydia trachomatis*, *Neisseria gonorrheae*, and *Ureaplasma urealyticum*. The mucosa is congested and inflamed during the acute phase. Biopsy is uncommon, so the experience of most surgical pathologists with urethritis is limited.

Reiter's syndrome is an important form of urethritis of unknown cause that occurs chiefly in men between 18 and 40 years of age in association with conjunctivitis and arthritis (Hoffman and Cheatum, 1978). Other urological manifestations include hemorrhagic cystitis and prostatitis. Symptoms persist for up to 4 weeks and the majority of patients relapse.

15.1.2 Polypoid urethritis (proliferative papillary urethritis)

Polypoid urethritis is similar to polypoid cystitis, consisting of papillary broad-based exophytic masses of edematous granulation tissue invested with inflamed or ulcerated urothelium, often with metaplastic changes (Figure 15.1).

It commonly occurs in association with indwelling catheter or calculi and usually resolves spontaneously after removal of the inciting agent. Polypoid urethritis may be confused with papillary urothelial neoplasms cystoscopically and pathologically (Schinella, Thurm and Feiner, 1974; Walker and Mills, 1989).

15.1.3 Malakoplakia

Although malakoplakia commonly affects the bladder, urethral involvement is rare (Damjanov and Katz, 1981; Sharma, Kagan and Shiels, 1981). It appears as an inflamed plaque or polypoid mucosal mass that mimics malignancy. The microscopic features are identical to those seen in bladder and prostatic involvement (Chapter 2), including the presence of Michaelis–Gutmann bodies.

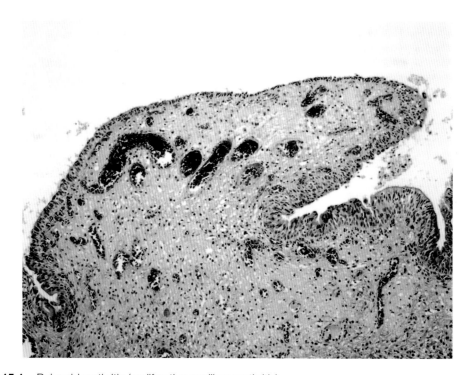

Figure 15.1 Polypoid urethritis (proliferative papillary urethritis).

15.1.4 Glandular and squamous metaplasia

Glandular and squamous metaplasia occur in the bladder and urethra as a result of chronic irritation from calculi, indwelling catheter, diverticuli, repeated instrumentation and urinary tract infection. Glandular metaplasia may appear as colonic-type goblet cells or typical mucin-rich columnar cells. Ectopic prostatic tissue may result from glandular metaplasia rather than ectopia. Squamous metaplasia is often seen with *Schistosoma haematobium* infection and with exstrophy. Both forms of metaplasia are considered by many to be precursors of carcinoma of the urinary tract, but the supportive evidence is weak for glandular metaplasia.

15.1.5 Nephrogenic metaplasia (nephrogenic adenoma)

This reactive proliferative lesion of small tubules and papillae can occur anywhere within the urothelial tract, thought to arise secondary to irritation and chronic inflammation. It usually arises in the bladder, but occasional cases have been reported in the urethra, sometimes mimicking adenocarcinoma (Bhagavan *et al.*, 1981). Occasional cases occur in a urethral diverticulum (Medeiros and Young, 1989), rarely in association with adenocarcinoma. Urethritis cystica, urethritis glandularis and von Brunn's nests frequently coexist; rarely, there may also be glandular metaplasia in the adjacent mucosa.

Architecturally, nephrogenic metaplasia is polypoid, with occasional infiltrating appearance at the base with involvement of the underlying prostatic stroma. The hallmark of nephrogenic metaplasia is the presence of hobnail or cuboidal cells lining small tubules or small papillae. The tubules have prominent basement membranes and the lumens often contain dark, eosinophilic, PAS-positive, diastase-resistant secretions. When the tubules are small, some cells may have features of signet-ring cells suggestive of infiltration. Nuclei tend to be round and regular, and contain small nucleoli. Mitotic figures are uncommon and atypical forms are lacking.

Nephrogenic metaplasia is considered benign, with no apparent malignant predisposition. However, it may predate or coexist with carcinoma, sharing a similar pathogenesis of chronic irritation.

15.2 POLYPS AND PAPILLOMAS

A variety of unusual and interesting polyps, polypoid masses and papillomas occur in the prostatic urethra (Walker and Mills, 1989). Important differential features include patient age, pathological findings in the adjacent mucosa and prostate, and the degree of cytological abnormality.

15.2.1 Congenital urethral polyp (fibroepithelial polyp)

This polyp arises in the prostatic urethra near the verumontanum (posterior urethral polyp) and is exclusively seen in boys, usually under 10 years of age (Bruijnes *et al.*, 1985; Foster and Garrett, 1986). Patients present with hematuria, obstructive symptoms and urethritis and cystitis. This polypoid mass of vascularized loose connective tissue and smooth muscle is covered by urothelium which is often eroded or ulcerated. Squamous metaplasia is common.

15.2.2 Prostatic urethral polyp (ectopic prostatic tissue; benign polyp with prostatic-type epithelium)

Prostatic urethral polyp is one of the most common causes of hematuria in adolescents and young adults (Figure 15.2) (Craig and Hart, 1975; Goldstein *et al.*, 1981; Lubin, Mark and Wirtschafter, 1984; Remick and Kumar, 1984; Satoh *et al.*, 1989).

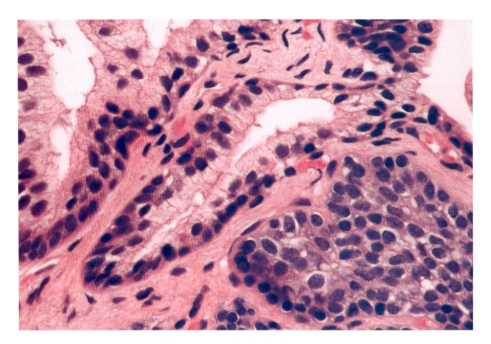

Figure 15.2   Ectopic prostatic tissue (prostatic urethral polyp).

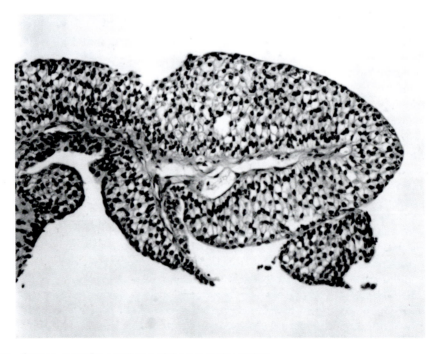

Figure 15.3   Benign urothelial papilloma of the prostatic urethra.

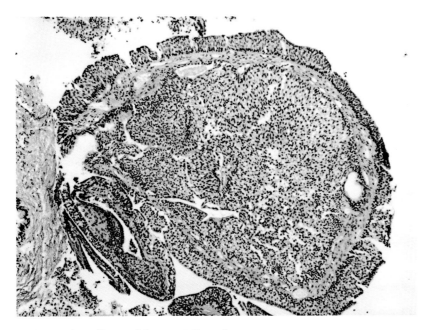

Figure 15.4   Inverted papilloma of the prostatic urethra.

It usually occurs in the prostatic urethra, but rarely arises in the distal urethra and bladder. The polyp may be focal or extensive, consisting of delicate papillae with fibrovascular stalks and prostatic epithelial lining without cytological atypia. The cells express prostate-specific antigen and prostatic acid phosphatase. The main differential diagnostic considerations in adults are ductal (endometrioid) adenocarcinoma of the prostate, papillary urothelial carcinoma and seeding of the prostatic urethra by papillary adenocarcinoma of the bladder or urachus.

15.2.3 Papilloma (urothelial papilloma)

Papilloma lies at the benign end of the spectrum of non-invasive papillary urothelial proliferations of the bladder and urethra (Figure 15.3).

We employ strict criteria for its diagnosis, following the recommendations of the World Health Organization (Mostofi and Price, 1973). These criteria include patient age under 50 years, single, less than 2 cm in greatest dimension, intact superficial (umbrella) cell layer, no more than seven cells in thickness and atypia which is no greater than that seen in grade 1 urothelial carcinoma; rare exceptions to one or more of these criteria are allowed if the remaining criteria are satisfied. Using these strict criteria, papilloma comprises less than 5% of papillary urothelial neoplasms. It is rare in the urethra.

Murphy, Beckwith and Farrow (1994) employ a more liberal definition of papilloma, which includes about half the cases that we and others consider grade 1 urothelial carcinoma. The expansion of the papilloma category is based on recognition that the recurrence rate for this tumor is low after excision and it rarely metastasizes. Regardless of nomenclature, patients should be followed clinically.

15.2.4 Inverted papilloma

This lesion rarely occurs in the urethra and may form an exophytic or endophytic mass similar to its counterpart in the bladder (Figure 15.4) (Renfer, Kelly and Belville, 1988).

Patients present with hematuria and lower-urinary-tract obstructive symptoms. Cystoscopically, inverted papilloma appears as a smooth-surfaced nodular polyp, which may be sessile or pedunculated. The lesion is usually 1–2 cm in diameter and single, but may rarely be as large as 8 cm in diameter or multiple, particularly in the bladder.

The 'typical' inverted papilloma is characterized by smoothly contoured invaginated cords and columns of urothelial cells with an intact urothelium on the luminal surface. The arrangement of the epithelial cells is virtually diagnostic, with outer basaloid cells of the cords showing peripheral palisading perpendicular to the prominent enveloping basement membrane and central cells arrayed in a parallel orientation. Central cells may show incomplete squamous metaplasia and microcystic change with PAS-positive material. The complex arborizing invaginations are in continuity with the overlying mucosa, and there is usually no significant cytological atypia. Mitotic figures are rarely observed. Stroma is usually scant and surrounds the endophytic epithelial cords rather than forming a central fibrovascular core as is seen in exophytic papillary urothelial tumors. The 'glandular' variant of inverted papilloma is similar to the typical pattern, but is composed chiefly of cystitis cystica and/or glandularis.

Mild cytological atypia and mitotic activity may be identified, but changes that approach those seen in grade 2 papillary urothelial carcinoma should raise the serious consideration of 'inverting' or nested variant of urothelial carcinoma, a rare variant that has been recently described in the bladder. 'Atypical' inverted papilloma accounted for 15% of cases in one large series. Inverted papilloma should not recur if entirely excised.

Malignant transformation has been rarely described in recurrences of inverted papilloma, but may represent underdiagnosis of 'inverted' carcinoma. It is also likely that inverted papilloma has been misinterpreted in

the past as low-grade urothelial carcinoma. Rare reports of malignancy in association with inverted papilloma have been noted, including papillary urothelial carcinoma arising in or adjacent to the papilloma.

The histogenesis of inverted papilloma is unknown but is related to metaplastic changes such as von Brunn's nest formation, cystitis cystica and cystitis glandularis.

15.2.5 Villous adenoma

Rare cases of villous adenoma have been described in the urethra which may represent a precursor of adenocarcinoma. This tumor is histologically identical to its counterpart in the colon and some display PSA and PAP immunoreactivity. One case arose in association with ductal adenocarcinoma of the prostate (Walker *et al.*, 1982).

15.3 OTHER NEOPLASMS

15.3.1 Condyloma acuminatum

Prostatic urethral involvement by condyloma acuminatum is very rare, usually occurring by extension from the penile urethra. Patients present with hematuria and irritative symptoms, but many are asymptomatic. The condyloma may be solitary, multifocal or diffuse, varying from papillary to flat. Typically, it consists of papillary or acanthotic flat mucosa with hyperplastic squamous epithelium. The cells display distinctive features of koilocytotic atypia, including abundant cytoplasm with perinuclear clearing ('halo') and shrunken eccentric hyperchromatic nuclei. The most common human papilloma serotypes in urothelial condylomata are 6, 11, 16 and 18; special studies such as immunohistochemistry, *in situ* hybridization and polymerase chain reaction may be diagnostically useful in difficult cases, but are not routinely employed (Murphy *et al.*, 1983; Del Mistro *et al.*, 1987; Melchers *et al.*, 1989). Treatment is variable, depending on the extent of the disease. Condyloma may be associated with squamous cell carcinoma.

15.3.2 Urothelial carcinoma (transitional cell carcinoma)

Urethral involvement by urothelial carcinoma and carcinoma *in situ* is usually associated with bladder involvement, present in up to 45% of cases of bladder cancer and diligent search for synchronous lesions should be made (Gowing, 1960; Wolinska *et al.*, 1977; Richie and Skinner, 1978; Schellhammer, 1983; Hermansen *et al.*, 1988; Orihuela, Herr and Whitmore, 1989; Hardeman and Soloway, 1990; Tobisu *et al.*, 1991). Urothelial carcinoma is discussed in Chapter 11.

15.3.3 Squamous cell carcinoma

Primary squamous cell carcinoma of the prostatic urethra is very rare and appears to have the same prognosis as adenocarcinoma; survival at 5 years appears to be worse than in cancer arising in the distal urethra, probably as a result of diagnosis at higher stage and the potential for prostatic stromal infiltration. The distinction of high-grade urothelial carcinoma and non-keratinizing squamous cell carcinoma is often difficult and of no apparent clinical value. Human papillomavirus type 16 is associated with urethral squamous cell carcinoma (Weiner, Liu and Walther, 1992).

15.3.4 Urethral adenocarcinoma, including those involving accessory glands

Primary adenocarcinoma of the urethra, Cowper glands or periurethral glands of Littre is rare and usually high-grade, with less than 50 reported cases (Keen *et al.*, 1970; Sacks *et al.*, 1975; Cantrell *et al.*, 1981; Saito, 1981; Silverman *et al.*, 1981; Lieber *et al.*, 1983; Bostwick, Lo and Stamey, 1984; Yachia and Turani, 1991;

Diaz-Cano *et al.*, 1992; Loo and Chan, 1992). Patients present with hematuria, dysuria, obstructive symptoms and irritative symptoms, and some have intractable urethritis.

The most common adenocarcinoma of the prostatic urethra is ductal (endometrioid) carcinoma (Chapter 9). Adenocarcinoma of Cowper glands is chiefly located in the bulbomembranous urethra, and periurethral gland adenocarcinoma usually occurs in the distal urethra rather than the prostatic urethra. The microscopic features are typical of adenocarcinoma at other sites. Separation from prostatic adenocarcinoma is difficult, particularly in large cancers with obstructive symptoms and prostatic involvement; PSA and PAP may occasionally be useful, with immunoreactivity in prostatic cancers but not always in cancers at these other sites.

Clear cell adenocarcinoma (mesonephric adenocarcinoma or glycogen-rich carcinoma) is a histological variant of adenocarcinoma with characteristic hobnail cells within glands with tubular, papillary, micropapillary, acinar or diffuse growth (Cantrell *et al.*, 1981; Assimos and O'Conor, 1984; Young and Scully, 1985; Hull *et al.*, 1987). The cells have abundant, clear, glycogen-rich cytoplasm and large nuclei. Luminal secretions are mucicarmiophilic but tumor cells usually have little or no mucin. Some cases display PSA and PAP immunoreactivity. This tumor probably arises by urothelial metaplasia rather than from müllerian or mesonephric origin. Patients occasionally have paraneoplastic hypercalcemia, similar to other clear cell adenocarcinomas (Saito, 1981). The main differential diagnostic considerations are nephrogenic metaplasia, metastatic clear cell renal cell carcinoma, prostatic adenocarcinoma following androgen deprivation therapy, ductal carcinoma with clear cell features and amelanotic melanoma. Prognosis depends on stage at presentation.

15.3.5 Malignant melanoma

Malignant melanoma involves the urethra more than any other site in the urinary tract, but there have been less than 50 reported cases (Weiss, Elder and Hamilton, 1982; Begun *et al.*, 1984; Sanders, Venable and Sanusi, 1986; Oldbring and Mikulowski, 1987; Manivel and Fraley, 1988; Pow-Sang *et al.*, 1988). Patients present with lower-urinary-tract obstructive symptoms and rarely with melanuria. The penile urethra and meatus are more commonly involved than the prostatic urethra, and cystoscopy reveals an ulcerated nodule or plaque-like mass, which may be pigmented.

Urethral melanoma usually has a lentiginous and radial growth pattern. The histological features are similar to melanoma at other sites, although it is more commonly amelanotic in the urethra. Prognosis is determined by the depth and extent; surgical treatment is recommended. The pathologist should report the status of surgical margins and the presence of satellite or skip lesions.

15.3.6 Other tumors and tumor-like conditions

Rare soft tissue tumors of the urethra include leiomyoma (Ohtani *et al.*, 1982), capillary hemangioma (Sharma *et al.*, 1981), and paraganglioma (Badalament *et al.*, 1991). Localized primary amyloidosis may form a mass simulating neoplasm (amyloidoma) (Vasudevan *et al.*, 1981; Dounis, Bourounis and Mitropoulos, 1985).

REFERENCES

Assimos, D. G. and O'Conor, V. J. Jr (1984) Clear cell adenocarcinoma of the urethra. *J. Urol.*, **131**, 540–541.

Badalament, R. A., Kenworthy, P., Pellegrini, A. and Drago, J. R. (1991) Paraganglioma of urethra. *Urology*, **38**, 76–78.

Begun, F. P., Grossman, H. B., Diokno, A. C. and Sogani, P. C. (1984) Malignant melanoma of the penis and male urethra. *J. Urol.*, **132**, 123–125.

Bhagavan, B. S., Tiamson, E. M., Wenk, R. E. *et al.* (1981) Nephrogenic adenoma of the urinary bladder and urethra. *Hum. Pathol.*, **12**, 907–916.

Bostwick, D. G., Lo, R. and Stamey, T. A. (1984) Papillary adenocarcinoma of the male urethra. Case report and review of the literature. *Cancer*, **54**, 2556–2563.

Bruijnes, E., de Wall, J. G., Scholtmeijer, R. J. and den Hollander, J. C. (1985) Congenital polyp of the prostatic urethra in childhood. Report of 3 cases and review of the literature. *Urol. Int.*, **40**, 287–291.

Cantrell, B. B., Leifer, G., DeKlerk, D. P. and Eggleston, J. C. (1981) Papillary adenocarcinoma of the prostatic urethra with clear-cell appearance. *Cancer*, **48**, 2661–2667.

Craig, J. R. and Hart, W. R. (1975) Benign polyps with prostatic-type epithelium of the urethra. *Am. J. Clin. Pathol.*, **63**, 343–347.

Damjanov, I. and Katz, S. M. (1981) Malakoplakia. *Pathol. Ann.*, **16**, 103–126.

Del Mistro, A., Braunstein, J. D., Halwer, M. and Koss, L. G. (1987) Identification of human papillomavirus types in male urethral condylomata acuminata by in situ hybridization. *Hum. Pathol.*, **18**, 936–940.

Diaz-Cano, S. J., Rios, J. J., Rivera-Hueto, F. and Galera-Davidson, H. (1992) Mixed cloacogenic carcinoma of male urethra. *Histopathology*, **20**, 82–84.

Dounis, A., Bourounis, M. and Mitropoulos, D. (1985) Primary localized amyloidosis of the urethra. *Eur. Urol.*, **11**, 344–345.

Elgamal, A., van de Voorde, W., van Poppel, H. *et al.* (1994) Immunohistochemical localization of prostate-specific markers within the accessory male sex glands of Cowper, Littre, and Morgagni. *Urology*, **434**, 84–90.

Foster, R. S. and Garrett, R. A. (1986) Congenital posterior urethral polyps. *J. Urol.*, **136**, 670–672.

Frazier, H. A., Humphrey, P. A., Burchette, J. L. *et al.* (1992) Immunoreactive prostate specific antigen in male periurethral glands. *J. Urol.*, **147**, 246–250.

Goldstein, A. M., Bragin, S. D., Terry, R. and Yoell, J. H. (1981) Prostatic urethral polyps in adults. Histopathologic variations and clinical manifestations. *J. Urol.*, **126**, 129–131.

Gowing, N. F. C. (1960) Urethral carcinoma associated with cancer of the bladder. *Br. J. Urol.*, **32**, 428–430.

Hardeman, S. W. and Soloway, M. S. (1990) Urethral recurrence following radical cystectomy. *J. Urol.*, **144**, 666–669.

Hermansen, D. K., Badalament, R. A., Whitmore, W. F. Jr *et al.* (1988) Detection of carcinoma in the post-cystectomy urethral remnant by flow cytometric analysis. *J. Urol.*, **139**, 304–307.

Hoffman, W. W. and Cheatum, D. E. (1978) Reiter's disease. *Urol. Surv.*, **28**, 197–205.

Hull, M. T., Eglen, D. E., Davis, T. *et al.* (1987) Glycogen-rich clear cell carcinoma of the urethra: an ultrastructural study. *Ultrastr. Pathol.*, **11**, 421–427.

Keen, M. R., Golden, R. L., Richardson, J. F. and Melicow, M. M. (1970) Carcinoma of Cowper's gland treated with chemotherapy. *J. Urol.*, **104**, 854–856.

Lieber, M. M., Malek, R. S., Farrow, G. M. and McMurty, J. (1983) Villous adenocarcinoma of the male urethra. *J. Urol.*, **130**, 1191–1193.

Loo, K. T. and Chan, J. K. (1992) Colloid adenocarcinoma of the urethra associated with mucosal in situ carcinoma. *Arch. Pathol. Lab. Med.*, **116**, 976–977.

Lubin, J., Mark, T. M. and Wirtschafter, A. R. (1984) Papillomas of prostatic urethra with prostatic-type epithelium. Report of 8 cases. *Mt Sinai J. Med.*, **51**, 218–221.

Manivel, J. C. and Fraley, E. E. (1988) Malignant melanoma of the penis and male urethra: 4 case reports and literature review. *J. Urol.*, **139**, 813–816.

Medeiros, L. J. and Young, R. H. (1989) Nephrogenic adenoma arising in urethral diverticula. A report of 5 cases. *Arch. Pathol. Lab. Med.*, **113**, 125–128.

Melchers, W. J., Schift, R., Stolz, E. *et al.* (1989) Human papillomavirus detection in urine samples from male patients by the polymerase chain reaction. *J. Clin. Microbiol.*, **27**, 1711–1714.

Mostofi, F. K. and Price, E. B. Jr (1973) *Tumors of the Male Genital System, Atlas of Tumor Pathology*, fascicle 8, second series, Armed Forces Institute of Pathology, Washington, DC, pp. 244–245.

Murphy, W. M., Beckwith, J. B. and Farrow, G. M. (1994) Tumors of the kidney, bladder, and related urinary structures, *Atlas of Tumor Pathology*, Armed Forces Institute of Pathology, Washington, DC, pp. 193–308.

Murphy, W. M., Fu, Y. S., Lancaster, W. D. and Jenson, A. B. (1983) Papillomavirus structural antigens in condyloma acuminatum of the male urethra. *J. Urol.*, **130**, 84–85.

Ohtani, M., Yanagizawa, R., Shoji, F. *et al.* (1982) Leiomyoma of the male urethra. *Eur. Urol.*, **8**, 372–373.

Oldbring, J. and Mikulowski, P. (1987) Malignant melanoma of the penis and male urethra. Report of 9 cases and review of the literature. *Cancer* **59**, 581–587.

Orihuela, E., Herr, H. W. and Whitmore, W. F. Jr. (1989) Conservative treatment of superficial transitional cell carcinoma of prostatic urethra with intravesicle BCG. *Urology*, **34**, 231–237.

Pow-Sang, J. M., Klimberg, I. W., Hackett, R. L. and Wajsman, Z. (1988) Primary malignant melanoma of the male urethra. *J. Urol.*, **139**, 1304–1306.

Remick, D. G. Jr and Kumar, N. B. (1984) Benign polyps with prostatic-type epithelium of the urethra and the urinary bladder. A suggestion of histogenesis based on histologic and immunohistochemical studies. *Am. J. Surg. Pathol.*, **8**, 833–839.

Renfer, L. G., Kelly, J. and Belville, W. D. (1988) Inverted papilloma of the urinary tract. Histogenesis, recurrence and associated malignancy. *J. Urol.*, **140**, 832–834.

Richie, J. P. and Skinner, D. G. (1978) Carcinoma in situ of the urethra associated with bladder carcinoma: the role of urethrectomy. *J. Urol.*, **119**, 80–81.

Sacks, S. A., Waisman, J., Apfelbaum, H. B. *et al.* (1975) Urethral adenocarcinoma (possibly originating in the glands of Littre). *J. Urol.*, **113**, 50–55.

Saito, R. (1981) An adenosquamous carcinoma of the male urethra with hypercalcemia. *Hum. Pathol.*, **12**, 383–385.

Sanders, T. J., Venable, D. D. and Sanusi, I. D. (1986) Primary malignant melanoma of the urethra in a black man: a case report. *J. Urol.*, **135**, 1012–1014.

Satoh, S., Ujiie, T., Kubo, T. *et al.* (1989) Prostatic epithelial polyp of the prostatic urethra. *Eur. Urol.*, **16**, 92–96.

Schellhammer, P. F. (1983) Urethral carcinoma. *Sem. Urol.*, **1**, 82–89.

Schinella, R., Thurm, J. and Feiner, H. (1974) Papillary pseudotumor of the prostatic urethra: proliferative papillary urethritis. *J. Urol.*, **111**, 38–40.

Sharma, T. C., Kagan, H. and Shiels, J. P. (1981) Malakoplakia of the male urethra. *J. Urol.*, **125**, 885–886.

Sharma, S. K., Reddy, M. J., Joshi, V. V. and Bapna, B. C. (1981) Capillary haemangioma of the male urethra. *Br. J. Urol.*, **53**, 277.

Silverman, M. L., Eyre, R. C., Zinman, L. A. and Corsson, A. W. (1981) Mixed mucinous and papillary adenocarcinoma involving male urethra, probably originating in periurethral glands. *Cancer*, **47**, 1398–1402.

Tobisù, K., Tanaka, Y., Mitzutani, T. and Kakizoe, T. (1991) Transitional cell carcinoma of the urethra in men following cystectomy for bladder cancer: multivariate analysis for risk factors. *J. Urol.*, **146**, 1551–1553.

Vasudevan, P., Stein, A. M., Pinn, V. W. and Rao, C. N. (1981) Primary amyloidosis of urethra. *Urology*, **17**, 181–183.

Walker, A. N. and Mills, S. E. (1989) Papillary and polypoid tumors of the prostatic urethra, in *Progress in Reproductive and Urinary Tract Pathology 1*, (eds I. Damjanov, A. H. Cohen, S. E. Mills and R. H. Young), Field & Wood, New York, pp.

113–114.

Walker, A. N., Mills, S. E., Fechner, R. E. and Perry, J. M. (1982) 'Endometrial' adenocarcinoma of the prostatic urethra arising in a villous polyp. A light microscopic and immunoperoxidase study. *Arch. Pathol. Lab. Med.*, **106**, 624–627.

Weiner, J. S., Liu, E. T. and Walther, P. J. (1992) Oncogenic human papillomavirus type 16 is associated with squamous cell carcinoma of the male urethra. *Cancer Res.*, 52, 5018–5023.

Weiss, J., Elder, D. and Hamilton, R. (1982) Melanoma of the male urethra: surgical approach and pathological analysis. *J. Urol.*, **128**, 382–385.

Wolinska, W. H., Melamed, M. R., Schellhammer, P. F. and Whitmore, W. F. Jr (1977) Urethral cytology following cystectomy for bladder carcinoma. *Am. J. Surg. Pathol.*, **1**, 225–234.

Yachia, D. and Turani, H. (1991) Colonic-type adenocarcinoma of the male urethra. *Urology*, **37**, 568–570.

Young, R. H. and Scully, R. E. (1985) Clear cell adenocarcinoma of the bladder and urethra. A report of 3 cases and review of the literature. *Am. J. Surg. Pathol.*, **9**, 816–826.

16

DNA PLOIDY ANALYSIS AND MOLECULAR BIOLOGY OF THE PROSTATE

There is a great need for studies of tissue biopsy samples that provide additional prognostic information beyond the usual light-microscopic findings. This chapter briefly surveys the current status of many of these markers in prostate cancer. Recent reviews provide details regarding methods and their limitations (Isaacs *et al.*, 1994; Netto and Humphrey, 1994; Ware, 1994; Bostwick, Pacelli and Lopez-Beltran, 1996). None of these markers is recommended for general use in practice by the College of American Pathologists, although DNA ploidy may be useful in specific clinical settings (Grignon and Hammond, 1995). This chapter is a brief introduction to this dynamic and rapidly expanding field, with emphasis on practical aspects in biopsy specimens such as DNA ploidy analysis.

16.1 DNA PLOIDY ANALYSIS (DNA CONTENT ANALYSIS)

DNA ploidy analysis of prostate cancer by flow cytometry and digital image analysis provides important prognostic information that supplements histopathological examination (Figure 16.1).

Patients with diploid tumors have a more favorable outcome than those with aneuploid tumors; for example, among patients with lymph node metastases treated with radical prostatectomy and androgen deprivation therapy, those with diploid tumors may survive 20 years or more, whereas those with aneuploid tumors die within 5 years (Zincke *et al.*, 1992). However, the ploidy pattern of prostate cancer is often heterogeneous, creating potential problems with sampling error. Most studies use matched benign or hyperplastic prostatic tissue as controls. Seminal vesicle tissue is unsuitable as a control because of the low but significant level of aneuploidy in the lining cells (Arber and Speights, 1991).

Flow cytometry is the most common method of DNA ploidy analysis, but is limited by the need for a large number of cells. The minimum amount of needle core tissue necessary to yield satisfactory results with flow cytometry is a 0.2 cm length of malignant acini, which corresponds to about 2500–5000 nuclei (Takai *et al.*, 1994). Digital image analysis overcomes this limitation and is gaining popularity despite a lack of standards for this method. Other methods such as fluorescence *in situ* can assess DNA ploidy for individual chromosomes. FISH requires less tissue, but is labor-intensive and expensive (Takahashi *et al.*, 1994).

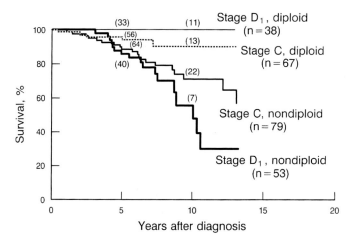

Figure 16.1 Postoperative probability of survival of pathological stage C and D1 prostatic carcinoma according to DNA ploidy pattern. (Source: reproduced with permission from Nativ *et al.*, 1989.)

16.1.1 Flow cytometry

DNA ploidy pattern by flow cytometry correlates with cancer grade (Nativ *et al.*, 1989; Montgomery *et al.*, 1990), tumor volume and stage (Jones *et al.*, 1990, 1992; Warzynski *et al.*, 1994). Most low-stage tumors are diploid and high-stage tumors are non-diploid, but numerous exceptions occur (Tribukait, 1993; Winkler *et al.*, 1988). The 5-year cancer-specific survival is about 95% for diploid tumors, 70% for tetraploid tumors and 25% for tumors with multiple aneuploid cell lines (Stephenson *et al.*, 1987; Deitch and deVere White, 1992; DeVere White *et al.*, 1992; Forsslund *et al.*, 1992; Van den Ouden *et al.*, 1993). Patients with diploid tumors have a more favorable outcome than those with aneuploid tumors; for example, among patients with lymph node metastases treated with radical prostatectomy and androgen deprivation therapy, those with diploid tumors may survive 20 years or more whereas those with aneuploid tumors die within 5 years (Zincke *et al.*, 1992).

An international DNA Cytometry Consensus Conference reviewed the literature in 1993 and concluded that the clinical significance and biological basis of DNA ploidy needed further investigation (Shankey *et al.*, 1993). At the Mayo Clinic, we routinely perform DNA ploidy analysis in radical prostatectomy specimens for cancer (Winkler *et al.*, 1988; Nativ *et al.*, 1989; Montgomery *et al.*, 1990; Zincke *et al.*, 1992).

16.1.2 Digital image analysis of needle biopsies

Digital image analysis (DIA) refers to the quantification of microscopic images of a cell by camera acquisition, digital conversion and spectrophometric and computer analysis of the image features. The Feulgen stain stoichiometrically binds to hydrolyzed nucleic acids, coloring nuclei blue according to the amount of DNA present. The concentration of DNA is directly proportional to the absorption at 620 nm.

High-grade PIN shows genetic instability, according to digital image analysis studies of nuclear DNA content in tissue sections and other studies (Petein *et al.*, 1991; Sakr *et al.*, 1992; Amin *et al.*, 1993; Crissman *et al.*, 1993; De La Torre *et al.*, 1993; Weinberg and Weidner, 1993; Baretton *et al.*, 1994; Takahashi *et al.*, 1994). Montironi *et al.* suggested that two successive phases occur (Montironi *et al.*, 1990); the first occurs in hyperplastic epithelium and low-grade PIN and is characterized by DNA duplication without nuclear division, resulting in euploidy (diploid (2N) or tetraploid (4N)); the second occurs only in high-grade PIN and cancer and results in the emergence of aneuploid elements (triploid, hyperdiploid, hypotetraploid and aneuploid). Similar results were reported by Petein *et al.*, who noted that the mean proliferative index and proportion of aneuploid cell nuclei in high-grade PIN were similar to cancer but differed significantly from hyperplastic epithelium and low-grade PIN (Petein *et al.*, 1991). Amin *et al.* (1993) found an incidence of 32% aneuploidy in high-grade PIN and 55% in carcinoma, somewhat lower than the results of Crissman *et al.* (57% and 62%, respectively; Crissman *et al.*, 1993). Weinberg and Weidner (1993) also noted concordance of DNA content in a small series of PIN and cancer, with the majority being diploid. Baretton and colleagues detected aneuploidy by image cytometry in 30% of cases of high-grade PIN and found that 70% of aneuploid cases were associated with aneuploid invasive carcinoma; conversely, only 29% of cases of aneuploid cancer were associated with aneuploid PIN (Baretton *et al.*, 1994). Berner and colleagues found that 68% of cases of high-grade PIN were aneuploid (Berner *et al.*, 1993).

We routinely perform DNA ploidy analysis by digital image analysis on needle biopsies or specimens with a limited amount of cancer and use flow cytometry only for radical prostatectomy specimens with abundant cancer. Concordance of static image analysis on needle biopsy and flow cytometry from radical prostatectomy specimens is 82% (Takai *et al.*, 1994).

16.1.3 Fluorescence *in situ* hybridization (FISH) ploidy

Fluorescence *in situ* hybridization (FISH) analysis of interphase cells with centromere-specific and region-specific probes is useful for the detection of numerical chromosomal anomalies in solid tumors, including prostatic carcinoma, which is often difficult for conventional cytogenetic analysis. When applied to histological sections, this method allows study of multiple foci of normal epithelium, AAH, PIN and carcinoma within a single prostate specimen and makes the evaluation of matched metastatic sites possible.

Genetic alterations are present in 9% of cases of AAH, according to a FISH ploidy study using centromere-specific probes for chromosomes 7, 8, 10, 12 and Y (Qian, Bostwick and Jenkins, 1995).

The overall frequency of numeric chromosomal anomalies in PIN and carcinoma foci is remarkably similar (50% and 51% respectively), suggesting that they have a similar pathogenesis (Emmert-Buck *et al.*, 1995). Overall, the mean number of abnormal chromosomes increased in PIN to carcinoma foci, and malignant foci contain more anomalies than paired PIN foci. These findings suggest that PIN is a precursor of carcinoma (Sakr *et al.*, 1994; Takahashi *et al.*, 1994; Bostwick, 1995; Emmert-Buck *et al.*, 1995).

Gain of chromosome 8 is the most frequent numeric anomaly in PIN and prostatic carcinoma (Emmert-Buck *et al.*, 1995), suggesting that alterations of this chromosome and/or a tumor suppressor gene(s) on the short arm may be important for the initiation or early progression of prostate cancer. FISH studies with centromere-specific probes for chromosomes 7, 8, 11 and 12 have shown that gains of chromosomes 7 and 8 are markers of tumor aggressiveness and prognosis (Takahashi *et al.*, 1994). The cumulative findings suggest that gain of chromosome 8 is a marker of clinically aggressive prostatic carcinoma. Chromosome 7 also appears to be important in cancer progression (Zitzelsberger *et al.*, 1994).

16.2 MOLECULAR BIOLOGY AND NEW BIOMARKERS

Molecular biology techniques require human tissue or serum for analysis (Figure 16.2).

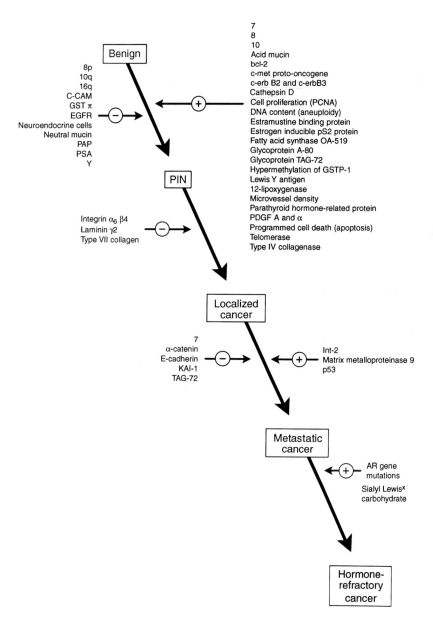

Figure 16.2 Genetic changes and other changes associated with progression of prostate cancer. Some bio-markers show upregulation or gain (+), whereas others are downregulated or lost (—). There is a prominent clustering of changes in expression for many biomarkers between benign epithelium and high-grade PIN, indicating that this is an important threshold for carcinogenesis in the prostate. A small number of other changes are introduced in the progression from high-grade PIN to localized cancer, metastatic cancer and hormone-refractory cancer. The model indicates the initial change in expression of a biomarker; most of these changes become magnified in subsequent steps. This model is based chiefly on studies of human prostatic tissue and excludes many biomarkers that have not been evaluated in PIN or different stages of cancer. (Source: reproduced with permission from Bostwick, Pacelli and Lopez-Beltran, 1996.)

Methods are being refined for use with scant specimens such as biopsies, recognizing that no additional tissue is obtained from patients treated by expectant management, radiation therapy, cryotherapy, androgen deprivation therapy and other non-surgical methods.

16.2.1 Allelic loss

Allelic loss is a common finding in high-grade PIN and prostatic adenocarcinoma, present in more than 50% of cases of cancer on chromosomes 8p, 10q and 16q (Bergerheim *et al.*, 1991; Sandberg, 1992; Bova *et al.*, 1993; MacGrogan *et al.*, 1994; Sakr *et al.*, 1994; Emmert-Buck *et al.*, 1995). One or more tumor suppressor genes appear to be present on 8p that may be involved in carcinogenesis (Bova *et al.*, 1993; MacGrogan *et al.*, 1994). Allelic loss appears to be more common in high-grade tumors (Mac-Grogan *et al.*, 1994). There is also loss of heterozygosity of chromosome Y in some cases of PIN and cancer (Alers *et al.*, 1995).

16.2.2 Tumor suppressor genes and oncogenes

Oncogenesis probably occurs through the selection of several genetic changes, each modifying the expression or function of genes controlling cell growth and differentiation. Overexpression of *p53*, a tumor suppressor gene on chromosome 17p, is present in up to 25% of high-stage prostate cancers but is rare in low-stage cancer, suggesting that it plays a role in late progression (Bookstein *et al.*, 1993; Effert *et al.*, 1993; Van Veldhuizen *et al.*, 1993; Fan *et al.*, 1994; Myers *et al.*, 1994; Hall *et al.*, 1995; Kubota *et al.*, 1995; Mirchandani *et al.*, 1995). The tumor suppressor gene *DCC* shows allelic deletion and loss of expression in 45% of cases, indicating that it is a frequent feature of prostate cancer (Gao *et al.*, 1993). There is upregulation of c-*met* proto-oncogene in PIN and cancer (Pisters *et al.*, 1995). Loss of expression of the retinoblastoma gene on chromo-

some 13q is seen in a minority of prostate cancers, usually in advanced stage (Bookstein *et al.*, 1990). Decreased expression of the tumor metastasis suppression gene *KAI1* may be involved in metastasis (Dong *et al.*, 1995). Activated oncogenes such as *ras* appear to be infrequent in early prostate cancer (Moul *et al.*, 1992; Kuhn *et al.*, 1993).

16.2.3 Growth factors

Peptide growth factors appear to control development of normal and neoplastic prostatic epithelium by acting as paracrine mediators of epithelial–stromal interaction and growth (Steiner, 1993). The epidermal growth factor (EGF) family of peptides includes EGF, TGF-alpha (transforming growth factor alpha), amphiregulin and other factors which act through the same transmembrane glycoprotein receptor and tyrosine kinase. Cancer cells synthesize of TGF-alpha, and this stimulates epithelial and fibroblastic proliferation (Myers *et al.*, 1993; Harper *et al.*, 1993; Maygarden, Strom and Ware, 1992; Cohen *et al.*, 1994; Robertson *et al.*, 1994; Turkeri *et al.*, 1994). Epidermal growth factor receptors are downregulated in PIN and cancer (Ibrahim *et al.*, 1993; Montone and Tomaszewski, 1993; Myers, Kudlow and Grizzle, 1993; Maygarden *et al.*, 1994; Robertson *et al.*, 1994; Turkeri *et al.*, 1994).

The transforming growth factor beta (TGF-beta) family of peptides, including TGF-beta$_1$ and TGF-beta$_2$, appear to be regulators of cell differentiation and proliferation (Myers, Kudlow and Grizzle, 1993; Thompson *et al.*, 1992; Eklov *et al.*, 1993). Expression of the TGF-beta receptor appears to be under negative androgenic regulation, suggesting that TGF-beta plays a role in cell death following androgen deprivation. The TGF-beta binding protein is produced in benign and hyperplastic tissue but not in malignant tissue (Eklov *et al.*, 1993). Members of the platelet-derived growth factor peptide family also appear to be upregulated with PIN and cancer (Fudge, Wang and Stearns,1994; Fudge, Bostwick and

Table 16.1 Micrometastases in patients with prostate cancer (RTPCR = reverse-transcriptive PCR for PSA mRNA sequence; PSA = prostate-specific antigen; PAP = prostatic acid phosphatase)

Site	Author and year	No. of cancer patients	Method of detection	Results
Lymph nodes	Deguchi et al, 1993	22	RTPCR and immunohistochemistry (anti-PSA)	Micrometastases by RTPCR in six patients (27.3%), including four with both histological and immunohistochemical confirmation
	Gomella et al, 1993	32	Immunohistochemistry (anti-PSA, PAP, and cytokeratin)	Micrometastases in one of 32 patients (3%)
	Moul et al, 1994	32	Immunohistochenistry (anti-PSA and cytokeratin)	Micrometastases in one of 32 patients (3%)
Bone marrow	Mansi et al, 1988	40	Immunohistochemistry (anti-PSA)	Micrometastases in 73% of patients with clinically metastatic cancer and 13% with clinically organ-confined cancer
	Wood et al, 1994	55	RTPCR and immunohistochemistry (anti-PSA)	Micrometastases in 65% of patients with extraprostatic organ-confined cancer; immunohistochemistry confirmed micrometastases in 79% of those with positive RTPCR
Serum	Hamdy et al, 1992	40	Flow cytometry and immunohistochemistry (anti-PSA)	PSA-positive cells in 47% of patients with stage non-D2 cancers and 100% with stage D2 cancer
	Moreno et al, 1992	12	RTPCR (anti-PSA)	PSA-positive cells in four of 12 patients with stage D cancer (33%)
	Katz et al, 1994	83	RTPCR (anti-PSA)	PSA-positive cells in 77.8% of patients with stage D cancers, and 38.5% with clinically organ-confined cancer

Stearns, 1995). The role of growth factors in prostatic adenocarcinoma has recently been reviewed (Steiner, 1993; Ware, 1994).

16.2.4 Other prostatic biomarkers

There are many other tumor markers in prostatic adenocarcinoma that may be clinically valuable, including Bcl-2 (Colombel *et al.*, 1993), cathepsin D (Makar *et al.*, 1994; Maygarden *et al.*, 1994; Ross *et al.*, 1995), tumor-associated glycoprotein TAG-72 (Brenner *et al.*, 1995), E-cadherin (Umbas *et al.*, 1992; Morton *et al.*, 1993), epithelial cell adhesion molecule C-CAM (Kleinerman *et al.*, 1995), prostate mucin antigen, prostate specific membrane antigen, telomerase (Kim *et al.*, 1994), matrix metalloproteinases (Hamdy *et al.*, 1994), type IV collagenase (Stearns and Wang, 1993; Boag and Young, 1994), glutathione S-transferase pi (Lee *et al.*, 1994), Nm23 and nuclear matrix protein PC-1 (Bostwick and Qian, 1994).

16.2.5 PSA-positive cells in the peripheral blood detected by polymerase chain reaction

Cells that express PSA mRNA (presumably cancer cells) can be detected in the peripheral blood by reverse transcriptase polymerase chain reaction studies of routine blood samples. In one study, circulating cells were identified in four of 12 patients with adenocarcinoma with pelvic lymph node metastases (Table 16.1) (Moreno *et al.*, 1992).

Katz *et al.* demonstrated the clinical utility of this test in predicting stage, and referred to it as 'molecular staging' (Katz *et al.*, 1994; Cama *et al.*, 1995). By comparison, circulating PSA-immunoreactive cells in the blood were identified by flow cytometry in all cases of adenocarcinoma with distant metastases and 47% of lower stage adenocarcinomas (Hamdy *et al.*, 1992).

REFERENCES

Alers, J. C., Krijtenberg, P. J., Vissers, K. J. *et al.* (1995) Interphase cytogenetics of prostatic adenocarcinoma and precursor lesions: analysis of 25 radical prostatectomies and 17 adjacent prostatic intraepithelial neoplasias. *Genes Chromosomes Cancer*, **12**, 241–250.

Amin, M. B., Schultz, D. S., Zarbo, R. J. *et al.* (1993) Computerized static DNA ploidy analysis of prostatic intraepithelial neoplasia. *Arch. Pathol. Lab. Med.*, **117**, 794–798.

Arber, D. A. and Speights, V. O. (1991) Aneuploidy in benign seminal vesicle epithelium: an example of the paradox of ploidy studies. *Mod. Pathol.*, **4**, 687–689.

Baretton, G. B., Vogt, T., Blasenbreu, S. *et al.* (1994) Comparison of DNA ploidy in prostatic intraepithelial neoplasia and invasive carcinoma of the prostate: an image cytometric study. *Hum. Pathol.*, **25**, 506–513.

Bergerheim, U. S. R., Kunimi, K., Collins, V. P. and Ekman, P. (1991) Deletion mapping of chromosomes 8, 10, and 16 in human prostatic carcinoma. *Genes Chromosomes Cancer*, **3**, 215–220.

Berner, A., Danielsen, H. E., Pettersen, E. O. *et al.* (1993) DNA distribution in the prostate. Normal gland, benign and premalignant lesions, and subsequent adenocarcinomas. *Anal. Quant. Cytol. Histol.*, **15**, 247–252.

Boag, A. H. and Young, I. D. (1994) Increased expression of the 72-kd Type IV collagenase in prostatic adenocarcinoma. Demonstration by immunohistochemistry and in situ hybridization. *Am. J. Pathol.*, **144**, 585–591.

Bookstein, R., Rio, P., Madreperla, S. *et al.* (1990) Promoter deletion and loss of retinoblastoma gene expression in human prostate carcinoma. *Proc. Nat. Acad. Sci. USA*, **87**, 7762–7766.

Bookstein, R., MacGrogan, D., Hilsenbeck, S. G. *et al.* (1993) p53 is mutated in a subset of advanced-stage prostate cancers. *Cancer Res.*, **53**, 3369–3373.

Bostwick, D. G., Pacelli, A. and Lopez-Beltran, A. (1996) Molecular biology of prostatic intraepithelial neoplasia. *Prostate*, **29**, 117–134.

Bostwick, D. G. and Qian, J. (1994) Current and proposed biologic markers in prostate cancer: 1994. *J. Cell Biochem. Suppl.*, **19**, 197–201.

Bova, G. S., Carter, B. S., Bussemakers, M. J. G. *et al.* (1993) Homozygous deletion and frequent allelic loss of chromosome 8p22 loci in human prostate cancer. *Cancer Res.*, **53**, 3869–3873.

Brenner, P. C., Rettig, W. J., Sanz-Moncasi, M. P. *et al.* (1995) TAG-72 expression in primary, metastatic and hormonally treated prostate cancer as defined by monoclonal antibody CC49. *J. Urol.*, **153**, 1575–1579.

Cama, C., Olsson, C. A., Raffo, A. J. *et al.* (1995) Molecular staging of prostate cancer. II. A comparison of the application of an enhanced reverse transcriptase polymerase chain reation assay for prostate specific antigen versus prostate specific membrane antigen. *J. Urol.*, **153**, 1373–1378.

Cohen, D. W., Simak, R., Fair, W. R. *et al.* (1994) Expression of transforming growth factor receptor in human prostate tissues. *J. Urol.*, **152**, 2120–2124.

Colombel, M., Symmans, F., Gil, S. *et al.* (1993) Detection of the apoptosis-suppressing oncoprotein Bcl-2 in hormone-refractory human prostate cancers. *Am. J. Pathol.*, **143**, 390–400.

Crissman, J. D., Sakr, W. A., Hussein, M. E. *et al.* (1993) DNA quantitation of intraepithelial neoplasia and invasive carcinoma of the prostate. *Prostate*, **22**, 155–162.

Deitch, A. D. and deVere White, R. W. (1992) Flow cytometry as a predictive modality in prostate cancer. *Hum. Pathol.*, **23**, 352–359.

De La Torre, M., Haggman, M., Brandstedt, S. *et al.* (1993) Prostatic intraepithelial neoplasia and invasive carcinoma in total prostatectomy specimens: distribution, volume and DNA ploidy. *Br. J. Urol.*, **72**, 207–213.

DeVere White, R. W., Deitch, A. D., Meyer-Haass, G. M. *et al.* (1992) Deoxyribonucleic acid ploidy in the irradiated prostate. *World J. Urol.*, **10**, 173–178.

Dong, J-T., Lamb, P. W., Rinker-Schaeffer, C. W. *et al.* (1995) KAI1, a metastasis suppressor gene for prostate cancer on human chromosome 11p11.2. *Science*, **268**, 884–886.

Effert, P. J., McCoy, R. H., Walther, P. J. and Liu, E. T. (1993) *p53* gene alterations in human prostate carcinoma. *J. Urol.*, **150**, 257–261.

Eklov, S., Funa, K., Nordgren, H. *et al.* (1993) Lack of the latent transforming growth factor Beta binding protein in malignant, but not benign prostatic tissue. *Cancer Res.*, **53**, 3193–3197.

Emmert-Buck, M. R., Vocke, C. D., Pozzatti, R. O. *et al.* (1995) Allelic loss on chromosome 8p12-21 in microdissected prostatic intraepithelial neoplasia (PIN). *Cancer Res.*, **55**, 2959–2962.

Fan, K., Dao, D. D., Schutz, M. and Fink, L. M. (1994) Loss of heterozygosity and overexpression of p53 gene in human primary prostatic adenocarcinoma. *Diag. Mol. Pathol.*, **3**, 265–270.

Forsslund, G., Esposti, P. L., Nilsson, B. and Zetterberg, A. (1992) The prognostic significance of nuclear DNA content in prostatic carcinoma. *Cancer*, **69**, 1432–1439.

Fudge, K., Bostwick, D. G. and Stearns, M. E. (1996) Platelet-derived growth factor A and B chains and the Alpha and Beta receptors in prostatic intraepithelial neoplasia. *Prostate*, (in press).

Fudge, K., Wang, C. Y. and Stearns, M. E. (1994) Immunohistochemistry analysis of platelet-derived growth factor A and B chains and platelet-derived growth factor alpha and beta receptor expression in benign prostatic hyperplasias and Gleason-graded human prostate adenocarcinomas. *Mod. Pathol.*, **7**, 549–554.

Gao, X., Honn, K. V., Grignon, D. *et al.* (1993) Frequent loss of expression and loss of heterozygosity of the putative tumor suppressor gene DCC in prostatic carcinomas. *Cancer Res.*, **53**, 2723–2727.

Grignon, D. J. and Hammond, E. H. (1995) College of American Pathologists Conference XXVI on clinical relevance of prognostic markers in solid tumors. Report of the Prostate Cancer Working Group. *Arch. Pathol. Lab. Med.*, **119**, 1122–1126.

Hall, M. C., Navone, N. M., Troncoso, P. *et al.* (1995) Frequency and characterization of p53 mutations in clinically localized prostate cancer. *Urology*, **45**, 4700–4705.

Hamdy, F. C., Lawry, J., Anderson, J. B. *et al.* (1992) Circulating prostate specific antigen-positive cells correlate with metastatic prostate cancer. *Br. J. Urol.*, **69**, 392–396.

Hamdy, F. C., Fadlon, E. J., Cottam, D. *et al.* (1994) Matrix metalloproteinase 9 expression in primary human prostatic adenocarcinoma and benign prostatic hyperplasia. *Br. J. Cancer*, **69**, 177–182.

Harper, M. E., Goddard, L., Glynne-Jones, E. *et al.* (1993) An immunocytochemical analysis of TGF-alpha expression in benign and malignant prostatic tumors. *Prostate*, **23**, 9–23.

Ibrahim, G. K., Kerns, B-J. M., MacDonald, J. A. *et al.* (1993) Differential immunoreactivity of epidermal growth factor receptor in benign, dysplastic and malignant prostatic tissues. *J. Urol.*, **149**, 170–173.

Isaacs, W. B., Bova, G. S., Morton, R. A. *et al.* (1994) Molecular biology of prostate cancer. *Sem. Oncol.*, **21**, 514–521.

Jones, E. C., McNeal, J., Bruchovsky, N. and deJong, G. (1992) DNA content in prostatic adenocarcinoma. A flow cytometric study of the predictive value of aneuploidy for tumor volume, percentage Gleason grade 4 and 5 and lymph node metastases. *Cancer*, **70**, 302–306.

Katz, A. E., Olsson, C. A., Raffo, A. J. *et al.* (1994) Molecular staging of prostate cancer with the use of an enhanced reverse transcriptase-PCR assay. *Urology*, **43**, 765–775.

Kim, N. W., Piatyszek, M. A., Prowse, K. R. *et al.* (1994) Specific association of human telomerase activity with immortal cells and cancer. *Science*, **266**, 2011–2015.

Kleinerman, D. I., Troncoso, P., Lin, S-H. *et al.* (1995) Consistent expression of an epithelial cell adhesion molecule (C-CAM) during human prostate development and loss of expression in prostate cancer: implication as a tumor suppressor. *Cancer Res.*, **55**, 1215–1220

Kubota, Y., Shuin, T., Uemura, H. *et al.* (1995) Tumor suppressor gene p53 mutations in human prostate cancer. *Prostate*, **27**, 18–24.

Kuhn, E. J., Kurnot, R. A., Sesterhenn, I. A. *et al.* (1993) Expression of the c-erbB-2 (HER-2/neu) oncoprotein in human prostatic carcinoma. *J. Urol.*, **150**, 1427–1433.

Lee, W.-H., Morton, R. A., Epstein, J. I. *et al.* (1994) Cytidine methylation of regulatory sequences near the Pi-class glutathione S-transferase gene accompanies human prostatic carcinogenesis. *Proc. Nat. Acad. Sci. USA*, **91**, 11733–11737.

MacGrogan, D., Levy, A., Bostwick, D. *et al.* (1994) Loss of chromosome 8p loci in prostate cancer: mapping by quantitative allelic balance. *Genes Chromosomes Cancer*, **10**, 151–159.

Makar, R., Mason, A., Kittleson, J. M. *et al.* (1994) Immunohistochemical analysis of cathepsin D in prostate carcinoma. *Mod. Pathol.*, **7**, 747–751.

Maygarden, S. J., Strom, S. and Ware, J. L. (1992) Localization of epidermal growth factor receptor by immunohistochemical methods in human prostatic carcinoma, prostatic intraepithelial neoplasia, and benign hyperplasia. *Arch. Pathol. Lab. Med.*, **116**, 269–273.

Maygarden, S. J., Novotny, D. B., Moul, J. W. *et al.* (1994) Evaluation of Cathepsin D and epidermal growth factor receptor in prostate carcinoma. *Mod. Pathol.*, **6**, 930–936.

Mirchandani, D., Zheng, J., Miller, G. *et al.* (1995) Heterogeneity in intratumor distribution of p53 mutations in human prostate cancer. *Am. J. Pathol.*, **147**, 92–101.

Montgomery, B. T., Nativ, O., Blute, M. L. *et al.* (1990) Stage B prostate adenocarcinoma. Flow cytometric nuclear DNA ploidy analysis. *Arch. Surg.*, **125**, 327–331.

Montironi, R., Scarpelli, M., Sisti, S. *et al.* (1990) Quantitative analysis of prostatic intra-epithelial neoplasia on tissue sections. *Anal. Quant. Cytol. Histol.*, **12**, 366–372.

Montone, K. T. and Tomaszewski, J. E. (1993) In situ hybridization for epidermal growth factor receptor (EGFR) external domain transcripts in prostatic adenocarcinoma. *J. Clin. Lab. Anal.*, **7**, 188–195.

Moreno, J. G., Croce, C. M., Fischer, R. *et al.* (1992) Detection of hematogenous micrometastasis in patients with prostate cancer. *Cancer Res.*, **52**, 6110–6112.

Morton, R. A., Ewing, C. M., Nagafuchi, A. *et al.* (1993) Reduction of E-cadherin levels and deletion of the alpha-catenin gene in human prostate cancer cells. *Cancer Res.*, **53**, 3585–3590.

Moul, J. W., Friedrichs, P. A., Lance, R. S. *et al.* (1992) Infrequent RAS oncogene mutations in human prostate cancer. *Prostate*, **20**, 327–333.

Myers, R. B., Kudlow, J. E. and Grizzle, W. E. (1993) Expression of transforming growth factor-alpha, epidermal growth factor and the epidermal growth factor receptor in adenocarcinoma of the prostate and benign prostatic hyperplasia. *Mod. Pathol.*, **6**, 733–737.

Myers, R. B., Oelschlager, D., Srivastava, S. and Grizzlem W. E. (1994) Accumulation of the p53 protein occurs more frequently in metastatic than in localized prostatic adenocarcinoma. *Prostate*, **25**, 243–248.

Nativ, O., Winkler, H. Z., Raz, Y. *et al.* (1989) Stage C prostatic adenocarcinoma. Flow cytometric nuclear DNA ploidy analysis. *Mayo Clin. Proc.*, **64**, 911–919.

Netto, G. J. and Humphrey, P. A. (1994) Molecular biologic aspects of human prostatic carcinoma. *Am. J. Clin. Pathol.*, **102**(Suppl 1), S57–S64.

Petein, M., Michel, P., Van Velthoven, R. *et al.* (1991) Morphonuclear relationship between prostatic intraepithelial neoplasia and cancers as assessed by digital cell image analysis. *Am. J. Clin. Pathol.*, **96**, 628–634.

Pisters, L. L., Troncoso, P., Zhau, H. E. *et al.* (1995) C-*met* proto-oncogene expression in benign and malignant prostate tissues. *J. Urol.*, **154**, 293–298.

Qian, J., Bostwick, D. G. and Jenkins, R. B. (1995) Chromosomal anomalies in atypical adenomatous hyperplasia and carcinoma of the prostate using fluorescence in situ hybridization. *Urology*, **46**, 837–842.

Robertson, C. N., Robertson, K. M., Herzberg, A. J. *et al.* (1994) Differential immunoreactivity of transforming growth factor alpha in benign, dysplastic and malignant prostatic tissues. *Surg. Oncol.*, **3**, 237–242.

Ross, J. S., Nazeer, T., Figge, H. *et al.* (1995) Quantitative immunohistochemical determination of cathepsin D levels in prostatic carcinoma biopsies. Correlation with tumor grade, stage,

PSA level, and DNA ploidy status. *Am. J. Clin. Pathol.*, **104**, 36–41

Sakr, W. A., Haas, G. P., Drozdowicz, S. M. *et al.* (1992) Nuclear DNA content of prostatic carcinoma and intraepithelial neoplasia (PIN) in young males. An image analysis study. *Mod. Pathol.*, **5**, 58A.

Sakr, W. A., Macoska, J. A., Benson, P. *et al.* (1994) Allelic loss in locally metastatic, multisampled prostate cancer. *Cancer Res.*, **54**, 3273–3277.

Sandberg, A. A. (1992) Chromosomal abnormalities and related events in prostate cancer. *Hum. Pathol.*, **23**, 368–380.

Shankey, T. V., Kallioniemi, O.-P., Koslowski, J. M. *et al.* (1993) Consensus review of the clinical utility of DNA content cytometry in prostate cancer. *Cytometry*, **14**, 497–500.

Stearns, M. E. and Wang, M. (1993) Type IV collagenase (M(r) 72,000) expression in human prostate: benign and malignant tissue. *Cancer Res.*, **53**, 878–883.

Steiner, M. S. (1993) Role of peptide growth factors in the prostate: a review. *Urology*, **42**, 99–110.

Stephenson, R. A., James, B. C., Gay, H. *et al.* (1987) Flow cytometry of prostate cancer: relationship of DNA content to survival. *Cancer Res.*, **47**, 2504–2507.

Takahashi, S., Qian, J., Brown, J. A. *et al.* (1994) Potential markers of prostate cancer aggressiveness detected by fluorescence in situ hybridization in needle biopsies. *Cancer Res.*, **54**, 3574–3579.

Takai, K., Goellner, J. R., Katzmann, J. A. *et al.* (1994) Static image and flow DNA cytometry of prostatic adenocarcinoma: studies of needle biopsy and radical prostatectomy specimens. *J. Urol. Pathol.*, **2**, 39–48.

Thompson, T. C., Truong, L. D., Timme, T. L. *et al.* (1992) Transforming growth factor Beta-1 as a biomarker for prostate cancer. *J. Cell Biochem. (Suppl)*, **16H**, 54–61.

Tribukait, B. (1993) Nuclear deoxyribonucleic acid determination in patients with prostate carcinomas: clinical research and application. *Eur. Urol.*, **23**, 64–76.

Turkeri, L. N., Sakr, W. A., Wykes, S. M. *et al.* (1994) Comparative analysis of epidermal growth factor receptor gene expression and protein product in benign, premalignant, and malignant prostate tissue. *Prostate*, **25**, 199–205.

Umbas, R., Schalken, J. A., Aalders, T. W. *et al.* (1992) Expression of the cellular adhesion molecule E-cadherin is reduced or absent in high grade prostate cancer. *Cancer Res.*, **52**, 5104–5109.

Van den Ouden, D., Tribukait, B., Blom, J. H. *et al.* (1993) Deoxyribonucleic acid ploidy of core biopsies and metastatic lymph nodes of prostate cancer patients: impact on time to progression. *J. Urol.*, **150**, 400–406.

Van Veldhuizen, P. J., Sadasivan, R., Garcia, F. *et al.* (1993) Mutant p53 expression in prostate carcinoma. *Prostate*, **22**, 23–30.

Ware, J. L. (1994) Prostate cancer progression. *Am. J. Pathol.*, **145**, 983–993.

Warzynski, M. J., Soechtig, C. E., Maatman, T. J. *et al.* (1994) DNA analysis by flow cytometry of paraffin embedded core biopsies of the prostate. *Prostate*, **24**, 313–319.

Weinberg, D. S. and Weidner, N. (1993) Concordance of DNA content between prostatic intraepithelial neoplasia and concomitant carcinoma. Evidence that prostatic intraepithelial neoplasia is a precursor of invasive prostatic carcinoma. *Arch. Pathol. Lab. Med.*, **117**, 1132–1137.

Winkler, H. Z., Rainwater, L. M., Myers, R. P. *et al.* (1988) Stage D1 prostatic adenocarcinoma: significance of nuclear DNA ploidy patterns studied by flow cytometry. *Mayo Clin. Proc.*, **63**, 103–112.

Zincke, H., Bergstrahl, E. J., Larson-Keller, J. J. *et al.* (1992) Stage D1 prostate cancer treated by radical prostatectomy and adjuvant hormonal treatment. Evidence for favorable survival in patients with DNA diploid tumors. *Cancer*, **70**(Suppl 1), 311–323.

Zitzelsberger, H., Szucs, S., Weier, H.-U. *et al.* (1994) Numerical abnormalities of chromosome 7 detected by fluorescence in situ hybridization (FISH) on paraffin-embedded tissue sections with centromere-specific DNA probes. *J. Pathol.*, **172**, 325–335.

INDEX

Note: page numbers in *italics* refer to tables, those in **bold** refer to figures; '*vs*' preceding subentry refers to differential diagnosis.